# Decision Making and Control for Health Administration

The Management of
Quantitative Analysis

SECOND EDITION

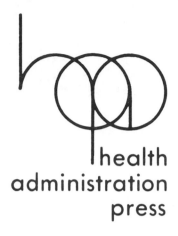

health
administration
press

# Decision Making and Control for Health Administration

## The Management of Quantitative Analysis

SECOND EDITION

D. Michael Warner
Don C. Holloway
Kyle L. Grazier

Health Administration Press 1984

**Library of Congress Cataloging in Publication Data**

Warner, D. Michael.
  Decision making and control for health administration.

  Bibliography: p.
  Includes index.
  1. Health services administration—Decision making.
2. Health services administration—Statistical methods.
3. Operations research. I. Holloway, Don C. II. Grazier,
Kyle L. III. Title.
RA394.W37    1984      362.1'068      83-22690
ISBN 0-914904-85-X

Grateful appreciation is extended to the copyright owners for permission to use portions of the following material:

"Scheduling Nursing Personnel According to Nursing Preference: A Mathematical Programming Application." *Operations Research,* Vol. 24, No. 5, 1976, pp. 842–56. Copyright 1976 by the Operations Research Society of America.

*Biometrika Tables for Statisticians,* Vol. 1 (Second Edition), pp. 130–1, 159–61. Copyright 1962 by the Biometrika Trustees.

"Staffing the Nursing Unit." Parts I and II. *Nursing Research,* Vol. 14, Nos. 3 and 4, Summer and Fall 1965. Copyright 1965 by the American Journal of Nursing Company.

"Development of Hospital Levels of Care Criteria." *Health Care Management Review,* Vol. 1, No. 3, Summer 1976, pp. 61–72. Copyright 1976 by Aspen Systems Corporation, 20010 Century Blvd., Germantown, Maryland 20767.

"Barriers to Appropriate Utilization of an Acute Facility." *Medical Care,* Vol. 14, No. 7, July 1976, pp. 559–573. Copyright 1976 by J. B. Lippincott Company.

"Methods for Quantifying Subjective Probabilities and Multi-Attribute Utilities." *Decision Sciences,* Vol. 5, 1974, p. 437. Copyright 1974 by the American Institute for Decision Sciences.

Health Administration Press
A Division of the Foundation of the
  American College of Healthcare Executives
1021 E. Huron Street
Ann Arbor, Michigan 48104-9990
(313) 764-1380

# Contents

# Illustrative Problems

# Preface

*The Curriculum in Quantitative Methods: A Task Force Report\** recommends a minumum of two quantitative courses for health administration curricula—one in statistics and one in operations analysis. The *Report* recommends that the operations analysis course provide "a basic understanding and familiarity *sufficient to support the [health] administrator's position as a sophisticated and involved consumer of operations analysis techniques.*" The *Report* added that the course should enable administrators to "identify problem areas which could benefit from the services of various kinds of operations analysis," to "formulate these problems" so that they are amenable to solution using operations analysis, to "communicate with the analyst," and to "evaluate the quality" of the analyst's work. In other words, the administrator should be able to *manage* staff operations analysts (we have chosen to call them *quantitative specialists*).

The *Report* was published at the same time that we began teaching operations analysis courses in health administration programs. The *Report* and its authors provided us with guidance at an important time in our careers. It suggested an approach quite different from that which we had been taught as quantitative specialists and different from the one we would otherwise have used. It was difficult to resist teaching a set of loosely related quantitative techniques applied (if at all) to a variety of industries and at a mathematical level appropriate only for quantitative specialists, especially since contemporary texts followed that pattern. Over the years we learned that, to respond to the *Report's* recommendations, we must present a conceptual frame-

*The Curriculum in Quantitative Methods: A Task Force Report.* Association of University Programs in Health Administration. Washington, D.C.

work at the mathematical level appropriate for the specialists' boss and with applications drawn from the health field. Our text emphasizes frameworks for decision making and control, the role of the manager in those frameworks, and successful applications to the health field. It uses only the mathematics (college algebra) that the manager needs to know in order to formulate problems, to communicate with quantitative specialists, and to evaluate their work.

Subsequent to publication of the *Report,* we have each served as Chairman of the Quantitative Methods Task Force and have gained a feeling for the general differences among operations analysis courses. The two most critical differences concern faculty experience and the relative emphasis on health services applications. We believe this text can be used with equal effect under these varying circumstances.

With the objective of preparing health administrators to manage the work of quantitative specialists, we have emphasized both the decision-making and control frameworks as well as specific techniques. A conceptual emphasis combined with illustrative problems and exercises based on real applications seems to us the optimum approach. Accordingly, we have furnished many exercises which specifically require techniques described in the text. Yet, since comparatively few real-world problems have "definite" answers and because most require reasoned assumptions, other exercises pose problems significantly different from those analyzed in the text and are designed as an applied extension of the text.

## Preface to the Second Edition

Since the first edition was published, we have received many suggestions for revisions which we have incorporated in this edition. In addition, we have added an author whose extensive experience with the first edition, and her own special expertise, led to several significant expansions of various chapters. Finally, she has added two new chapters of special relevance to recent developments in the field of health administration. Chapter 8 addresses the administrator's need to be familiar with management information systems, and Chapter 10 examines the rapidly growing area of external regulation and how it affects decision making and control.

# Acknowledgments

Two members of the original Quantitative Methods Task Force have been especially influential and helpful in the development of our approach to the subject. We are especially indebted to John R. Griffith and David B. Starkweather for their contribution to the Task Force, their willingness to share ideas and teaching materials, and for providing us with direction. In addition, we wish to thank Professor Griffith for his insightful critique of an earlier version of the manuscript.

During our participation on the Task Force, its members influenced our thinking and provided valuable perspective. We appreciate their contribution and wish to especially thank Joni Steinberg for providing feedback about our ideas.

C. West Churchman designed and jointly taught a course with D.C.H.; his insights and influence are deeply appreciated. We recommend his book, *The Systems Approach* (Dell, 1968), to our students.

We are indebted to Jerry Rose and Vandankumar Trivedi for their valuable comments on earlier versions of the manuscript.

R. K. Dieter Haussmann, George P. Huber, Joseph D. Restuccia, and Harvey Wolfe have generously granted us permission to quote from their works.

D.M.W. wishes to thank Judy Oehring, Bobbie Harris, and Martha Clegg for typing several drafts of his chapters, his students at Duke University for the often painful "real-time editing" which they contributed in using an early draft of the text, Jo Mauskopf for her careful proofing of the final draft, and his wife Polly for numerous hours of proofreading and for her patience in indulging a sometimes crabby companion.

D.C.H. wishes to thank Kathleen Buckley and Cherilyn Harris

for their assistance and support in preparing the manuscript, Sidney Weinstein for her helpful editing, and his students at Berkeley who worked every exercise, provided feedback on unclear presentations, challenged our thinking, and discovered subtle errors. He wants Barb to know that he will always have loving memories of the good times they shared while he was not working on this book.

Finally, although we wrote our chapters individually (D.M.W. on planning and decision making and D.C.H. on measurement and control), we each learned from the other. The exchange of ideas will be a most memorable part of our collaboration.

The preceding was the acknowledgment to the first edition. Since that edition appeared in 1978, many users (both professors and students) have provided valuable comments and suggestions, for which we are grateful and which we have included in this edition. One of these users provided so many good ideas that we asked her to join us in preparing this edition: D.M.W. and D.C.H. are especially grateful and indebted to Kyle Grazier for organizing the second edition and contributing many of the changes and additions.

K.L.G. would like to thank D.M.W. and D.C.H. for the opportunity to participate in their collaboration, Donna Carroll for her typing skill and her patience, and, most of all, William A. G'Sell for his continued personal and professional support.

# Part I

# Introduction

*Health administration (or management) is a broad discipline incorporating many responsibilities and requiring a variety of concepts and approaches. The quantitatively oriented concepts and techniques presented in this text are not a substitute for management: they offer an overall approach to management and some useful concepts and techniques for managerial decision-making and control. To provide an understanding of how the approach of this text applies to health administration or management, Part I consists of two chapters that give both an overview of the general approach and a description of the environment within which health administrators face decision-making and control problems.*

# 1

# Administrative Decision Making and Control

## 1.1 Introduction

Much of what health administrators and planners do can be considered either decision making or control. Very generally, decision making involves choosing among alternative ways to meet objectives, while control entails making sure objectives are being met and will continue to be met. These definitions of decision making and control leave much unsaid. What alternatives should be considered? What effect will each alternative have on achieving the objectives? What should be measured to determine if the objectives are being met? What role should the health administrator or planner take in the decision making and control process, and what roles should others play?

Most of this book describes methods for forecasting the effect that individual alternatives will have on achieving certain objectives, and methods for measuring to what extent such objectives are being met. But the preliminary decisions of which objectives are appropriate in each case, and which alternative actions should be considered for meeting those objectives, are much more important, and much more troublesome. There are usually multiple objectives to be addressed, and usually these objectives conflict with one another. Individual alternative actions usually serve only a subset of the objectives (often only one), and are usually detrimental to another subset. Thus some scheme for considering each alternative's effect on all important objectives is necessary. To illustrate, consider the following typical problem confronting health administrators.

The administrator of a satellite outpatient clinic has discovered that some patients are complaining because of the time they must wait, and others are being asked to return on another day or to go to another facility. Since one objective of the clinic is to meet the demand for its services and another is to limit the time patients must wait to an acceptable level, the administrator decides to investigate.

**Control Problem:** How can the administrator ensure that the clinic is meeting the demand for its services and keeping the time its patients must wait at an acceptable level?

The administrator begins her study by contacting several of the physicians. These physicians indicate that the facility is too small. They claim there are not enough examining rooms to see all patients arriving at the clinic at certain times of the day. They also believe that a different arrangement of the rooms, involving making some smaller and some larger, is needed. They maintain that these are the reasons patients have to wait or be turned away.

**Resource-Size Decision:** What size (in number of examining rooms) should the clinic be to adequately meet its demand?

**Procedure Decision:** Would the room arrangement the physicians want be better than the present one?

The administrator is reluctant to "solve" the problem by expanding the facility, noticing that examining rooms are empty at certain times of the day. The head nurse explains that they are empty because there are not enough physicians and nurses to staff the rooms at those times of the day. He maintains that hiring more staff would solve the problem.

**Resource-Size Decision:** How much physician time and nurse time should be available at specific times of the day to meet demand?

Checking with the nurse practitioner employed at the facility, the administrator is told that physicians are not making use of the nurse practitioner's skills. There are plenty of nursing staff members but they are performing clerical duties, and plenty of physicians but they are performing nursing functions. The nurse practitioner assumes that practitioners' doing more nursing would solve the problem.

**Procedure Decision:** What tasks should each type of professional perform?

The clinic receptionist points out to the administrator that patients tend to arrive between eleven in the morning and two in the afternoon, and again between four and six in the evening. At other times of the day, relatively few patients come to the clinic. It would ease the pressure on the clinic if at least *some* patients were given appointments to arrive during the off-peak hours. The receptionist believes scheduling patients for non-peak hours would solve the problem.

**Scheduling Decision:** When should patients be scheduled so that staff and facilities will be available?

Now, it occurs to the administrator that perhaps the staff is taking its lunch hour some time between eleven and two. Upon inquiring, she discovers that the staff takes half-hour lunch breaks, usually whenever they can be squeezed in. Frequently, patients have to wait for the staff to return from lunch.

**Scheduling Decision:** How should staff members be scheduled so that they are available when patients arrive? Would rescheduling lunch breaks help solve the problem?

As the investigation proceeds, the administrator discovers that a third-party payer has been questioning whether several patients have received medically necessary services. The third-party payer threatens to deny payment unless provided with further justification for the services.

**Control Problem:** How can the administrator ensure that patients are receiving only medically necessary services?

If unnecessary services are being provided or if the same services could be provided in a facility other than the clinic, the demand might be reduced, and the reduced demand might help solve the clinic's problems. Even if waiting times could be reduced to acceptable levels by addressing one or more of the above steps, how can the administrator be sure the problem will not happen again?

**Control Problem:** How can the administrator control the clinic so that it will continue to achieve its objectives?

Besides the difficulty of dividing the administrator's investigation into separate problems, two "megaproblems" underlie the administrator's plight. The first is determining the appropriate objectives for the clinic. The second megaproblem is, given that appropriate objectives are known, where should one begin? It seems that the whole process begins as a control problem, but should the scheduling, procedure, or resource size decisions be tackled first? Must they all be considered simultaneously? Let's look at these two megaproblems separately.

## 1.2 THE APPROPRIATE OJECTIVES MEGAPROBLEM

The physicians see the appropriate objectives of the clinic as the provision of enough examining rooms so that patients may be seen quickly. The head nurse sees the objectives as the provision of adequate staff so that patients will be seen quickly. The administrator also views seeing patients quickly as an objective, but she regards controlling costs as an important objective as well; often this cost objective begins to conflict with the others. She is also likely to see maintaining a certain volume of service, on which revenue for the clinic is based, as an objective. The third-party payer (on behalf of the community) sees the objective of the clinic as serving only those patients who cannot be served better (less expensively) elsewhere, and serving only those patients who medically need care. Both of these community views may conflict with the administrator's objective of revenue maintenance.

To determine which of the above objectives are "appropriate," we need some scheme that relates and balances the views of the different participants. One approach, and the one underlying the philosophy of this book, is the systems approach. The systems approach is a conceptual aid to unraveling the potentially confusing interrelatedness of the objectives and activities of our clinic example. If we begin by *thinking* of a different system's being associated with each of the different objectives offered by the clinic's staff, what results is the complex of *imbedded interdependent systems and subsystems* of Figure 1.1.

The physicians are viewing the medical care process system: their "problem" is not enough examining rooms to meet the needs of their system. The head nurse is viewing the nursing care system:

*Figure 1.1*

*The Community Health Service System*

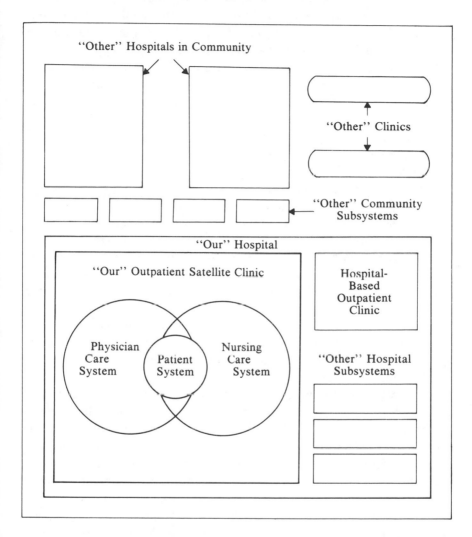

his "problem" is insufficient personnel. The administrator is viewing the clinic system: her "problems" involve maintaining revenue, controlling cost, and meeting demand. The third-party payers (and the community) are viewing the community health service system; their "problems" are to obtain appropriate care at lowest possible cost.

These "smaller" systems are all subsystems to larger ones. Even the community health service system is a subsystem. (To what?)

A major concept of "systems thinking" requires that a subsystem not be considered independently of its parent system, or indeed of its grandparent and other ancestral systems. One must also view the system as interdependent with its siblings—e.g., the medical care system and the nursing care system. The danger of ignoring the family ties leads quite easily and often to solutions which may improve performance for that subsystem, but which do not serve the objectives of the parents or siblings. For example, providing more examining rooms certainly solves the medical care system's problem but may well result in wasted resources in terms of the clinic system and the community system. There are many other examples of possible dangers of non-systems thinking in this example and in most any example you consider. (What are some?)

The systems approach seems to demand that we look at the *whole complex* of systems of Figure 1.1 (which includes only a fraction of the actual systems involved) *simultaneously* to make even the smallest objective-oriented decision about any of the systems. This of course is not feasible. But fortunately there is a way to include parent and sibling systems implicitly in an analysis of a subsystem. The systems approach says that we can look at even the smallest subsystem if we carefully *define that subsystem's objectives in terms of how the subsystem plays its part in meeting its parent's and siblings' objectives.* Its parent's and siblings' objectives must in turn have been defined in terms of *their* parent's (and siblings') objectives, etc. Thus the important link between systems lies in the establishment of each system's objectives. To analyze the satellite outpatient clinic, we must first establish its objectives in terms of how it serves the objectives of the hospital and, in turn, the objectives of the community health service system. Thus the medical care subsystem must adopt cost control, medically necessary care, and appropriate patient placement for medical care into its objectives. The clinic must adopt appropriate patient placement and medically necessary care into its objectives (the third-party payer will require this). By "appropriate" or "systems" objectives for a subsystem we mean objectives that have been defined in terms of how a subsystem helps meet its larger family's objectives.

This method of establishing objectives does three things. First, it provides a framework for *describing* the relationship between multiple, conflicting objectives. (It also tends to encourage the *listing* of all objectives that should be considered.) Second, it provides (at this point conceptually) a method to *balance* the objectives and *combine* them in a way that considers their relationship. Third, by its definition of appropriateness, it offers a way to analyze a subsystem without having to analyze completely the systems of which it is a part. We will see that the first step of any decision or control problem is to establish carefully the "appropriate" or "systems" objectives.

Let's look at another example of the effect of systems thinking. Independent of its surrounding community, a hospital's objectives might include: *providing high quality care; meeting demand; maintaining high utilization of beds;* and *maximizing revenue*. To consider the hospital as a subsystem of community health services we must first carefully examine the latter system's objectives. These might include *meeting the health care needs of the community with high quality care at the lowest possible cost*. (Both the hospital's and the community's objectives have been greatly simplified for this example, of course.) The effect of the systems approach is to change the hospital's objectives to serve the parent system's objective of *eliminating unneeded hospital stay* (in direct conflict with maximizing utilization), and *reducing cost* (an incentive only indirectly felt without the systems approach). *High quality* and *meeting demand* remain, but if the same quality care can be provided elsewhere in the parent system (community) at lower cost, then the systems approach may lead to reducing utilization of inpatient beds in favor of outpatient treatment—a direct conflict with the objectives of hospitals in overbedded communities.

This approach to identifying appropriate objectives requires us to be practical. How can we ever be sure we have identified the objectives of a system such that they help meet the objectives of all of the larger systems above it? How do we know when we are on the "top" system that matters? The answers are we can't, and we don't. From a practical standpoint, therefore, we normally go several systems "above" until we estimate that the system under analysis has relatively little effect on even "higher" systems.

Even after determining the appropriate objectives, we are left with the second megaproblem: which of the several different problems do we analyze first?

## 1.3 THE WHERE-TO-START MEGAPROBLEM

Let's accept that patients are waiting too long. Is the problem that the facility is too small; or that there is not enough staff; or that the staff's skills are not being fully utilized; or that patients are not scheduled appropriately; or that the staff is not scheduled appropriately; or that some of the same services should be provided at another clinic; or that the other clinic is in a bad location; or that unnecessary services are being provided; or that the current situation of long waiting lines and turned-away patients should have been predicted so that changes could have been incorporated in previous plans? Or are patients waiting and being turned away as a result of the systems approach (the clinic has defined its objectives in terms of a "higher" system, and this level of patient wait actually helps the higher system more closely achieve its objectives)?

If the administrator had quickly concluded that the facility should be expanded, or that a patient scheduling system should be installed, the solution to the problem of long waiting times and turned-away patients might have been needlessly expensive, the problem might not have been solved at all, or worse, the solution might have created difficulty for the clinic's parent systems. Looked at another way, it seems that she must wait to find out how large the clinic will be and who the patients will be before she begins working on the scheduling of personnel or patients. On the other hand, her ability to schedule patients might affect the number of examining rooms needed. All of the other decisions are similarly linked: solving one changes another.

The "best" approach would be to make all of the decisions simultaneously, but this is seldom practical or possible. One possible approach is to establish priorities: assuming cost-effectiveness is an objective, first work on decisions which would most effectively reduce waiting time and turned-away patients for each dollar spent. For example, if a *patient* scheduling system cost $2,000 to install and $200 per month to operate, and the average waiting time for patients was predicted to be reduced from 60 minutes to 20 minutes, then the cost of reducing the average waiting time 1 minute would be $110 in the first year ([2000 + (12 × 200)] ÷ 40 minutes). If a *personnel* scheduling system cost $50 for each minute that it reduced average waiting time, then scheduling personnel would receive higher priority than scheduling patients. (When available, the text will provide the costs and benefits derived from implementing solutions to problems we use as examples.)

Of course, it is not that simple. If rescheduling staff could reduce the average waiting time by 5 minutes at most, perhaps the cost per minute of waiting time that would be eliminated by scheduling patients would then be increased because the total waiting time could no longer be reduced another 20 minutes. The facility might have to be expanded to do that. The megaproblem has surfaced again.

This solution to the where-to-start problem was a cost-benefit analysis (dollars per minute of waiting time eliminated). The next question is how much money to spend on the cost-benefit analysis. We are then back to deciding how the clinic's objectives fit into the community's goals. For example, suppose that money were spent to decide which problem to start with, rather than simply working on the problem that is intuitively most important. Perhaps the money would have been better spent on an outpatient hemodialysis unit.

Unfortunately, there is no quantitative method to help us here. There is, however, a hierarchy of approaches depending mainly on time, cost, and the relative importance of the objectives involved. More often than not, the question of where to start will need to be defined by listing all possible places to start, and sequencing them as intelligently as possible. This will require help from physicians, nurses, patients, receptionists, third-party payers, other facility administrators, planners, financial managers, and quantitative specialists. It will be possible in some cases to make two (or even three) decisions at once. In other cases, a "back and forth" or iterative approach might be necessary, in which first the patient scheduling decision is tentatively made, the number of examining rooms decision is made, the scheduling decision is re-made with the new number of examining rooms, etc. The process is often more management art than management science.

Although our example describes a clinic that could not meet its demand, similar problems occur when there is not enough demand for available resources. Does the problem stem from the facility's or the staff's being too large, or the staff's being overskilled, or from patients' not being scheduled when they could be, or from staff's being scheduled when there are no patients, or from the clinic's not providing a service that it should, or from the clinic's being in a bad location, or from health professionals' perceiving "need" while consumers do not, or from the administrator's having failed to predict that excess resources would occur so that changes could have been incorporated in previous plans?

## 1.4 DECISIONS VERSUS TECHNIQUES

We should point out a related danger here, concerning the relationship between the decisions illustrated by the outpatient clinic and the techniques to assist in making them. These decisions occur so frequently that some quantitative specialists have concentrated on one type of decision (scheduling patients, for example) and have developed techniques applicable to similar decisions in a wide range of health facilities. At times, the techniques become so associated with the decisions that specialists and managers begin thinking in terms of the technique, and become technique-oriented rather than decision-oriented. Specialists or managers who become very familiar with a technique have a natural inclination to use it. They then are tempted to lose their objectivity and decide that the real problem is a patient scheduling problem, not because it seems to have the greatest potential to minimize waiting time or turned-away patients, but because they understand *that* problem (and the way to solve it) so well. Certainly they should not be criticized for understanding a problem and the technique for its solution, but someone (the administrator) has to be responsible for deciding which problem should receive priority and be attacked first.

## 1.5 OTHER EXAMPLES

At this point we can introduce a classification of decisions based on three general types:

**Resource-Size Decisions**—choosing the amount of resources to provide in order to meet demand. In most cases, the decision is how much demand to meet or, more to the point, how much *not* to meet.

**Procedure Decisions**—*given* a level of demand to meet, choosing the best (usually lowest cost) way to meet it.

**Scheduling Decisions**—choosing the arrangement or manipulation of a *given* level of resources and/or a *given* level of demand to best meet objectives.

At this point we may also include a more precise definition of a control problem.

**Control Problem**—choosing measures of performance for monitoring systems and, when necessary, choosing among the above three decisions (in addition to organizational design alternatives) such that systems continue to achieve objectives.

The decisions and control problems of the clinic example were labeled according to the above classification, and the reader may now want to review that example before continuing.

To see the difference between the types of decisions, and to see that the problems of the satellite clinic occur in all health service systems, consider other facilities and their subsystems. Within a community or planning area, a patient could be receiving health services while located in an acute facility, an acute-based skilled nursing facility (SNF), a free-standing (not acute-based) SNF, a surgicenter (either acute-based or free-standing), an intermediate care facility (ICF), a nursing home, a physician's office, his own home with home health agency support, or in the outpatient clinic.

**Resource-Size Decision:** What size should each of these facilities or agencies be?

Within the acute facility alone, a patient could be located in the intensive care unit (ICU), coronary care unit (CCU), rehabilitation unit, psychiatric unit, surgical suite, recovery room, radiology department, obstetric unit (labor, delivery, newborn), pediatric unit, medical-surgical unit, or emergency room.

**Resource-Size Decision:** What size should each hospital unit be?

The size of a facility or hospital unit required to meet demand is in part dependent on what service it provides that the others do not. The decision is not just what one acute facility should provide compared to another acute facility, but also what services a free-standing SNF should provide compared to an acute-based SNF, or compared to the acute facility itself, or an ICF, or a home health agency.

**Procedure Decision:** What services should each facility provide?

Within an acute facility, specialty units have been differentiated by the services each provides, even though they may also provide similar services.

**Procedure Decision:** What services should each unit provide—different from any other? What basic services should they all provide?

But deciding what services each facility should provide to meet demand is in part dependent on where in the community or planning area the facility is located—or in the case of establishing new facilities, where in the community or planning area they *will* be located.

**Scheduling (or Location) Decision:** In order to meet demand, where should services (facilities) be located?

These facilities, agencies, or hospital units are heavily dependent on physicians, nurses, and other personnel to deliver their health services.

**Resource-Size Decision:** How much physician time, nurse time, and other staff time should be available to meet the demand for health services?

The time required of physicians, nurses (registered nurses [RNs], licensed practical nurses [LPNs], or nurses aides), and other staff to meet the demand for their services is in part dependent on what tasks and procedures each performs that other professionals do not.

**Procedure Decision:** What services should each type of professional perform?

As when determining the facilities' sizes, the amount of physician time, nurse time, or other staff time required to meet demand is dependent on when it is available and when it is needed.

**Scheduling Decision:** When should physicians, nurses, and other staff (as well as facilities themselves) be scheduled so that the demand for their services will be met?

**Scheduling Decision:** When should patients classified as "nonurgent" or "elective" be scheduled so that the staff and facility will be available?

In some situations there are alternative ways to provide a service—using X-ray machine A or X-ray machine B, for example, or automating a procedure instead of doing it manually, or doing a procedure solely within the facility as opposed to sharing it with other facilities. Prepaid health plans must decide whether to provide a service themselves or to contract with another provider.

**Procedure Decision:** What is the best way to provide a service when selecting between alternative methods that achieve the same purpose?

Once a decision has been made to meet a certain amount of demand for a service using a certain sized facility, with a certain number of medical, nursing, or other staff, at certain times of the day and week, and in certain locations within the planning area, the health administrator or planner's work is only half done. She must assure that the system is meeting its budget, assure quality of care, and assure that services are being provided in the most economical setting.

> **Control Problem:** How can the health administrator or planner control her system's budget, quality, and utilization?

## 1.6 ORGANIZATION OF TEXT

The remaining chapters present concepts and techniques with which to approach the types of decision and control problems introduced in this chapter. We will see that some concepts and techniques are useful for all types of problems, while others are more suited to a subset of problems. The concepts of the systems approach are so important to decision making and control that they should become "second nature" when approaching decision and control problems. All objectives should be put to the systems approach test of whether they indeed serve the objectives of parent and grandparent systems. It would be preferable to include a discussion of the two megaproblems—the appropriate objectives and where to start—each time we examine the formulation and solution of a particular problem. Unfortunately, this will not be possible because of space. The responsibility of considering the two megaproblems will have to remain with the reader. The examples that will be used will illustrate typical objectives and typical places to start, thereby *presupposing* solutions to the two megaproblems. That is, the examples will usually have objectives already defined, and we will normally deal with only one problem type at a time. Thus it is important that the reader critically consider how the objectives were established, and how the particular problem being used to demonstrate a concept and/or technique interrelates with other decision and control problems.

In Chapter 2 we present frameworks for decision making and control which will be used to structure the problems of the later chapters and provide useful ways to approach them. The concepts and techniques of the later chapters play definite parts in the framework, allowing an overall view of quantitative decision making and control.

Part II, *Analysis for Decision Making*, has four chapters, each chapter similar in that resource-size decisions, procedure decisions, and scheduling decisions are presented. Each chapter differs in the degree of complexity and degree of uncertainty incorporated in the analyses. Chapters 3 and 4 consider simple analyses—ones in which there are only a few variables, a few available alternatives to be evaluated, and few, if any, difficult to quantify objectives. Chapters 5 and 6 consider more complex analyses. Chapters 3 and 6 consider deterministic analyses—ones in which it is assumed events will occur for certain, while chapters 4 and 5 consider stochastic analyses—ones in which uncertainty is incorporated. In this way, the level of mathematical background increases so that managers and planners might expect to perform the type of analyses in Chapters 3 and 4 themselves, but must rely on quantitative specialists for many of the methods discussed in Chapters 5 and 6. The methods presented in Part II are formulated using the decision-making framework presented in Chapter 2.

Part III, *Forecasting and Measurement*, presents concepts that are fundamental to both Parts II and IV. They are included after Part II so that their fundamental relationship can be motivated by the decision-making chapters of Part II. The methods presented are for the most part straightforward, even if detailed, and managers or planners might perform some of the forecasting and measurement themselves, or at least be highly involved in the process. Again, Part III could easily be presented before Part II.

Part IV, *Regulation and Control*, begins with a review of the reimbursement and payment systems that are evolving as a result of increasing regulatory activity, both within and outside of hospitals. Next, the application of the process and structural requirements of cybernetic control to two important areas for health administrators is described. Chapter 11 discusses how admission-scheduling and nurse-staffing systems make use of the decision techniques described in Chapters 5 and 6. However, the daily scheduling of admissions and the daily reallocation of nurses is added. Chapter 12 analyzes the problem of physician peer review using the concepts of measurement and cybernetic control. Although controlling physician performance is admittedly a complex problem, experience with applying these concepts has shown them to be particularly useful in this situation.

Similar to the megaproblem of choosing a problem with which to start, the order of Parts II, III, and IV is somewhat arbitrary. Control could come before decision or vice versa. Measurement and forecasting are fundamental concepts to both decision making and control and could precede both. Any of the parts could precede the others: the reader should try to keep in mind how they interrelate in terms of the where-to-start megaproblem.

## Exercises

1.1 Choose a health care delivery system with which you are familiar and identify its subsystems. Next, specify their objectives. What is the relationship between these subsystems' objectives and your system's objectives? Which objectives require trade-offs to be made?

1.2 Now identify the systems of which your system is a subsystem and specify their objectives. Are your system's objectives in conflict with its parent systems'? How would you change your system's objectives? How might the new objectives affect your system's operations?

1.3 Identify a subsystem and its parent in the health field where the goals of the subsystem are likely to be significantly different if the subsystem is regarded as an independent system rather than as a subsystem. What are likely goals for the subsystem in each case?

## Additional Reading

Churchman, C. W. *The Systems Approach*. New York: Dell Publishing Co., 1968.

Bonder, Seth. "Operations Research Education." *Journal of the Operations Research Society of America* 19 (November 1971): 796–809.

Donabedian, Avedis. "Program Objectives" (Chapter II). *Aspects of Medical Care Administration*. Cambridge, Mass.: Harvard University Press, 1973.

Grundy, F. and Reinke, W. A. *Health Practice Research* (Chapter 1). Geneva, Switzerland: World Health Organization Public Health Paper S1, undated.

# 2

# Frameworks for Quantitative Decision Making and Cybernetic Control

## 2.1 INTRODUCTION

Once the administrator of the last chapter has solved the where-to-start megaproblem and decided to begin by analyzing a particular resource size, procedure, or scheduling decision or control problem, how should she go about it? There is more to quantitative decision making and cybernetic control than a collection of concepts and techniques: there must be overall *approaches*, general enough so that they are applicable to all decision and control problems. The approaches must thus be problem-oriented rather than technique-oriented, where quantitative concepts and techniques are called on by the approaches as they are needed.

In this chapter we develop two such approaches, which we call *frameworks:* one for decisions and one for control problems. Throughout the remainder of the text, these frameworks will provide the foundation for our approach to decisions and control problems, and we will introduce specific concepts and techniques as they are called for by a particular type of problem, or the treatment of that problem.

A fundamental concept of the quantitative decision-making framework is modeling, and before introducing the decision framework we must introduce this concept. Broadly, modeling is the representation of a real world structure or process in a different medium. Analysis of the *model* leads to inferences about the real world. The most intuitively pleasing models are physical, such as fractional scale models of buildings or ships. Physical models are useful for observing easily and inexpensively assessed structural characteristics of the model and then projecting these characteristics to its full size, real world counterpart. Such models can be of existing real world structures or, more often, of hypothetical or proposed structures. The type of modeling we will use is quite similar to physical modeling. Our representations are usually of real world *processes* and the representation medium is mathematical rather than physical. The purpose is exactly the same: to project the model's characteristics, observed through manipulation of the model, to the real world situation, avoiding expensive (and often impossible) manipulation of the real world itself. The quality of inferences from the model is of course less than the information gained by manipulating the real world itself. One of our major concerns with modeling will be the extent to which inferences from a model may validly be applied to the real world.

Consider the satellite outpatient clinic again. After the careful consideration described in Chapter 1, suppose the manager decided that the first step toward reducing patient waiting time and turnaway should be increasing the facility's size. To keep the problem simple, suppose there are only four alternatives: add no examining room, add 1 room, add 2 rooms, or add 3 rooms. Further, suppose her objective is *to reduce patient waiting time without spending unnecessary money*. Her decision would be easier, though not solved, if she knew exactly how much patient waiting time would be reduced by each room addition. A mathematical model of the type we will develop in Chapter 5 would simulate the flow of patients in the clinic, allowing her to add rooms one by one to the model and to observe the patients' waiting time generated by the model. She could then (carefully) project the model's waiting times to the real world situation.

Models don't make decisions for the administrator, but they do play an important role in our decision framework. In most cases, modeling makes available more information about the possible *consequences* of alternative actions. In some cases, its role lies in more precisely predicting such consequences. In a few cases, modeling may help the administrator *choose* that one or those few alternatives which best meet specified criteria. Modeling, however, should only be viewed as an aid to decision making.

## 2.2 THE DECISION-MAKING FRAMEWORK

We will use the following resource-size decision to develop and illustrate the decision framework.

**Problem:** Balham, a community of 60,000, has two general acute hospitals, each with about 250 beds. Each has its own obstetric services. (Hospital A has 4 labor, 3 delivery, and 36 postpartum beds; Hospital B has 3 labor, 3 delivery, and 30 postpartum beds.) The 14 obstetric physicians in the community are members of medical staffs of both hospitals and usually admit to the hospital of the patient's choice. Though neither hospital has sufficient facilities to handle all deliveries in Balham, each operates at about 40 percent occupancy in the postpartum units. Balham, as a community, is generally overbedded: both hospitals run occupancies on their medical and surgical units of about 70 percent.

For physician and patient convenience (and safety), the obstetric physicians want the two services merged into either Hospital A or B. Neither hospital, however, wants to give up services to the other. There is some talk of merging another service (for example, pediatrics) to the hospital that would lose its OB unit. After several months, the physicians become impatient and suggest that if obstetrics is not merged soon, they themselves will simply admit all patients to one of the hospitals, using the other only when the first is full.

Representatives from both hospitals, from the area planning authority, and from the obstetric physicians, form a task force charged with analyzing the problem and making a recommendation within three months.

There are four steps to the decision framework we will develop:

Step 1: Problem and Model Formulation

Step 2: Quantification

Step 3: Solution

Step 4: Sensitivity Analysis

Step 1: Problem and Model Formulation

Many observers would conclude that the issues of the OB merger problem are essentially political and that most of the problem cannot be quantified. An important part of Step 1 is to separate the quantifiable aspects of the decision from the nonquantifiable.

First, however, the *system objectives* (i.e., objectives that pass the "systems test" of Chapter 1) *must be identified*. For the OB merger problem the objectives would probably include the following:

Medical: *Meeting demand with high-quality services.*

Political: *Both hospitals' survival, and physician convenience.*

Economic: *Cost of operating the two present facilities versus cost of merging services at Hospital A or Hospital B.*

(There are likely many more but these will serve for our example.)

After identifying which objectives are to be served, we must then *identify the alternatives available and the constraints* imposed by the environment. In our example, the alternatives might include:

—Do nothing.

—Do not merge but do something to placate the physicians.

—Merge at Hospital A, providing $L$ labor beds, $D$ delivery beds, and $P$ postpartum beds.

—Merge at Hospital B, providing $L$ labor beds, $D$ delivery beds, and $P$ postpartum beds.

Again, there are likely to be many more alternatives. Note that the last two are actually *sets* of alternatives, each element of the set specifying actual numbers for $L$, $D$ and $P$ (e.g., $L = 4$, $D = 3$, $P = 36$).

Constraints might include a maximum amount of money that could be spent, or a maximum number of beds that could be provided at one or the other of the two hospitals. An important implied constraint is that all demand must be met, although as we will see below, "must be met" will need to be defined more specifically.

After identifying alternatives and constraints, we must next establish a *measure of performance* for each objective. The measure of performance is simply a more precise statement of how we will measure the performance of each alternative against these objectives.

We might measure the medical objectives in terms of the number of patients we would expect to be served in overcrowded facilities, or to be turned away—for example, the number of patients arriving to find all labor beds filled, or being ready to deliver and finding all delivery beds filled, etc. To meet *all* demand (i.e., to have *no* probability of overcrowding or turnaway) would mean building beds used only once a year, or once every two years; this would have definite economic consequences. Thus we must consider the medical and economic objectives, together. Moreover, the political objectives must be considered with the other two: physician convenience cannot be provided at *any* economic cost, nor at the cost of not meeting patient demand.

Conceptually, these three factors are tied together by an *objective function*, an expression relating the objectives to the alternatives. Let's use cost to tie the three objectives together. To do so, we must expand the meaning of "cost" to include more than just dollar cost for some of the objectives. Our overall objective will be to minimize total "cost," or the *combined* medical, political, and economic costs involved in choosing one of our alternatives. At this point let's define specific numbers of beds for merging at either hospital, and label our alternatives $X_1$, $X_2$, ..., $X_6$ as in Figure 2.1. The objective function for the Balham example can be stated

Minimize TOTAL COST $(X)$ = MEDICAL COST $(X)$ + POLITICAL COST $(X)$

+ ECONOMIC COST $(X)$,

where Medical Cost $(X)$, for example, means that medical cost is a function of which alternative $X$ we take—$X$ could be $X_1$, $X_2$, etc. We will call $X$ our *decision variable*; it is variable because it can take on the different values $X_1$, $X_2$, etc.

Two of the objective function's three terms can be divided into elements more amenable to measurement. We can divide medical costs into two factors: $N_L(X)$, the annual *number* of patients who arrive to find the labor facilities full (underserving), and $C_L$, the *cost* per such episode. We do the same for delivery ($N_D(X)$ and $C_D$) and postpartum ($N_P(X)$ and $C_P$). Medical costs would then be stated

MEDICAL COST $(X) = C_L \cdot N_L(X) + C_D \cdot N_D(X) + C_P \cdot N_P(X)$.

Under alternatives $X_1$ and $X_2$ these terms would be zero, since there

*Figure 2.1*

*Alternatives for OB Merger*

$X_1$ Do nothing

$X_2$ Placate physicians

$X_3$ Merge at Hospital A providing 4 labor, 3 delivery, and 38 postpartum beds

$X_4$ Merge at Hospital A providing 6, 5, and 43 beds, respectively

$X_5$ Merge at Hospital B with bed complement of $X_3$

$X_6$ Merge at Hospital B with bed complement of $X_4$

is not overcrowding at present. These terms may become positive for $X_3$ through $X_6$, however, depending upon how many beds are provided.

The economic cost term can be broken down into $C_C(X)$ = cost for building (or converting, as the case may be) and $C_S(X)$ = cost (or savings) of providing additional (or less) equipment and staff. The economic costs would then be stated as

$$\text{ECONOMIC COST } (X) = C_C(X) + C_S(X).$$

This cost will probably not change under $X_1$ or $X_2$, but is likely to be an important factor of $X_3$ through $X_6$.

The political term is difficult to break down further, and for the time being we leave it as is. The total cost equation can now be rewritten as that of Figure 2.2.

### Figure 2.2

### Objective Function for OB Merger

Minimize TOTAL COST $(X)$ =

$C_L \cdot N_L(X) + C_D \cdot N_D(X) + C_P \cdot N_P(X) +$           (Medical cost)

POLITICAL COST $(X)$ +           (Political cost)

$C_C(X) + C_S(X)$           (Economic cost)

Where

$C_L$ = cost per episode for labor "underserving,"
$N_L(X)$ = annual number of patients underserved at labor as a function of which
       alternative $(X)$ is taken,
$C_D$, $N_D(X)$, $C_P$ and $N_P(X)$ are similarly defined for delivery and postpartum,
$C_C(X)$ is cost of building or converting beds, and
$C_S(X)$ is the cost (or, if negative, savings) of additional (or reduced) staff and
       equipment.

This is Step 1: describing the problem; identifying objectives, alternatives, and constraints; and formulating a general model. We have looked at this step in some detail because it is here that the health administrator's primary responsibility lies. The health administrator's ability to perceive the relevant objectives, to identify alternatives and constraints, and to appreciate dividing the more easily quantified from the nonquantifiable elements of the problem is essential to successful quantitative decision making.

Step 2: Quantification

The model of Figure 2.2 is not in a form that allows the best alternative to be readily identified. The second step of the decision framework is to replace the symbols of the Step 1 model with *specific numbers and/or functions*—we call this quantification.

Consider the $C_C(X)$ and $C_S(X)$ terms of our model (Figure 2.2). For these terms, we need estimates from architects, construction firms, and accountants concerning the costs to modify or build beds; and estimates from nurses, physicians, industrial engineers, accountants, etc., concerning the cost to staff and equip the modified or newly constructed facilities. Since the decision will affect the costs for some time (arbitrarily let's assume 10 years), these costs may need to be amortized over such a horizon to give annual costs as in Figure 2.3. (An alternative would be to estimate the present value of such costs for the next 10 years for each alternative.) Quantification for the $C_C(X)$ and $C_S(X)$ terms involves quantifying as far as possible what the functions will equal for each alternative.

We will see in Chapter 5 that the $N_L(X)$, $N_D(X)$, $N_P(X)$ functions

### Figure 2.3

### Quantification of Terms in Objective Function

| $X$ | Alternative | $C_C(X)$ | $C_S(X)$ | $C_C(X) + C_S(X)$ |
|---|---|---|---|---|
| $X_1$ | Do nothing | 0 | 0 | 0 |
| $X_2$ | Placate physicians | 0 | 0 | 0 |
| $X_3$ | Merge at Hospital A providing 4 labor, 3 delivery, and 38 postpartum beds | \$ 20,000 | −\$820,000 | −\$800,000 |
| $X_4$ | Merge at Hospital A providing 6, 5, and 43 beds, respectively | \$ 80,000 | −\$480,000 | −\$400,000 |
| $X_5$ | Merge at Hospital B with bed complement of $X_3$ | \$ 80,000 | −\$280,000 | −\$200,000 |
| $X_6$ | Merge at Hospital B with bed complement of $X_4$ | \$120,000 | \$ 80,000 | +\$200,000 |

*A negative sign in these columns denotes a *savings* associated with undertaking that alternative.

can be quantified by a technique called simulation, which involves forecasting the demand for OB facilities in the future, estimating the distribution of service times (the amount of time a patient occupies a facility) in labor, delivery, and postpartum, and building a computer model of the facility. Each alternative is then "implemented" in the computer model, and the number of turnaways at labor, delivery, and postpartum are "observed" for the simulated facility. We will then infer that, if we were to implement an alternative in the real world facility, we would get the same number of turnaways as we "observed" for the simulated facility. (We will examine other ways to quantify the number of turnaways $N_L(X)$, $N_D(X)$, and $N_P(X)$ in Chapters 3, 4, and 5.) Quantification for these functions thus means assigning numbers to them in the form of Figure 2.4.

*Figure 2.4*

*Number of Turnaways by Alternative*

| Alternative | Number of Patients Arriving to Find Facilities Full | | |
|---|---|---|---|
| $X$ | $N_L(X)$ Labor | $N_D(X)$ Delivery | $N_P(X)$ Postpartum |
| $X_1$ | 0 | 0 | 0 |
| $X_2$ | 0 | 0 | 0 |
| $X_3$ | 13 | 14 | 128 |
| $X_4$ | 3 | 4 | 8 |
| $X_5$ | 13 | 14 | 128 |
| $X_6$ | 3 | 4 | 8 |

The cost per episode components ($C_L$, $C_D$, and $C_P$) and the political costs of each alternative are not directly quantifiable by the types of techniques we will examine. One approach is to do our best to assign costs subjectively to these terms. Again, the argument could appear here that since we cannot objectively quantify *every* component of the objective function, why quantify *any* of it? The answer is in the third step.

Step 3: Solution

It is at this step that a preliminary solution is determined. A solution means deciding which alternative is "best." In our case, suppose we first summarize the quantified (in Step 2) and "nonquantifiable" components of each alternative as in Figure 2.5 (Alternative $X_2$ is omitted to simplify the analysis).

*Figure 2.5*

*Full Quantification of Objective Function*

| | Alternative | Medical | Political | Economic |
|---|---|---|---|---|
| | $X_1$: Do nothing | 0 | Obstetric staff unsatisifed; may take action to use only one hospital | 0 |
| Merge at Hospital A | $X_3$: Provide 4 labor, 3 delivery and 38 postpartum beds | Each year, 13 labor, 14 delivery, and 128 postpartum patients arrive to find facilities full (i.e., are underserved) (Total = 155) | Hospital B may suffer financial problems | Save $800,000 a year |
| Merge at Hospital A | $X_4$: Provide 6, 5, and 43 beds, respectively | 3 labor, 4 delivery and 8 postpartum "underserved" patients per year (Total = 15) | Hospital B may suffer financial problems | Save $400,000 a year |
| Merge at Hospital B | $X_5$: (Same as $X_3$) | Same as $X_3$ | None | Save $200,000 a year |
| Merge at Hospital B | $X_6$: (Same as $X_4$) | Same as $X_4$ | None | *Cost* $200,000 more each year |

Now an important benefit of quantification, and the way around the nonquantifiable components, can be seen. Given that the decision *must* be either $X_1$, $X_3$, $X_4$, $X_5$, or $X_6$, the decision can be reduced to a sequence of pairwise comparisons with quantifiable versus nonquantifiable components. For example, the first comparison could be between $X_3$ and $X_4$. Is the reduction in "underserved" patients (from 155 in $X_3$ to 15 in $X_4$) "worth" the $400,000 a year more that it will cost (in reduced savings) to effect the reduction? (Only two alternative configurations, $X_3$ and $X_4$, are included, although it is often possible to expand the concept to any number.) Instead of having to put a dollar cost on underserving a patient, we need only decide if the cost of underserving 140 (155 − 15) patients is more or less than the cost to avoid it: $400,000. Suppose we decide that $X_4$ is preferable to $X_3$. This means that the cost of underserving one patient is *at least* $400,000 ÷ 140 = $2,857. (Right?)

If $X_4$ is preferable to $X_3$, then $X_6$ must be preferable to $X_5$ since it is the same comparison, and we next need to choose between $X_1$, $X_4$, and $X_6$. The choice between $X_4$ and $X_6$ is again between a quantifiable component, $600,000 a year ($400,000 + $200,000), and a nonquantifiable component, the financial difficulties of Hospital B. Again, it is a "more than or less than" decision rather than a case of quantifying the cost of financial difficulties of Hospital B into a single dollar term. Let's say we choose $X_6$ over $X_4$. Then avoiding the financial difficulties of Hospital B "is worth" at least $600,000.

The final decision is whether it is worth more or less than $200,000 a year to avoid the conflict with the obstetric physicians ("avoid the conflict" includes all the true benefits to both the physician and patient in merging).*

Step 4: Sensitivity Analysis

How confident are we in our solution? Where could we have gone wrong? Decision making is a dynamic process, and in the quantification step it is likely that we will identify objectives, alternatives, and constraints left out in Step 1, and it is certain that we will make many compromises in quantification because of time and cost. Some of these—the new objectives and new alternatives and

---

*We use the above pairwise comparison sequence only as an example of the concept of "pricing out" or "costing out" the effect of adopting alternatives. Although it works as a solution technqiue in this simplified example, it neither guarantees that the best solution will be found nor is it easy to perform in many situations, and the chapters that follow present other, more general, methods of solution.

constraints—can be included as we go along in the first three steps, sometimes requiring backtracking to a previous step.

But there comes a time when we must face the question of how much the compromises made in quantification affect the quality of the result of the analysis (the decision). Another way to look at this is how *sensitive* the results are to

—assumptions made in model formulation (e.g., linearity, independence, length of decision horizon, etc.),

—an error in the number of forecasted deliveries,

—an error in estimation of construction costs,

—an error in estimating the $N_L$ $(X)$, $N_D$ $(X)$, and $N_P$ $(X)$, and

—any number of other errors in the quantification step.

It is at Step 4, at sensitivity analysis, that a serious examination of assumptions and compromises made in prior steps is carried out, often resulting in a loop back to Step 2 (or even Step 1). For some compromises, we hope we will find the results relatively insensitive. For example, we may find that the same alternative would be chosen even if there were a 20 percent error in the $C_S$ $(X)$ function. On the other hand, if the results are very sensitive to the number of forecasted deliveries (i.e., a different alternative is better with a small change in the number of deliveries), it indicates that more time (and money) should be spent on the forecast. By systematically examining the sensitivity of each component of the decision process we begin to obtain a feel for the "quality" of the decision and are guided on how to improve the quality with more effort.

We will attempt to apply this decision-making framework throughout the examples of the next four chapters. This is not a "case" text, however, and certain parts of the framework will be emphasized more than others in a given example. It is the reader's responsibility, then, to keep the full decision-making framework in mind when we examine the concepts and techniques of the next four chapters.

## 2.3 THE CYBERNETIC CONTROL FRAMEWORK

The administrator's profession is based on the assumption that he can steer systems in ways that will achieve desired performance— i.e., that he can control systems. The decision-making framework developed in the previous section is a *part* of the control process in two important ways. First, it identifies objectives and measures of performance that are used to monitor the performance of the system being controlled. Second, the decision-making framework specifies the steps and logic that allow the administrator to return a system's performance back to desired levels, or to prevent the system's performance from deviating too far from these levels.

But the decision-making framework is not enough to maintain desired system performance. There is a control *process* that specifies the steps required to maintain desired performance and a set of *structural* requirements that specifies abilities that must exist in the system being controlled, and in its parent system, in order to carry out the control process. Both the process *and* structure describe the cybernetic control framework. As will be seen, most of the structural requirements are met by going through the decision-making framework.

The essence of cybernetic control is that systems should be designed to control their own performance. This is in contrast to other control strategies that rely solely on employing laws or rules supported by positive or negative sanctions. Consider the structural requirements necessary to allow the OB system in Balham to control its own performance.

Requirement 1: Explicit Performance Measures

In order to achieve its objectives, the OB system in Balham (which would include the units in both hospitals) must have its measures of performance and the desired levels of those measures of performance *explicitly* stated.

The task force was formed to analyze the OB merger decision primarily because of a shift in objectives. The majority of the obstetric physicians wanted the two services merged into either Hospital A or B so they would no longer have to travel back and forth between hospitals. The health planners wanted to participate on the task force because of the size of the separate OB units. The standard set by the American College of Obstetrics and Gynecology is that at least 2,000 births per year should occur in each separate facility. It is thought that 2,000 or more births lead to higher quality, first because specialized equipment necessary for quality care can be justified, and second, because peer review among physicians and nurses can take place. In Balham, there were 2,300 births last year, split between the two hospitals. Merging would presumably increase quality.

What triggered the analysis of the OB merger decision was the discrepancy between what the physicians, planners, and administrators implicitly wanted, and what was actually happening. They each used a different objective and a different measure of performance, but the result was the same—desired performance was not being achieved: physicians were inconvenienced, the OB units each delivered fewer than 2,000 births per year, and, on the average, the OB units were less than 70 percent full.

Recall the discussion of the effect of the systems approach in Chapter 1. What *should* the performance measures be, and what *should* the desired performance levels be? The objectives of the larger systems—the hospital, the community, etc.—must first be identified, and the performance measures (and levels) that serve the larger system's objectives must then be identified. For example, the analysis of the OB merger decision led to a community objective and performance measure—to minimize the number of patients who arrive when there is no bed (for labor, delivery, or postpartum).

As the analysis of the OB merger decision was conducted, the task force began making the performance measures and desired levels more explicit. These explicit statements become the basis for control; and without such explicit statements, the OB system in Balham would not be able to continue to achieve "systems" objectives.

Requirement 2: Feedback

The Balham OB system must be able to obtain feedback about actual performance. This feedback is essential to increase the probability that the objectives will be achieved and maintained after the decision is made. Without feedback about physicians' satisfaction, number of births in the facility, occupancy rate, and number of patients who arrive when all beds are full, it is unlikely that the OB system will continue to achieve its objectives (i.e., be in control). *Deliberate arrangements* must be made so that feedback is provided; it does not occur naturally.

There is no guarantee that a good decision will lead to a good outcome. As a result, there are very few "one-time" decisions—most are sequential decisions made in response to feedback about actual performance compared to desired performance. If, after the merger at Hospital B, feedback indicates that the desired level of performance is not being met, the decision may have to be modified, the original size of the unit at B may have to be reconsidered, the desired level of performance compromised, or other steps taken.

The notion of feedback implies that it reaches the administrator in time for corrective action. "Late" feedback may be used by the administrator to forecast future performance, but when the system being controlled is complex and uncertain, "late" feedback is likely to describe performance that no longer exists. Naturally the definition of "late" depends on how rapidly the system being controlled changes.

### Requirement 3: Problem-Solving Capacity

The OB administrator's role must be such that he has the capacity to generate alternatives and make decisions that will cause the system to return to its desired state. This requires the administrator to be able to use the *decision-making framework*. The types of decisions that may need to be made include those discussed in Chapter 1: resource-size decisions, procedure decisions, and/or scheduling decisions. If feedback indicates that desired performance *is* being achieved, the "decision" would be to make no changes unless the manager anticipates problems ahead that could be alleviated by making changes now.

Since Step 1 of the decision-making framework requires that the objectives, performance measures, and desired performance levels be reconsidered, these might also be changed at this point.

### Requirement 4: Forecast

The OB process operates in an environment that includes many uncertainties which could prevent the system from continuing to achieve its objectives. Recall that in the merger decision, the analysis attempted to anticipate (1) the number of women who will arrive for delivery, (2) construction and personnel costs, (3) the financial consequences to each hospital of each alternative, and (4) the physicians' satisfaction with each alternative. Such forecasting at decision time is inexact, but necessary for planning.

Because forecasting is an inexact process, and because of the complexity of the OB system, forecasting cannot stop after the decision has been made. An effective control system must continue to anticipate changes in the environment that may cause the obstetrics system to fail to maintain its objectives, so that corrective action can be taken before the system goes out of control.

### Requirement 5: Learn Environment

As a result of Steps 3 and 4, the manager must become knowledgeable about the system's environment—about other hospitals, about women's preferences for giving birth at home, about third-party payer restrictions (pay for only 3 days of stay if no complications), about Chamber of Commerce efforts to attract new industry to the community, etc. It is not enough to understand the OB system well. To be able to continue to have it achieve desired performance, the administrator must also understand its environment so that future performance is anticipated and decisions are made that prevent future problems.

Requirement 6: Back-Up Support

Finally, some form of back-up support is required if the system fails to achieve its objective: managers with more experience, more expertise, more authority, different attitudes, etc., must be available. This means the manager of the OB system must know when to obtain back-up support, and his supervisor (or administrator of the hospital) must know when to intervene. If, for example, the occupancy rate remains below 50 percent, the facility may be too large. Part of the facility could be converted for other uses, and the manager of the OB system would need support from the hospital administrator to undertake such a conversion. If, on the other hand, the OB merger results in too few beds, and four women arrive each month to find no beds available, the number of beds may have to be increased. Again, the OB manager requires back-up support to acquire additional resources.

It is left as an exercise to consider what would happen to the OB system if, one at a time, each structural requirement were missing. We will see that if one is missing, it will be difficult (if not impossible) for the OB system to continue to achieve its objectives when interrupted by an unpredicted event.

Once the structural requirements are met, the cybernetic control process puts them together as illustrated in Figure 2.6. Desired performance is compared to actual performance (Box 1). Future performance is anticipated using past experience and knowledge of the environment (Box 2). In light of anticipated future performance, decisions are made and problems solved in order to maintain desired performance (Box 3). Desired performance levels may be adjusted (dotted line). As services are delivered, unanticipated events occur that affect actual performance (Box 4). This effect is detected when actual performance is fed back and compared to desired performance (Box 5). This process for the Balham OB system is illustrated in Figure 2.7.

## 2.4 FORECASTING AND MEASUREMENT

Forecasts and measurements serve both the decision-making and control frameworks, while the frameworks provide guidance as to

Figure 2.6

The Cybernetic Control Framework

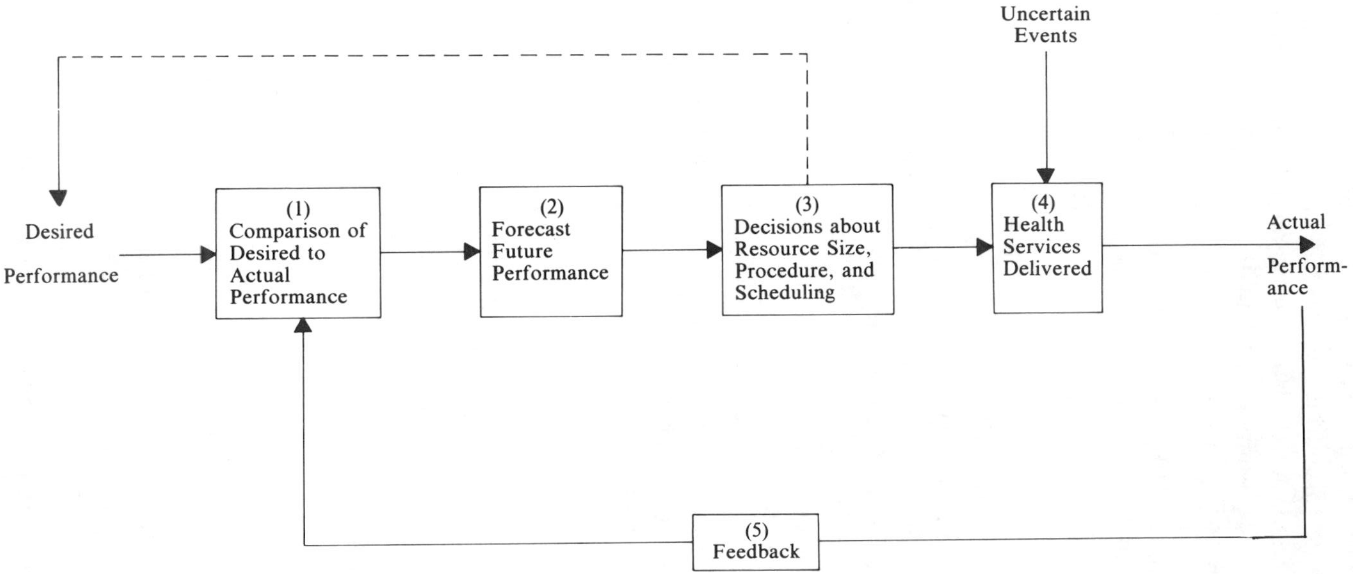

*Figure 2.7*

## OB Merger in the Cybernetic Control Framework

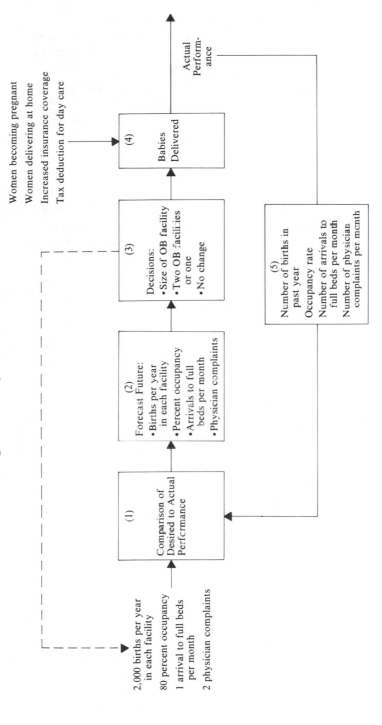

which forecasts and measurements to make. It is therefore important to have a clear understanding of these concepts, the difference between them, and to appreciate how they serve decision making and control.

Measurement is assigning a number to a system according to a rule, in such a way that the number represents the quantity of an attribute of the system. Measurements can only be made on actual, existing systems. For example, some of the measurements used in the decision-making framework as applied to the OB merger decision are listed in Table 2.1. The attribute in Column 1, for the system in Column 2, is measured using the rule in Column 3, resulting in the observation in Column 4. Most of the measurements in Table 2.1 are straightforward—so straightforward that they are often overlooked as measurements of an attribute. Others are complicated by the fact that there may not be agreement that they in fact measure the attribute which they are supposed to measure.

Counting beds to measure the "size" of the facility, or counting filled beds and calculating the occupancy rate to measure "utilization" of the facility, are straightforward measurements. But what about counting the numbers of hospitals in a community to measure "accessibility," or the number of beds to measure "availability," or the number of patients arriving to find filled beds to measure "underserving," or the number of births per year in a facility to measure "quality," or the number of complaining physicians to measure physician "satisfaction." Although these measures may not seem valid, they may be perfectly good for the way they were used in the OB merger decision. Chapter 9 will readdress this question: what would be valid measures of accessibility, availability, underserving, quality, and satisfaction; and how could their validity be evaluated?

All of the measurements in Table 2.1 were made on the existing OB system. Figure 2.5, Row 1, summarizes the *measurements* on the *existing* system made to evaluate the medical, economic, and political costs of doing nothing. What about the other rows in Figure 2.5? Those alternatives do not now exist, and we cannot make "measurements" on them. We are forced to *forecast* what the numbers would be if the alternatives did exist.

Consider an example: Measurement 2 in Table 2.1—number of acute hospitals. Our measurement is 2 acute hospitals. What is our forecast for 5 years? Still 2 acute hospitals? Or will there be 1? Or 3? The point is that when in our decision-making and control frameworks we assume there will still be 2 hospitals in 5 years, it is a forecast and not a measurement. Consider Measurements 14, 15 and 16 in Table 2.1—costs for construction, equipment, and staff.

## Table 2.1
## Measurements for OB Merger

| Attribute (1) | System (2) | Rule (3) | Number (4) | Unit (5) |
|---|---|---|---|---|
| 1. Size | Balham | Count people | 60,000 | People |
| 2. Accessibility | Balham Health Service | Count hospitals | 2 | Acute hospitals |
| 3. Availability | Balham Health Service | Count beds | 500 | Beds in acute hospitals |
| 4. Availability | Balham Health Service | Count physicians | 14 | OB physicians |
| 5. Size | Hospital A labor room | Count beds | 4 | Labor beds |
| 6. Size | Hospital A delivery room | Count beds | 3 | Delivery beds |
| 7. Size | Hospital A postpartum unit | Count beds | 36 | Postpartum |
| 8. Utilization | Hospital A or B postpartum unit | Count filled postpartum beds each day for one year | 5,184 | Patient days per year |
| 9. Utilization | Hospital A or B postpartum unit | Divide patient days per year by number of postpartum beds times 365. | 40 | % OB occupancy |
| 10. Utilization | Hospital A or B | Same as above for hospital | 70 | % hospital occupancy |
| 11. Degree of underserving | Hospital A or B labor room | Count patients | 0 | Patients arriving to find all labor beds filled |

## Table 2.1 (Continued)
### Measurements for OB Merger

| Attribute (1) | System (2) | Rule (3) | Number (4) | Unit (5) |
|---|---|---|---|---|
| 12. Degree of underserving | Hospital A or B delivery room | Count patients | 0 | Patients arriving to find all delivery beds filled |
| 13. Degree of underserving | Hospital A or B postpartum suite | Count patients | 0 | Patients arriving to find all postpartum beds filled |
| 14. Construction cost today | Hospital A or B OB unit | Count dollars | * | Cost for construction |
| 15. Equipment cost today | Hospital A or B OB unit | Count dollars | * | Cost for equipment |
| 16. Staff cost today | Hospital A or B | Count payroll dollars | * | Cost for staff |
| 17. OB demand | Balham Health Service | Count births | 2,300 | Births last year |
| 18. Quality | Hospital A OB unit | Count births | 1,090 | Births last year |
| 19. Quality | Hospital B OB unit | Count births | 1,210 | Births last year |
| 20. OB physician satisfaction | Balham | Count complaining physicians | 8 | Complaining OB physicians |

* These measurements were not reported.

We can measure the cost today, but using that cost measurement in our decision making would be an obvious mistake with the current inflationary trend. We are required to forecast (estimate) costs in the future, taking into account whatever we can about cost increases.

Consider preparing the list in Table 2.1 for last year, the year before, and so on for 15 years back. This would be a measurement process, since the system existed. Having such past measurements may aid in forecasting the future. The necessary assumption is that some trend in the past may continue into the future. In Chapter 7 we will investigate making forecasts based on the measurement of past behavior of a system, to which we will add all other information available—both objective and subjective.

Measurement and forecasting play an important role in both decision and control. The problem- and model-formulation step in the decision-making framework relies heavily on measurement and forecasts to establish that a problem exists and to describe the problem in a manner amenable to solution. It is in the second step—quantification—however, that these two concepts play the major role. Sensitivity analysis involves evaluating measurements and forecasts made in previous steps, and in many cases it results in re-measurement and re-forecasting certain components of the decision. Measurement is essential for determining if a system is in control, and forecasting performance is essential for predicting if (and when) it may fall out of control.

## 2.5 THE ADMINISTRATOR'S ROLE

While the task force of the OB merger example has overall *responsibility* for analyzing the decision, it is unlikely that it will *perform* all parts of the quantitative analysis itself. For some aspects of the analysis, it will rely on quantitative staff specialists. These staff specialists could be members of an in-house staff or outside consultants. What roles will the administrator and his staff specialist play in the decision-making and control framework?

Let's return to the OB merger problem and to our decision-making and control frameworks. The first step of the decision-making framework is often almost entirely the responsibility of the administrator. While a number of measurements and forecasts might be required to define the scope of the problem, and these may be performed by a staff specialist, the administrator must take the dominant role in identifying objectives (established by his board), suggesting alternatives, and defining constraints. This step guides the rest of the analysis and is essential to effective management. This is not to say that the staff specialist should not be included in formulation of the problem and model—only that he should take an advisory role.

It is at the second step—quantification—that the staff specialist usually assumes a larger role. The techniques of quantification usually involve either a significant amount of time, or a certain amount of quantitative expertise, or both. For both reasons, the administrator's time and skills are better utilized here as a manager of the staff specialist. Thus, important skills for the administrator include a conceptual knowledge of the quantitative techniques used in this step, an ability to recognize when certain techniques should be used, how much it costs in time and money to use them, and an ability to evaluate the results of their use, which includes appreciation of the necessary assumptions made for their use.

Since more often than not the solution step involves trading off quantified and nonquantifiable elements in the objectives, the administrator again assumes the dominant role in Step 3. It is he who is responsible for representing the interests of the nonquantifiable elements of the objective. Again, the staff specialist is important in an advisory capacity.*

The fourth step—sensitivity analysis—is a joint effort of the administrator and his staff specialists. The administrator must appreciate the quality of the analysis he is buying and be able to evaluate the analysis in terms of its sensitivity to design, quality of data, assumptions, and compromises in quantification. Then he must be able to ask the appropriate questions of the staff specialists, who in turn would provide the answers.

Some of the structural requirements for the cybernetic control framework are met as the decision-making framework is employed: measures of performance become explicit, decisions that solve problems are made, future demand and future system performance are forecast, and measurements of the environment are made. The roles of administrator and quantitative staff specialist for decision-making activities do not change in the control framework. The control framework may indicate the need for additional measures of performance to be constructed (quality of nursing care, for example), and quantitative specialists would construct such measures and perform tests of reliability and validity. However, the administrator is the one who ultimately must decide whether the performance measure will be used for what it was intended.

---

*There are a few rather sophisticated techniques used for the solution of models where the most important elements can be quantified; with the use of these, the staff specialist plays a more involved role.

In addition, the reports that provide feedback are often computer generated. The quantitative specialist would arrange for the reports, but the administrator should specify the most usable format for decision making and request appropriate graphs and tables. Since the administrator should manage the quantitative staff specialist, it goes without saying that the administrator is responsible for making sure the decision-making and cybernetic control frameworks are implemented appropriately. (For further discussion of implementation, see the Munson and Hancock reference at the end of the chapter.)

The presentation of concepts and techniques in the remaining chapters follows this assumption of the interlinking roles of the administrator and the staff specialist. Some of the techniques are straightforward and can be performed quickly. For these, which the administrator might choose to perform himself, the presentation includes a fair amount of detail. Other techniques are straightforward but require a considerable amount of the administrator's time to perform. Finally, some of the techniques involve a considerable amount of mathematical expertise, and these are presented at a more conceptual level, emphasizing the type of knowledge that an administrator would need to manage effectively the staff specialists performing the technique, and to evaluate its use.

## 2.6 CONCLUSION

There are many factors integral to the decision and control problems we will be analyzing that are difficult, and often impossible, to quantify. Indeed, these factors in the health field are often the most important; for example, improving patient care, increasing patient or physician convenience, avoiding turned-away patients, and saving lives. Two questions arise that we should keep in mind throughout our examination of quantitative decision making and control:

1. How much should we try to quantify?

2. How can quantitative decision making and cybernetic control be useful when everything cannot be quantified?

It is the nature of all the decisions we will analyze that there is a trade-off involved; usually it is money paid out (costs) versus the benefits we can expect from such an outlay. In order to make a decision, the benefits must ultimately be expressed in the same measurement units as the costs. Since costs are in dollars (net, present valued, or any other type—but still dollars), making the decision ultimately requires that benefits be expressed in dollars as well, either explicitly or by inference. Some benefits can be easily converted to dollars—manpower saved, in-patient days avoided, equipment purchase avoided, etc. The value of other benefits—reduced turnaways, reduced patient waiting time, etc.—may be determined by the values we, the parties responsible for the decision, place on such benefits. What *can* be quantified here are the physical benefits—the *number* of reduced turnaways, the *number* of minutes wait reduced, etc.

In answer to the first question, we will quantify to the extent that the value of the results of quantification, in terms of improved decision making and control, exceeds the cost of further quantification. In answer to the second, the quantitative decision and control processes allows us to quantify as far as possible (at least in most cases up to the physical benefit), leaving only those factors which the manager believes are not quantifiable. Quantitative decision making and control then allows the manager to focus sharply on the *values* he is imputing to the unquantifiable factors through his decisions, because he can compare them with the factors which are quantified in dollar terms (the imputed value to underserving in our OB example is an excellent illustration).

In our example, the health administrator's role has been crucial in several ways. First, he needed to conceptualize the problem in terms of the decision-making framework. Second, he needed to separate the quantifiable components from the unquantifiable ones. Third, he needed to provide and manage the technical resources (staff specialists) to measure, forecast, and quantify. This included appreciating and evaluating the limitations and the results of the analysis. Fourth, he needed to compare the quantifiable with the unquantifiable components to make a decision. Last, he needed to control the system after the decision was implemented.

## Exercise

2.1 Consider the OB system for six different situations; in each, assume one of the six structural requirements for cybernetic control is missing (implicit measures of performance, no or late feedback, no problem-solving ability, no anticipation of the future, no knowledge of the environment, and no back-up support). What would happen in each case if the *un*anticipated event was that one-half of all births begin to occur in the home because having babies at home is the "thing to do."? (Assume deliveries in the home are done as often now as in your own community.)

**Additional Reading**

Munson, Fred C. and Hancock, Walton M. "Implementation of Hospital Control Systems." In *Cost Control in Hospitals*, edited by John R. Griffith, Walton M. Hancock, and Fred C. Munson. Ann Arbor, Michigan: Health Administration Press, 1976.

# Part II

# Analysis for Decision Making

*The decision-making problems discussed in Part I can be approached on several levels of sophistication, depending on how important the problem is, how valuable a more sophisticated analysis is, and how much time, data, and money are available to solve it. Part II develops four levels of sophistication for analyzing decision-making problems. The levels progress from less to more sophisticated along two dimensions: simple to complex, and deterministic to stochastic. For the most part, a decision-making problem can be analyzed at any of the four levels, although some problems fall more naturally to certain levels than others.*

# 3

# Simple Deterministic Analysis

## 3.1 INTRODUCTION

What distinguishes a simple deterministic analysis from other types of analyses? First, a deterministic analysis is one in which the decision is treated as if there were no uncertainty involved. For example, consider the decision of determining the appropriate number of laboratory technologists to provide in order to meet a given level of demand (a resource size decision). If the analysis assumes that demand for laboratory tests will be *exactly* 200 tests every day, and that a typical lab technician can perform *exactly* 10 tests every hour, we would consider the analysis a deterministic one. On the other hand, if the analysis takes into account that demand is a random variable which followed a normal distribution with mean 200 and standard deviation 20, and/or that the number of examinations per hour that a technologist could perform was a random variable distributed normally with mean 10 and standard deviation 2, we would call the analysis a stochastic one.

"Simple" has particular meanings for our purposes. For deterministic analyses, a simple analysis is one in which there are only a few unknowns and/or a few available alternatives to be evaluated for each unknown. For example, the analysis of the technologist decision above becomes complex if we now consider four levels of skill (head technologist, senior technologist, junior technologist, lab secretary), each of which can substitute to some degree for some of the tasks of the others (more unknowns), and we try to determine the number of *hours* of each skill class needed each day of the week (more alternatives per unknown). When there are a large number of unknowns and/or alternatives, we are faced with a complex but deterministic analysis. In this case we can sometimes use a special modeling technique called Mathematical Programming, discussed in Chapter 6. (For the stochastic analysis, "simple" has a slightly different meaning, which we address in the next chapter.)

Another important distinction between simple and complex analyses is that in the latter, objectives are difficult to quantify. The decision process is much more straightforward when it involves a procedure decision, such as whether to use automated or non-automated equipment (or whether to contract for services or to provide them yourself) if we want to minimize the cost of producing exactly 200 lab tests per day. It becomes much more complex when it involves the resource-size decision of how much demand *should* be met. The latter requires a complex analysis to balance the dollar cost of providing and maintaining resources versus the complex "cost" of not being able to meet all demand in a timely fashion.

Most decisions that a health administrator or planner faces are stochastic and complex. It is, however, often desirable (because of cost) or mandatory (because of time and unavailable data) that the administrator *analyze* a complex stochastic decision as if it were simple and/or deterministic. Thus our simple/complex, deterministic/stochastic characterization is applied to the *analysis* of the decision rather than to the decision itself. We will see that any decision can be analyzed as if it were simple or complex, deterministic or stochastic, although some decisions are more amenable to a simple and/or deterministic analysis than others. We will treat some decisions first as if they were simple and deterministic, and later as if complex and stochastic.

As we work through examples in these four chapters, the reader should keep carefully in mind the simplifying assumptions implied by treating the decisions as simple or deterministic, how the assumptions limit the applicability of the results of the analysis, how the analysis could be done if the assumptions were not made, and how much more it might cost (in time and money) not to make them.

## 3.2 RESOURCE-SIZE DECISIONS

When treated as deterministic, simple resource-size decisions are largely *measurement* and *forecasting* problems, which we discuss in Chapters 7, 8, and 9.

**Problem:** The Balham community of population 60,000 has decided to build and staff a pediatric primary care walk-in clinic. The resource size decisions are:

1. How many examining rooms will be needed?
2. How many physicians will be needed?
3. How many other staff members will be needed?
4. How often should the clinic be open?

Assume that we have forecasted a point estimate for demand (number of visits per week). The deterministic analysis reduces to determining *service times*—the amount of each resource a visit will consume. Suppose we have decided independently to run the clinic 8 A.M. to 4 P.M. on weekdays and 8 A.M. to 12 noon on Saturdays. (Our old where-to-start megaproblem reappears: should this resource-size decision be made independently of the other resource-size decisions?) Addressing the number of examining rooms decision, we would first determine the average time per visit that an examining room is used. (If examining room usage differed significantly by type of patient, a weighted average might be calculated.) Suppose we determine (either by direct observation or from published "standards") that the average examining room service time is 20 minutes per visit. Suppose further that we have predicted that the clinic will average 400 visits per week. On the average we will need 8,000 minutes per week and since the clinic will be open 44 hours (2,640 minutes) per week, we need 3 examining rooms *if they are used at 100 percent utilization.* Of course such high utilization is not possible for several stochastic reasons that we cannot ignore: (1) the actual number of weekly visits will be stochastic about the average, (2) demand will be stochastic by day of week, and (3) the service time is also stochastic.

Stochastic effects such as these usually render the deterministic treatment of resource-size decisions unsatisfactory, and a stochastic treatment is necessary. A deterministic method which attempts to include the effect of stochastic factors *indirectly* assumes (or attempts to measure) an appropriate utilization (or occupancy) rate for the resource. This may be the utilization rate for a clinic of similar type and size in another community, or the average of several clinics. The disadvantages of this method should become apparent from an example. Suppose we have settled on an "appropriate" utilization rate of 60 percent for examining rooms, based on the rate of a larger adult clinic in a nearby community. We will still need 8,000 minutes of examining rooms per week, and each examining room will be available 2,640 minutes per week. Since each room will be used only 60 percent of the time,

$$\text{Rooms needed} = \frac{8,000}{2,640 \times .6} = 5.05 \text{ or } 5.$$

The problem with such an analysis is that questions such as How long will patients wait?, How many patients will not be seen the same day they walk in?, and Could the clinic get by with only 4 rooms without significantly affecting wait and turnaway? are not answered. To address these questions, a stochastic analysis that *directly* takes into account the stochastic demand and service time is required, and we will return to that problem in the next two chapters.

The general relationship, of which the above is an example, is

Units of resource needed

$$= \frac{\text{Number of units of service demanded}}{(\text{Capacity of each unit of resource}) \times (\text{Utilization})}.$$

A common example of the general relationship is the case of the number of beds required in a given hospital, which takes the form

Beds required = Admissions per year (per 1,000 population)

$\times$ Average length of stay

$\times$ Population (in 1,000s)

$\div$ (365 $\times$ Occupancy).

(Since Patient days = Admissions per year (per 1,000 population) $\times$ Average length of Stay $\times$ Population (in 1,000s), it may take the form

$$\text{Beds required} = \frac{\text{Patient days (per year)}}{365 \times \text{Occupancy}},$$

which is more closely analogous to the general form.)

The determination of the terms on the right side of the above relationship involves measurement and forecasting problems of the types discussed in Chapters 7, 8, and 9. A great deal of work has been done in developing methods for such determinations (usually called measurement or forecasting of service areas), and the interested reader is referred to the Griffith reference at the end of this chapter.

A resource-size decision that can be treated deterministically with apparent success is the nurse-staffing decision, although we will return to this decision in later chapters with both a stochastic treatment and a more complex deterministic treatment. The nurse-staffing decision involves how many full-time-equivalent nursing personnel positions of each skill class (Registered Nurse (RN), Licensed Practical Nurse (LPN), and Nurse's Aide (AIDE)) should be funded for each nursing unit. The decision can be reduced to how many nursing hours of each skill class should be provided for each shift in each nursing unit. Demand for nursing care services per patient is usually assumed to depend on such factors (among others) as (1) the patient's care level—e.g., low care, intermediate care, high care; and (2) the patient's service—e.g., medical, surgical. Thus "standards" of the form $S_{ijk}$ can be derived such that $S_{ijk}$ is the number of minutes of skill $i$ nursing care needed for patients of care level $j$ and service $k$. The determination of the $S_{ijk}$ is a measurement problem of the type discussed in Chapter 9.

The total number of, say, RN ($i = 1$) minutes needed would be be

$$R = \sum_{j} \sum_{k} S_{1jk} \cdot X_{jk}$$

where $X_{jk}$ is the *average* number of patients of care level $j$ and service $k$ who are expected to be on the unit. There are several reasons why the deterministic treatment might be felt justifiable for *this* resource size problem:

1. If the unit is large and usually serves patients of similar ages, care levels, and service, the variance of the *total* number of RN nursing minutes demanded may not be outside the range of the ability of RNs to increase their output for short periods of time (either by doing more or by eliminating or delaying certain tasks).

2. For those days when demand does exceed the (extended) capacity, a nurse reallocation system (discussed in Chapter 11) can be employed to adjust temporarily the number of nurses among units in the hospital to meet demand.

There are other resource-size decisions which may be treated as deterministic. The important considerations are: (1) the implications of the simplifying assumptions necessary to treat a stochastic decision as if it were deterministic, (2) how much more information a stochastic treatment would yield, (3) how much a deterministic analysis reduces our ability to maintain control, and (4) how much a stochastic analysis (if possible at all) will "cost" in terms of money and time. We will be able to get a feel for these types of considerations when we begin to treat resource-size decisions as stochastic in later chapters, and in the control framework.

## 3.3 PROCEDURE DECISIONS

**Problem:** Demand in the radiology department in your hospital has reached and exceeded capacity to the extent that it is clear the facility will have to be expanded to meet projected increases of 500–1500 examinations a month (mostly outpatient). There are two alternatives: *M*—the *make* alternative—involves leasing two additional examining rooms (with equipment) and hiring another radiologist and two additional technicians to do only outpatient exams; or *B*—the *buy* alternative—requires your contracting on a per-exam basis for outpatient exams with a private radiologist group located in a building adjacent to the hospital. (The rooms of the make alternative would be leased from the private radiologist group.)

The major difference in the two alternative procedures is the high fixed cost of alternative *M*, and the high variable cost of alternative *B*. Fixed cost is that portion of cost that does not depend on the amount of output involved (output = X-ray exams in our case). Variable cost is that portion of cost that varies directly with the level of output. The fixed costs of alternative *M* include leasing the rooms and equipment and paying the radiologist's and technicians' salaries. Assume that to perform up to 1500 additional examinations a month, you must pay the additional radiologist $7,000 per month, and each of the two technicians $1,000 per month. Each of two rooms (with equipment) also rents for $1,000 per month. Variable costs include those costs that vary continuously with the level of output, such as supplies and film in the make alternative, and the charge per exam in the buy alternative. Assume these costs are $10 per examination for the make alternative.

The fixed cost and variable cost of the make alternative are related to output as solid lines in Figure 3.1 and add together to equal the total cost of the make alternative.

Suppose that you can contract with the private group for a charge of $22 per examination. The total cost of the buy alternative is shown

*Figure 3.1*

*Total Costs of Make and Buy Alternatives*

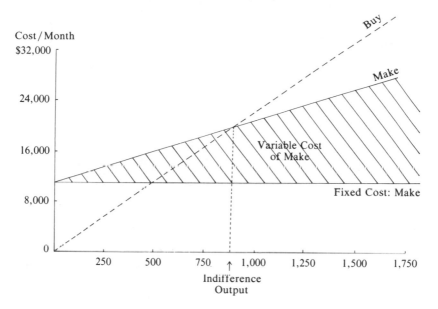

as a dotted line in Figure 3.1. Since there is no fixed cost in the buy alternative, total cost = variable cost.

## The FCVC (Fixed Cost/Variable Cost) Model

Our model for the FCVC problem will, in general, be

$$\text{Minimize } TC(X) = FC(X) + VC(X)$$

where $X$ stands for an alternative (e.g., $X = M = make$ and $X = B = buy$), $TC(X)$ is the total cost of alternative $X$, $FC(X)$ and $VC(X)$ are the fixed and variable cost of alternative $X$, respectively. For a *given* level of output, the solution is straightforward.

For output = 1,000 examinations per month:

$$TC(M) = FC(M) + VC(M)$$

$$= 11,000 + (1,000)(10) = \$21,000$$

$$TC(B) = FC(B) + VC(B)$$

$$= 0 + (1,000)(22) = \$22,000.$$

Thus at 1,000 exams a month, the make decision is better (less

*Table 3.1*

*Calculation of Indifference Level of Output*

| Output | TC(M) | TC(B) | TC(M) − TC(B) |
|--------|-------|-------|---------------|
| 0 | 11,000 | 0 | 11,000 |
| 250 | 13,500 | 5,500 | 8,000 |
| 500 | 16,000 | 11,000 | 5,000 |
| 750 | 18,500 | 16,500 | 2,000 |
| 1,000 | 21,000 | 22,000 | − 1,000 |
| 1,250 | 23,500 | 27,500 | − 4,000 |
| 1,500 | 26,000 | 33,000 | − 7,000 |

expensive). The solution to the FCVC model is so straightforward that we can easily solve the model for many levels of output, as calculated in Table 3.1.

The Break-Even or Indifference Point

At low levels of output, the buy decision is more attractive, but as output increases, the make decision becomes the more attractive. The level of output at which $TC(M)$ and $TC(B)$ are equal is called the break-even point, or the indifference point. Graphically, it occurs where the $TC$ lines cross. Algebraically, it can be determined by setting $TC(M) = TC(B)$, and solving for the level of output, $y$:

$$TC(M) = TC(B)$$

$$11,000 + 10y = 0 + 22y$$

$$11,000 = 12y$$

$$y \text{ (breakeven)} = 917 \text{ examinations}/\text{month}.$$

For levels of output lower than 917, the buy decision is preferred, and for levels above 917, the make decision is preferred.

**The FCVC Decision in the Decision-making Framework**

Before considering problems and extensions with the basic FCVC model, it will be useful to put the FCVC problem in the decision-making framework outlined in Chapter 2.

Step 1: Problem and Model Formulation

In this case, the problem and model are well defined already. The objective is to minimize cost; the decision variables $(X)$ are the two (or possibly more) alternatives; and the model is

$$\text{Minimize } TC(X) = FC(X) + VC(X).$$

("Minimize" means choose the $X$ which minimizes $TC$.)

Step 2: Quantification

This step is also straightforward, in that we have only one relationship: the simple addition of $FC$ and $VC$ to make $TC$. The value of the functions are given:

$$FC(M) = 11,000$$

$$VC(M) = \$10 \text{ per examination}$$

$$FC(B) = 0$$

$$VC\ (B) = \$22 \text{ per examination.}$$

In practice, this step would involve estimating the number of radiologists, technicians, and rooms (and equipment) needed for each level of output (or for the likely ranges of output). Such estimation would involve measuring output rates per day of the radiologist, rooms, and technicians and would require investigating legal restrictions and quality considerations. This step would also involve investigating probable salaries and fringe benefits (and increases) of radiologists and technicians, investigating room leasing prices, adequacy of equipment, cost of supplies, etc. For the buy alternative, it would only be necessary to negotiate for charge per examination. An important part of this step would be to include forecasts of possible changes in these costs for the planning horizon.

Step 3: Solving the Model

For a *given* level of output, this simply involves comparing $TC(M)$ to $TC\ (B)$ and choosing the smaller. We may also wish to "solve" the model for *all* levels of output, which for our example is done by calculating the indifference point.

Step 4: Sensitivity Analysis

For our example, this would involve investigating the sensitivity of the solution to

—the actual level of output,

—the salary of the radiologist(s),

—the salary of the technicians,

—the cost to lease the rooms and equipment,

—the supplies expense of the make alternative, and

—the cost per examination of the buy decision.

The sensitivity of the solutions to the level of output is clearly shown in Figure 3.1, Table 3.1, and the indifference point. Since the salary of the radiologist makes up the largest part of the fixed cost of the make alternative, the solution is most likely very sensitive to the actual salary that must be paid. For example, suppose it is not clear exactly what salary would be negotiated, but it is likely to be no less than $5,000 per month and no more than $9,000 per month. Figure 3.2 gives the sensitivity of the indifference point to such a range in radiologist monthly salary. If it is *known* that additional demand will be greater than 1,083 examinations a month, we can say that the solution is insensitive to the radiologist's salary within the $5,000–$9,000 range, since, even at $9,000, the make alternative is superior. The same can be said if demand is *known* to be less than 750, since the buy decision is superior even if the salary is as low as $5,000 month. If demand can be in the 750 to 1,083 interval, the solution is sensitive to the radiologist's salary, and in order to make the decision deterministically, more information (i.e., a smaller range for the salary) is required. The same analysis should be done

*Figure 3.2*

*Sensitivity of Indifference Point to Radiologist's Salary*

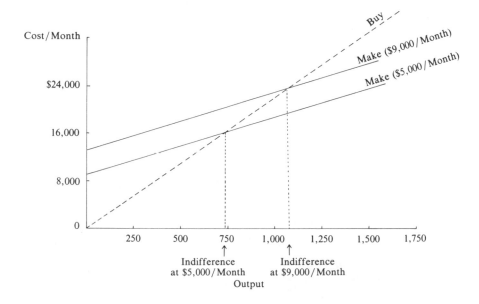

for each of the major items in the model, especially the price per examination of the buy alternative. Here, as in Step 2, the possible increases (or decreases?) in the cost over time should be carefully considered.

### Extensions of the Basic FCVC Decision

Often fixed cost is fixed only over a range of output and is actually related to output in a *stepwise* fashion. For our example, suppose that for up to 750 additional examinations per month, the make alternative would require one additional radiologist, two technicians, and two rooms. For between 750 and 1,250 exams per month, the make alternative would require still another technician and one more room. For between 1,250 and 1,750 exams per month, there would need to be still another room and technician, plus one-half additional radiologist at $4,000 per month. Figure 3.3 displays the step-wise relationship of cost to output.

Suppose further that for the buy alternative, it would be necessary to hire two carriers to transport patients, reports, etc., a secretary, and other fixed costs amounting to $4,000 a month. With the hospital supporting $4,000 of the buy alternative in this way, the charge per examination from the private group would be $20 per exam. Figure

*Figure 3.3*

*Make or Buy Decision with Step Fixed Cost*

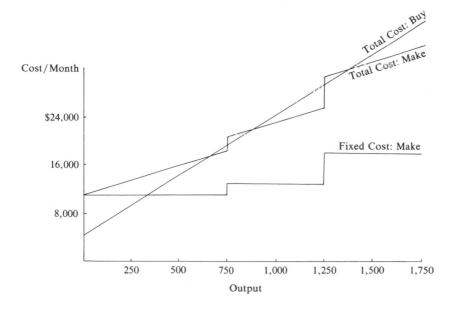

3.3 shows that now there are several indifference points; these must be carefully interpreted since each is valid only for a certain range of output.

Another possibility is a step-wise relationship between output and the charge per exam of the buy alternative (a quantity discount). Suppose the private group offers you rates as follows:

| | | |
|---|---|---|
| 0–499 | examinations/month | $25 per examination |
| 500–999 | examinations/month | 20 per examination |
| 1,000–1,499 | examinations/month | 18 per examination |
| 1,500+ | examinations/month | 16 per examination |

Figure 3.4 combines the new total cost of the buy alternative with the make alternative. Again there are several points where the two total cost lines cross.

There are many other factors that would be considered which up to this point we have treated as external to the analysis, but which in practice must be included. These include questions of the relative quality of the output from each alternative, including patient and physican convenience, and the amount of control over quality

*Figure 3.4*

*Make or Buy Decision with Step Fixed Cost and Quantity Discount*

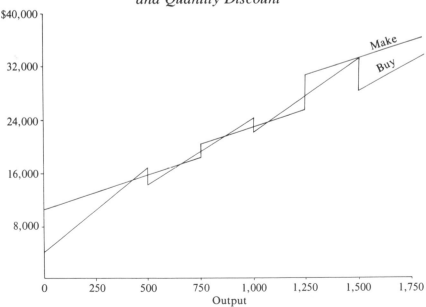

and convenience that the hospital wants and will in fact have. Also important is the length of the salary commitment for the make alternative and the length of the contract of the buy alternative, and, most important, what is likely to happen after such commitment and contracts expire. The "optimal" length of the contract is a related decision.

Finally, it may be appropriate to consider a combination of the two alternatives as follows: $X = C$ (a third alternative) is to use the make decision for the first 1,250 additional exams, and then use the buy decision for exams over 1,250, even at $25 per exam, thereby avoiding hiring the additional one-half radiologist for the make decision. There are many other possible combinations which could be treated within the framework of the basic FCVC model.

## 3.4 SCHEDULING DECISIONS: INVENTORY

The inventory decision involves the trade-off between the costs of *ordering* an item, and *carrying* the item in inventory (storage).

**Problem:** The daily demand for a certain item used by all patients is very stable, and for our purposes we can assume it remains constant at 180 units per day. Since it costs $40 to *order* any amount of the item from 1 to 40,000 units from the supplier (the *ordering* cost does not include the price paid per item, but it includes the cost of making the order, communicating with the supplier, arrangement of payment, taking delivery, etc.), it seems to make sense always to order the largest amount (40,000). However, it costs $.01 per item per day to *store* the items (this includes cost of warehouse, utilities, warehouse personnel, insurance, etc.). In addition, there is the *investment* cost of the cash tied up in inventory of 10 percent per year, with the price being $6 per item. These carrying (storage and investment) costs seem to suggest keeping as little in storage as possible. The problem then is to determine the optimal number of units to order (the lot size) each time an order is placed.

There are several assumptions we will make initially about the inventory decision, and then later in this chapter and in the next chapter we will investigate relaxing these assumptions.

1. We have only one item to consider; this item can be considered independently of other items to be inventoried.

2. Demand for the item is deterministic, i.e., "known" to be (for our example) exactly 180 per day.

3. Demand for the item is constant. Note that demand could be deterministic but not constant. For example, demand could be known to be exactly 191 on Mondays, 212 on Tuesdays, etc.

4. The amount of time between placing the order and the arrival of the order is deterministic. This time is called the "leadtime." We will initially assume it to be 0, then allow it to be positive, and finally allow it to be stochastic in the next chapter.

5. The price of the item does not depend on the size of the order (i.e., no quantity discount).

So far we have described the problem. The remainder of the first step of our decision process is to identify objectives, an objective function, the decision variables, and constraints.

Our objective is to minimize cost, and the decision variable is $Q$ = how many items to order each time we order. ($Q$ is called the lot size, and we are dealing with the "lot size problem.")

The objective function is

Minimize $TC(Q)$ = Ordering cost $(Q)$ + Carrying cost $(Q)$

where $TC(Q)$ refers to total cost's being a function of the decision variable $Q$. At this stage our only constraint is that $Q$ must be less than or equal to 40,000:

$$Q \leq 40,000.$$

The annual ordering cost is equal to the number of orders placed per year times the cost per order. If we let $U$ = the annual usage of the item (for our example $U = 180 \times 365 = 65,700$), we can note the annual number of orders by $U/Q$. Letting $C$ be cost per order, the annual ordering cost is

$$C(U/Q).$$

The carrying cost has two components: the cost to warehouse the items and the cost of the monetary investment in inventory. To specify these we must know the average amount of inventory in stock during the year. Refer to Figure 3.5. Note that at time $T_o$,

*Figure 3.5*

*Inventory Level over Time*

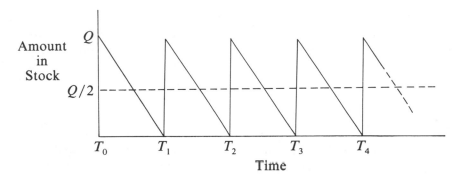

just when an order arrives, the amount in inventory increases from 0 to $Q$. (It should be clear that with deterministic demand and lead time the orders should always be planned to arrive just as the inventory reaches zero.) As time increases, the inventory drops to zero, when another order arrives at $T_1$. The average inventory is thus $Q/2$.

Letting $W$ = the cost per item per year to warehouse an item, the warehousing portion of the average carrying cost will be $WQ/2$. (It may be that space for the whole $Q$ items will have to be reserved for this item at all times, in which case this cost would be $WQ$. Using $WQ/2$ implies that other items can be stored in the space vacated as this item is used up.) Letting $p$ be the price paid per item and $i$ the annual investment cost, the average investment portion of carrying cost will be $ipQ/2$. Our objective function is thus to

$$\text{Minimize } TC(Q) = CU/Q + WQ/2 + ipQ/2$$

$$\text{subject to } Q \leq 40,000.$$

Step 2 of the decision process is to *quantify* the parameters of the model. In this case, all necessary information is given by the problem:

$$C = \$40 \text{ per order}$$

$$U = 365 \times 180 = 65,700 \text{ items per year}$$

$$W = (365 \times \$.01) = \$3.65$$

$$i = .10$$

$$p = \$6$$

so that

$$TC(Q) = \frac{(40)(65,700)}{Q} + \frac{3.65}{2}Q + \frac{(.1)(6)}{2}Q.$$

The third step is to solve the model for optimal $Q$—the $Q$ which minimizes $TC(Q)$. There are two methods of solution available. The first we can call the trial and error or approximation method, and the second is the use of calculus.

Trial and Error Solution

This solution technique, as the name suggests, proceeds by trying different values of $Q$ in the objective function, picking that one which minimizes $TC(Q)$. Table 3.2 shows the result of trying six values of $Q$: $Q = 1000$ is the best of the six tried. There may be

*Table 3.2*

*Trial and Error Calculation of Optimal* Q

| Trial | (1) | (2) | (3) | (4) | (5) | (6) |
|-------|-----|-----|-----|-----|-----|-----|
| $Q$ | 400 | 700 | 1,000 | 1,300 | 1,600 | 1,900 |
| $CU/Q$ | 6,570 | 3,754 | 2,628 | 2,021.5 | 1,642.5 | 1,383 |
| $WQ/2$ | 730 | 1,277.5 | 1,825 | 2,372.5 | 2,920 | 3,467.5 |
| $ipQ/2$ | 120 | 210 | 300 | 390 | 480 | 570 |
| $TC(Q)$ | 7,420 | 5,241.5 | 4,753 | 4,784 | 5,042.5 | 5,420.5 |

a $Q$ which gives a lower $TC$ than $Q = 1,000$, and one shortcoming of the trial and error technique is that the exact optimal may not be identified. Note in this case, however, that $TC(Q)$ is relatively insensitive to the $Q$ around $Q = 1,000$, so that we can assume that $Q = 1,000$ is not significantly far, in terms of $TC(Q)$, from the optimal $Q$.

Calculus Solution

An exact (optimal) solution of the lot size problem can be derived from the fact that the extreme points of a continuous function are where the function's first derivative is equal to zero, and an extreme point is a minimum if the second derivative is greater than zero at that point.

$$\text{Since } TC = CU/Q + \frac{W + ip}{2} Q,$$

$$dTC/dQ = \frac{-CU}{Q^2} + \frac{W + ip}{2} \quad \text{and}$$

$$d^2 TC/dQ^2 = \frac{2CU}{Q^3}.$$

The extreme point is where

$$\frac{CU}{Q^2} = \frac{W + ip}{2}, \text{ or}$$

$$Q^2 = \frac{2CU}{W + ip}, \text{ or}$$

$$Q = \sqrt{\frac{2CU}{W + ip}}.$$

Since $2CU/Q^3$ is positive for all positive $Q$, the above point is a minimum. Substituting values from our example gives

$$Q = \sqrt{\frac{(2)(40)(65,700)}{3.65 + (.1)(6)}} = \sqrt{\frac{5,256,000}{4.25}} = \sqrt{1,236,705.882}$$

$$= 1,112.$$

The total cost at the optimal $Q$ is

$$TC(1,112) = (40)(65,700)/1,112 + (3.65)(1,112)/2 + (.1)(6)(1,112)/2$$

$$= 2,363.31 + 2,029.4 + 333.6 = \$4,726.31$$

so that our approximation solution, in this case, is not far off. (This is *not* necessarily true for the use of the approximation solution technique in all cases, as we shall see.) In general, for the lot size inventory problem, $TC(Q)$ is relatively insensitive to $Q$ around the optimal $Q$ (see Figure 3.6). Note also from Figure 3.6 that it is better to err on the high side of optimal $Q$ than the low side, as $TC(Q)$ rapidly rises to the left of optimal $Q$ after a short flat period, while the curve rises much more slowly to the right.

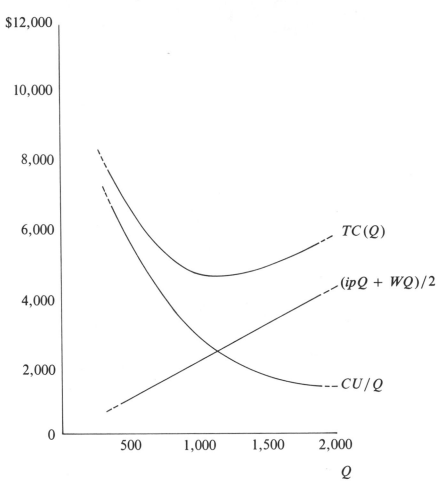

*Figure 3.6*

*Inventory Costs as a Function of* Q

The final step in the decision process is the investigation of the sensitivity of the results of the analysis (the optimal $Q$ and the $TC(Q)$ for our problem) to

1. errors and/or changes in the parameters of the model (the $W$, $C$, $U$, $i$, and $p$) and

2. the relationships implied by the assumptions made about the process in developing the model.

We will investigate the latter in the following section and in the next chapter.

Already we have investigated the sensitivity of $TC(Q)$ to $Q$. Since the values of $C$, $U$, $W$, $i$, and $p$ are, at best, estimates of actual values, it is important that we be aware of how errors in the estimates or changes in these values affect total cost. Consider changes in the demand $U$. If demand is overestimated by 20 percent, then actual demand will be $(.8) \times (180) \times (365) = 52,560$. Using $Q = 1,112$,

$$TC(1,112) = (40)(52,560)/1,112 + 2,029.4 + 333.6$$

$$= 1,890.65 + 2,363$$

$$= 4,253.65.$$

If we had known demand was to be 52,560, we would have calculated optimal $Q$ as

$$Q = \sqrt{\frac{(2)(40)(52,560)}{4.25}} = \sqrt{989,364.71} = 994.67,$$

and our actual cost would have been

$$TC(995) = (40)(52,560)/995 + (3.65)(995)/2 + (.6)(995)/2$$

$$= 2,112.96 + 1,815.88 + 298.5$$

$$= 4,227.34.$$

The percent change in $TC$ as a result of a 20 percent overestimate of demand is $(4,253.65 - 4,227.34)/4,253.65 = .01$, or only a 1 percent error. Table 3.3 gives the sensitivity of $TC(Q)$ to larger errors in the estimate of demand, showing that the effect on optimal $TC$ is quite insensitive to errors in $U$. Similar tables could be constructed for $C$, $w$, $i$, and $p$. If the error in $TC$ is found to be quite sensitive to a parameter, it suggests that careful attention be paid to the estimate of that parameter, which might include collecting more data for its

## Table 3.3

### Sensitivity of Inventory Cost to Demand

| If $U$ is . . . | 60% | 80% | 120% | 140% | of estimate . . . |
|---|---|---|---|---|---|
| $U$ | 39,420 | 52,560 | 78,840 | 91,980 | |
| $Q$ optimal | 861 | 995 | 1,218 | 1,316 | |
| $TC(1,112)$ | 3,784 | 4,253 | 5,199 | 5,672 | |
| $TC$(optimal) | 3,660 | 4,227 | 5,177 | 5,592 | |
| % Error in $TC$ | 3% | 1% | .4% | 1% | |

estimation. It may also suggest efforts to influence the value of the parameter.

### Relaxing Assumptions

An extremely important part of the sensitivity analysis is the investigation of the effect, on the model and its results, of the assumptions made at its development stage. Generally, such assumptions limit the extent to which the model represents the real world and, in turn, might limit the applicability of the results from the model to the real world.

The most limiting assumptions for the inventory model were those concerning the deterministic nature of the model. We will investigate relaxing these in the next chapter.

The easiest assumption to relax is Assumption 5: "The price of the item does not depend on $Q$." If $p$ does depend on $Q$, then we may define price as $p(Q)$ (a function of Q), and simply substitute the function $p(Q)$ for $p$ in the $TC(Q)$ equation, and add $p(Q) \times U$ as a term, since it is no longer constant. For example, suppose $p(Q) = 6 - Q/20,000$. That is, the more we order, the lower the price. The price ranges from \$6 if we order one, to $6 - 40,000/20,000$ = \$4 if we order 40,000. Now

$$TC(Q) = CU/Q + WQ/2 + i(6 - Q/20,000)Q/2$$

$$+ (6 - Q/20,000)U.$$

Solving by approximation is the same process as before. Since $p(Q)$ is a continuous function of $p$, we may also use calculus to determine the optimal $Q$. More likely, $p(Q)$ will be a step function of $Q$, in which case the approximation solution technique is applicable but calculus is not.

If demand for the item is deterministic but not constant (Assumption 3), the problem becomes much more complex. Note that no longer should $Q$ be constant from month to month, as we expect it to be higher when demand is higher and lower for lower demand. The model appropriate for relaxing this assumption is beyond the scope of this text, and the interested reader is referred to the Naddor reference at the end of Chapter 4. The important concept for our purpose is to what extent we may use the constant demand model for the situation of nonconstant demand, or how sensitive are the model's results to this assumption. As we would expect, the model is relatively insensitive to slight changes in demand (for example, monthly indices of the range .85 to 1.15), and thus the model developed above for constant demand could be used as an approximation.

Finally, if we consider more than one item at a time (Assumption 1), our model must be modified to reflect the extent to which the items compete for space (and possibly for investment capital). Consider two items, $a$ and $b$. The problem is to find optimal lot sizes for each item, designated by $Q_a$ and $Q_b$, respectively. Suppose item $a$ requires $S_a$ cubic feet for storage and item $b$ requires $S_b$ cubic feet. Suppose further that there are only $F$ cubic feet available to store both. Let us finally assume that we cannot store one item in the space reserved to store the other, so that we will need $S_a Q_a + S_b Q_b$ cubic feet at all times. Thus we have the constraint

$$S_a Q_a + S_b Q_b \leq F.$$

Our objective function becomes

$$TC(Q_a, Q_b) = \frac{C_a U_a}{Q_a} + W_a Q_a + \frac{C_b U_b}{Q_b} + W_b Q_b + \frac{i(p_a Q_a + p_b Q_b)}{2},$$

subject to

$$S_a Q_a + S_b Q_b \leq F,$$

$$Q_a \leq 40,000, \text{ and}$$

$$Q_b \leq \text{maximum allowable } Q_b.$$

Although the above may be solved with the approximation technique, it is not hard to see that many more than twice as many solutions should be "tried" than in the single item case. The number of possible solutions that should be tried grows very quickly with an increase in the number of decision variables ($Q$'s), and a special technique called mathematical programming, the subject of Chapter 6, is applicable to such problems for their solution. Chapter 11 will reconsider inventory in the control framework.

## A "Noninventory" Example

Inventory models can be applied to problems other than the traditional item-storage type.

> **Problem:** A community health clinic uses 120 physician associates (PAs). The final six weeks of the PAs' training is at the clinic itself, consisting of an intensive on-site training program. The program costs the clinic $8,000 to put on, independent of how many PAs are being trained. The PAs

stay with the clinic an average of three years; thus the clinic needs to train $120/3 = 40$ new PAs a year. The attrition of the 40 departing PAs is constant over the year, and the hiring of their replacements must correspond to the attrition. If a PA is hired before he can be used, he can work essentially as a nurse, but his salary is $3,000 more per year than a nurse, and the clinic must pay this extra $3,000. How many training sessions should the clinic put on per year? Or, how many PAs should be trained in each session?

Let $Q$ be the number to be trained at each session. Thus $40/Q$ is the number of training sessions, and the training (ordering) cost is

$$(8,000)(40)/Q \quad \text{(analogous to } CU/Q\text{)}.$$

The "unnecessary" salary of $3,000 will be paid to the average number of PAs who have been hired but who are working temporarily as nurses. As before, the average number is $Q/2$, and thus the "carrying" cost is

$$(3,000) \, Q/2.$$

Thus,

$$TC(Q) = (8,000)(40)/Q + 3,000 \, (Q)/2.$$

The equation could be solved by approximation or calculus. The calculus gives

$$\frac{dTC(Q)}{d(Q)} = \frac{-320,000}{Q^2} + 1,500$$

$$Q = \sqrt{320,000/1,500} = \sqrt{213.33} = 14.6 \text{ or } 15.$$

The approximation solution is left to the student as an exercise.

## 3.5 SCHEDULING DECISIONS: TASK SEQUENCING (PERT/CPM)

Quite often a project is made up of many interrelated tasks which, when undertaken in a particular sequence, lead to the completion of the project. The Program Evaluation and Review Technique (PERT) or Critical Path Method (CPM) model is useful in planning and scheduling the sequencing of the individual tasks, and in reviewing the progress of the project as a whole. Note that we are not concerned here with the "best" of several available projects, but only how best to undertake the project once it has been selected.

**Problem:** In beginning a new community outpatient clinic (the "project"), the following tasks have been identified as components of the project. (There are certainly many, many more tasks, but these are enough for our purpose.)

1. Find and Lease Space for Clinic.

2. Hire Radiologist and Lab Director.

3. Purchase Radiology and Lab Equipment.

4. Remodel the Space.

5. Install Equipment.

6. Hire Nurses and Other Personnel.

7. Train Personnel.

8. Design and Implement Publicity Campaign.

9. Final Preparations.

(The underlined words will represent the tasks in the discussion below.) The problem concerns *when* each task should begin in order that the project be completed in the least amount of time. (We will look at the *cost* of the project later in the chapter.)

The first step in the PERT analysis is to specify two things about each task: (1) an estimate of how long it will take and (2) its sequence in relation to other tasks—specifically, which other tasks must be completed before it can begin. For our example, suppose the following is established:

| Task | Time to Complete (in weeks) | Predecessor Tasks |
|---|---|---|
| 1. Space | 14 | — |
| 2. Radiologist | 16 | — |
| 3. Equipment | 12 | 2 |
| 4. Remodel | 6 | 1, 2 |
| 5. Install | 2 | 3, 4 |
| 6. Nurses | 5 | — |
| 7. Train | 4 | 6 |
| 8. Publicity | 11 | — |
| 9. Final | 3 | 5, 7, 8 |

(This sequencing is of course much simplified from the actual process but again it will serve our purpose here.)

The second stage in the analysis is to build the PERT model or network, which graphically shows the necessary sequencing of the tasks. This is best done by beginning at the end of the project and working backwards. But first, let us define an

> *event* as the end of one or more tasks and the beginning of one or more other tasks that must be preceded by the ending task(s).

The *last event* (we will denote events with circles) is *End*.

The tasks which terminate in the end event are those that precede no other tasks.

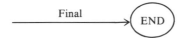

Thus, when the Final preparations are completed, the project is completed. Now, before we can begin Final preparations we must have Installed the equipment, Trained the personnel, and Publicized the clinic.

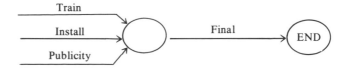

This defines a new *event*—the ending of Install, Train, and Publicity and the beginning of Final. Note now that we must purchase the Equipment before it can be Installed, and we must also have it Remodeled. Thus, we can end Equipment and Remodel in the event that begins Install.

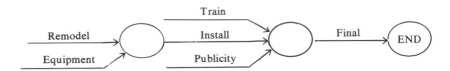

*Figure 3.7*

*PERT Network Diagram*

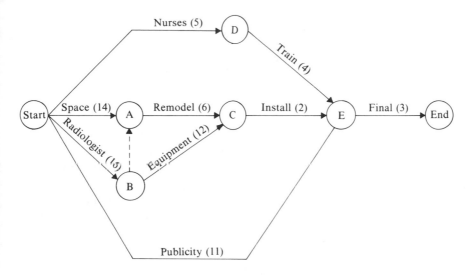

Proceeding in the same fashion with all other tasks leads to a PERT network—Figure 3.7. The names of the events are arbitrary (except for Start and End). Note that the entire network begins with one event (Start) and ends with one event (End). The time of each task is shown in Figure 3.7 just after its name in parentheses. The dummy task (denoted by a dotted line) from event B to event A is used to show that Radiologist must precede Remodel, but Space does not need to precede Equipment (as defined in the problem). The event defined as

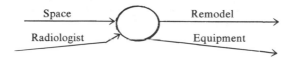

would be incorrect, since it implies that Space also must precede Equipment, which is not true in our example. Another use of a dummy task is in a case in which two tasks begin at one event and end together at another event. Although this could be shown as

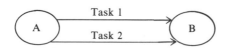

we will see below that it is preferable to use a dummy task.

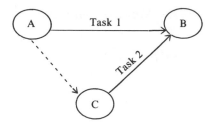

A dummy task requires no time or resources, so the two diagrams are equivalent.

These two steps of the analysis are roughly analogous to the first two steps of our decision process: we have described the problem, identified the decision variable (in this case, the appropriate starting time of each event), defined the objective function (minimize time to completion of the project), and built the model (the network).

The third step in the analysis is to "solve" the network—in this case, to determine the appropriate starting times for each task. This is done by determining the following for each event:

> *Earliest Starting Time (EST):* the earliest time an event can happen, given that all other preceding events occur at their earliest starting time; and

> *Latest Starting Time (LST):* the latest time the event can occur without causing a delay in the completion of the entire project.

For our example, event B can occur as soon as task Radiologist is completed. EST for B is thus 16. Event A can occur as early as the time of the longest path (in time) to reach A. (Why the longest path?) The two paths to A are Space (14), and Radiologist + Dummy (16 + 0). Thus, the EST for A is 16. The EST for C is the longest path to reach it: EST of A plus Remodel (16 + 6), or EST of B plus Equipment (16 + 12). Thus EST of C is 28.

The EST for a large number of tasks (100 or so) can be simply determined by following these steps:

1. Begin at the Start event and write 0 in the left side of the event circle as in Figure 3.8. This is the EST for the event.

2. Working from left to right, add the time for the next

## Figure 3.8

### Earliest Start Times (ESTs)

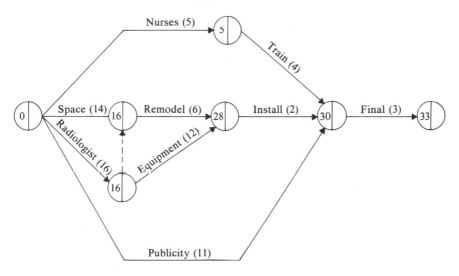

task to the number in the left side of the event circle preceding the task, and write this new sum in the left side of the event circle ending the task. When two or more tasks end at one circle, use the *largest* value. In the example below, 16 + 12 = 28 is larger than 16 + 6 = 22, so 28 is written in the ending circle.

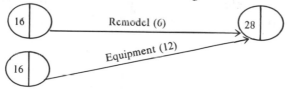

3. Continue Step 2 until the EST is placed in the left side of every event, as shown in Figure 3.8.

The minimum completion time for the entire project is 33 weeks. Thus, the latest starting time (LST) of End is 33. The latest starting time of event E is "LST of End less the time of Final" = 33 − 3 = 30. (Why?) The latest starting time of D is 30 − 4 = 26. Again, the LST can be simply determined for all tasks:

4. In the End event circle, show the LST as equal to the EST by writing the EST on the right side of the circle. (See Figure 3.9.)

*Figure 3.9*

*Latest Start Times and Slack*

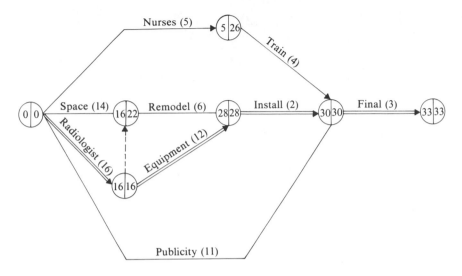

5. Working from right to left, subtract the time for each task from the number in the right side of the event circle ending the task and write this result in the right side of the preceding event circle. When two or more tasks begin at the same event circle, use the *smallest* value. For example, $28 - 12 = 16$ is smaller than $22 - 0 = 22$, so 16 is written in the event circle **B**.

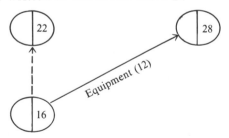

6. Continue Step 5 until the LST is placed in the right side of every event as shown in Figure 3.9.

By subtracting the LST (right side) from the EST (left side), the *slack* time for an event is determined. The *critical path* is the path through the events with no slack. In Figure 3.9, it is shown by the double lines. All tasks making up the critical path are critical, in the sense that any delay in beginning or delay in finishing them will result in delaying the project as a whole. Conversely, those tasks not on the critical path have some slack time available. The amount of slack for a task is defined as the

LST of event that ends the task

*minus* the EST of event that begins the task

*minus* the time to complete the task.

Thus, for example,

Slack Nurses = LST of D − EST of Start − 5 = 26 − 0 − 5 = 21.

Other task slack is shown in Figure 3.10. As expected, all critical path tasks have zero slack. Slack is better associated with *subpaths*

*Figure 3.10*

*Slack Times for Tasks*

| Tasks | Slack |
|---|---|
| 1. Space | 22 − 0 − 14 = 8 |
| 2. Radiologist | 16 − 0 − 16 = 0 |
| 3. Equipment | 28 − 16 − 12 = 0 |
| 4. Remodel | 28 − 16 − 6 = 6 |
| 5. Install | 30 − 28 − 2 = 0 |
| 6. Nurses | 26 − 0 − 5 = 21 |
| 7. Train | 30 − 5 − 4 = 21 |
| 8. Publicity | 30 − 0 − 11 = 19 |
| 9. Final | 33 − 30 − 3 = 0 |

of one or more tasks off the critical path than it is with individual tasks. For example, the slack of the subpath Nurses + Train is 21: if Nurses is started X weeks late, then Train has only 21 − X weeks slack, and vice versa. Some subpaths have only one task, such as Publicity.

It is difficult to visualize the time relationships on the PERT network diagram and, therefore, difficult to see how the slack time can be used. A Gantt chart (named after the person who thought of plotting tasks versus time) shows how long a task takes, when the task could start (EST), and when it must start (LST). Figure 3.11 illustrates the chart for our example.

To draw the chart, start from the last task and work backward. In this way, the tasks are shown in the LST position. Draw in the

*Figure 3.11*

*Gantt Chart for PERT Network*

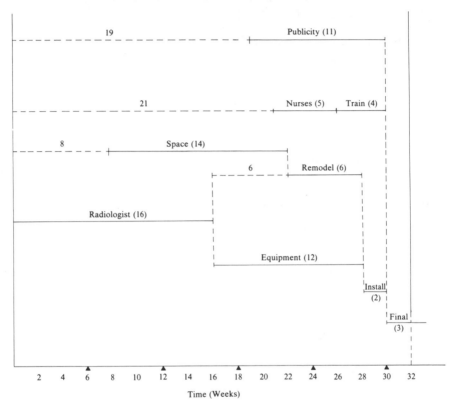

tasks on the critical path first (Final-Install-Equipment-Radiologist). Draw in the remaining tasks and place a vertical dotted line to show the relationship between activities. For example, Publicity, Training, and Install are connected to Final by one vertical dotted line, while Remodel is shown connected to Install. Finally, draw horizontal dotted lines to show slack time. For example, Publicity can be started immediately, but need not start for 19 weeks. If Remodel is begun at its EST, then Space only has 2 weeks' slack. The reason for moving the tasks back and forth in their slack time is to try to level out the work load.

The arrows along the bottom of the chart indicate the times when the project's progress will be checked. Perhaps the critical path has changed and the minimum time to completion needs to be recalculated.

## PERT/Probability

Even though the focus of this chapter is on deterministic analysis, PERT analysis can be viewed stochastically as well. Let us modify the list of tasks and time presented early in Section 3.5—see Table 3.4.

### Table 3.4

### Estimates of Time Required to Complete Tasks

| x<br>Tasks | o<br>Optimistic<br>Estimate | p<br>Pessimistic<br>Estimate | m<br>Most<br>Probable | $T_{exp}$ | T | σ | $σ^2$ |
|---|---|---|---|---|---|---|---|
| 1. Space | 8 | 20 | 14 | 14.00 | 14 | 2.00 | 4.00 |
| *2. Radiologists | 12 | 18 | 16 | 15.60 | 16 | 1.00 | 1.00 |
| *3. Equipment | 6 | 15 | 12 | 11.50 | 12 | 1.50 | 2.25 |
| 4. Remodel | 5 | 8 | 6 | 6.16 | 6 | .50 | .25 |
| *5. Install | 1 | 5 | 2 | 2.30 | 2 | .66 | .44 |
| 6. Nurses | 3 | 7 | 5 | 5.00 | 5 | .66 | .44 |
| 7. Train | 2 | 5 | 4 | 3.80 | 4 | .50 | .25 |
| 8. Publicity | 10 | 15 | 11 | 11.50 | 11 | .83 | .69 |
| *9. Final | 2 | 5 | 3 | 3.20 | 3 | .50 | .25 |

$$\Sigma = 8.05 \quad \Sigma = 9.58$$

*Critical path tasks

PERT used in this manner assumes that the time required for each activity is a random variable described by a particular probability distribution, beta. This distribution has a slight tail to the right; its expected mean and standard deviation are approximated by:

$$T_{exp}(x) = \frac{o + 4m + p}{6}$$

$$σ(x) = \frac{p - o}{6},$$

where

$T_{exp}$ = expected time of activity, given the beta distribution;
$x$ = activity;
$o$ = optimistic time estimate for the task;
$m$ = most probable time estimate for the task; and
$p$ = pessimistic time estimate for the task.

Using these equations, we are able to calculate the expected duration of a task and the deviation of that time from the expected time. The expected time of the project is the sum of the expected times of the activities along the critical path (Table 3.5). We are also able to calculate the time variance in the completion of the project ($\sigma^2$ project) by adding the variances of the tasks along the critical path (assuming, quite boldly, that the activities are independent and thus their variances are additive). By considering all the distributions of the activities, we allow an assumption of normality based on the central limit theorem. Given a normal distribution, the $Z$ statistic may quite easily be used to predict the probability that the project will be completed prior to or on a specified date. For example, your analysis has revealed an expected project duration of 32.6 weeks. The hospital administrator would like to know the probability that the clinic will be operating in 36 weeks or less. Standardizing $T_{exp, project}$ to the $Z$ statistic and referring to a table of the normal distribution, you find the following:

$$P\ (T_{project} \leq 36) = P\ (Z \leq \frac{36 - T_{exp,\ project}}{\sigma_{project}})$$

$$P\ (Z \leq \frac{36 - 32.6}{1.98}) =$$

$$P\ (Z \leq 1.71) = .95.$$

Thus, there is a 95 percent chance that the project will be done in 36 weeks or less.

If the project designer or the administrator is uncomfortable making deterministic estimates of task completion times, modifying those times to accommodate an optimistic and pessimistic estimate adds another dimension of control.

*Table 3.5*

*Expected Time of the Project with Variances*

| Critical Path Tasks | $\sigma$ | $\sigma^2$ | $T_{exp}$ | |
|---|---|---|---|---|
| 2. Radiologists | 1.00 | 1.00 | 15.6 | |
| 3. Equipment | 1.50 | 2.25 | 11.5 | |
| 5. Install | .66 | .44 | 2.3 | |
| 9. Final | .50 | .25 | 3.2 | |
| | $\Sigma =$ 3.94 | $\Sigma =$ 32.6 | $= T_{exp,\ project}$ | |
| | $\sigma_{project} =$ 1.98 | | | |

### PERT/Cost

We have worked above under the implied assumption that the task completion time is fixed, with no opportunity for influencing it. Conceivably (and quite likely for most PERT problems), some of the tasks in our example could be expedited if more resources are used. For example, the Equipment task might be accelerated by using more expensive shipping methods, making special handling arrangements, etc. Suppose we assume

| Equipment could be reduced to... | if we were willing to spend... |
| --- | --- |
| 11 weeks | $1,000 |
| 10 weeks | $3,000 |
| 9 weeks | $8,000 |

But why should we spend extra unless we receive benefit? The benefit in this case is reduced time to complete the project. In order to evaluate the alternative of expediting a task, we must change our objective function to minimize *cost* rather than time (thus PERT/Cost). In addition, we change our decision variable to express not only the starting time of each task, but also how much to spend on speeding up each task. Suppose that the following is known.

| If project is completed in... | the reduction in time is worth... |
| --- | --- |
| 32 weeks | $2,000 |
| 31 weeks | $5,000 |
| 30 weeks | $6,000 |
|  | $7,000 |

We would spend money to reduce time until the next increment in reduction of time costs more than it benefits. In our example, the first week's time reduction costs $1,000 but is worth $2,000; thus it would be undertaken. A second week's time reduction costs $2,000 and is worth $3,000, so it is also undertaken. The third week's time reduction costs $5,000 and is worth only $1,000, so it would not be undertaken.

Two circumstances can make large PERT/Cost problems very difficult to analyze by hand, although easily manageable using widely available computer programs. First, notice that after Equipment is reduced to 6 weeks, a further reduction takes it off the critical path, making such a reduction "worth" nothing. Second, if all tasks can potentially be expedited, *and* if reducing the time of each task by one week is worth an equal amount, then the first time reduction would be undertaken on the critical task whose reduction costs the least to implement. The second reduction may be on another task, etc. Throughout the analysis, tasks become critical and noncritical as they and other tasks are reduced in time.

Perhaps the administrator would like to investigate the possibility of finishing the project earlier than the originally calculated schedule. The process of reducing the overall completion time for the project is known as *crashing*.

There are, of course, costs involved in crashing a project; crashing an activity such as Remodeling the Space might require absorbing the cost of additional workers or designers and overtime payments for labor. These can be estimated just as the costs of the normally completed project are estimated (Table 3.6). Assessing the impact of crashing a project requires that one PERT chart be prepared for the project under normal conditions and another under fully crashed conditions (Figure 3.12), including all the costs of each crashed activity. (It should be noted that fully crashed conditions might reveal a different critical path if activities not on the critical path under normal project conditions are crashed beyond their slack time.)

## Table 3.6

### Costs Incurred in Crashing a Project

| Tasks | Normal Conditions | Fully Crashed | Crash Cost Per Week | × Weeks | = | Cost |
|-------|-------------------|---------------|---------------------|---------|---|------|
| 1. Space | 14 | 8 | 100 | 6 | | 600 |
| *2. Radiologists | 16 | 12 | 200 | 4 | | 800 |
| *3. Equipment | 12 | 6 | 200 | 6 | | 1,200 |
| 4. Remodel | 6 | 5 | 300 | 1 | | 300 |
| *5. Install | 2 | 1 | 100 | 1 | | 100 |
| 6. Nurses | 5 | 3 | 200 | 2 | | 400 |
| 7. Train | 4 | 2 | 200 | 2 | | 400 |
| 8. Publicity | 11 | 10 | 300 | 1 | | 300 |
| *9. Final | 3 | 2 | 200 | 1 | | 200 |
| | | | | | $\Sigma =$ | 4,300 |

*Critical path tasks

Figure 3.12

*PERT Network under Fully Crashed Conditions*

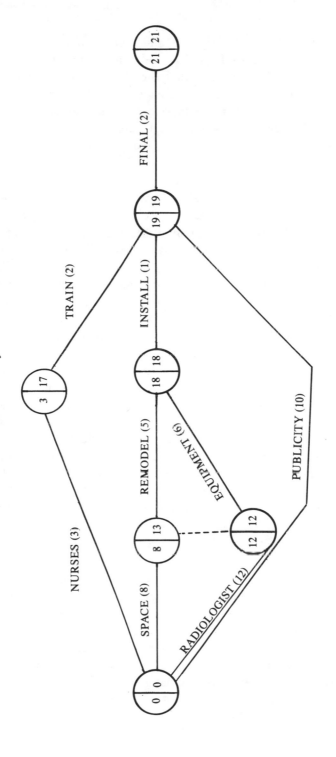

Project completion time under crashed conditions has been reduced to 21 weeks from 33 weeks under normal conditions. But at what cost? If we assume that the 33-week project will cost $50,000, then we can calculate the cost of a crashed project as $50,000 + $4,300, or $54,300. But suppose you, as project manager, wanted to know the least costly manner of completing the project within the time period between 21 weeks and 33 weeks. As before, the critical path still determines the tasks which affect the completion time. You must therefore examine the tasks on the critical path to determine which ones might be crashed at the lowest cost. While a simple illustration of this technique will be presented here, the adaptation of PERT/CPM under normal and fully crashed conditions to a computer-based linear programming analysis simplifies the computational tasks involved.

In choosing the least costly route to finish our project within, say, 26 weeks, the first step is to determine which task on the critical path is the least costly to crash. Installation of Equipment can be fully crashed for $100. (In a case in which multiple activities have the same costs, the activity which most reduces the length of time of the project is selected.) Crashing Install adds $100 to project costs and reduces duration of the project to 32 weeks. Final Preparation has the next least crashing costs, at $200 and a one-week time reduction. Only two tasks remain on the critical path. If hiring the Radiologists is a fully crashed task at a cost of $800 and a project time reduction of four weeks, then buying Equipment need be only partially crashed, by one week at a cost of $200. The project will be completed within 26 weeks, as specified, at a cost of $100 + $200 + $800 + $200 + $50,000 = $51,300, which is less than the total cost of crashing all activities.

In review, we should regard PERT as having two major functions: decision making and control. The decision function includes carefully dividing projects into tasks and specifying their completion times and sequence. It also entails scheduling tasks by their EST, LST, and slack and identifying which tasks are time-critical and which are not. This function can also help us to choose the appropriate resources to dedicate to the completion of each task (PERT/Cost).

The control function will be discussed in Chapter 11. Briefly, explicit goals are identified for each task (the EST and LST), and, as the project proceeds, regular reviews of performance against goals can be made. Note also that the remainder of the project can be re-analyzed by PERT at any stage of its progress, incorporating new information.

**Exercises**

3.1 The HMO you are administering must decide whether to provide radiology services itself, or to contract for them with the hospitals in its service area. You have discussed the "contract" option with several of the administrators and estimate that they would agree to a charge of approximately $24 per examination for a one-year contract. You estimate that you could hire a radiologist for between $8,000 and $9,200 per month and a technician for $1,000 per month; lease a suite of rooms for $1,000 per month; and lease radiology equipment for $1,000 per month. You have forecasted demand for exams to average 900 per month—with a 95 percent confidence interval of between 840 to 960 exams per month. You estimate you need one radiologist, two technicians, one suite of rooms, and the radiology equipment in order to provide between 840 and 960 exams per month. The supplier for film and other radiology supplies gives you cost estimates that indicate your variable costs will be about $9 per exam, but could go as high as $12 per exam.

   a. Perform a sensitivity analysis for the extremes in the radiologist's salary ($8,000–$9,200) and variable cost ($9–$12).

   b. List the important qualitative considerations.

   c. Taking both quantitative and qualitative considerations into account, would you do it yourself or contract for service? Why?

3.2 A meat-packing firm offers to provide you with portion-ready meat and poultry items (i.e., raw meat cut to your specifications for preparation in your kitchens). Your hospital has been employing a butcher and purchasing whole beefs, lambs, etc. Investigation reveals the following:

   —The butcher is employed full-time at a salary of $6,500 plus $1,000 in fringe benefits.

   —The average cost of usable meat on carcasses is 60¢/lb.

   —The average cost of cuts actually used, if purchased according to the packer's offer, is 75¢/lb.

   a. Formulate a total cost equation for the cost of meat purchasing and processing under each alternative. (Assume that you will be able to terminate the services of the butcher.)

   b. Solve the equations for the annual usage in pounds at which you are indifferent as to purchase of portion-ready cuts or purchase of carcasses.

c. What arguments could you use to justify the portion-ready alternative if annual usage was 60,000 pounds? What is the cost imputed to your justification of portion-ready over the present method?

3.3 As administrator of a 300-bed hospital, you are considering converting to disposable utensils instead of the nondisposable ones presently used in dietary. Through time studies found in published literature, you find that:

—Man-time associated with cleaning and handling nondisposable utensils per meal-equivalent (i.e., including nourishments) costs $.10.

Other facts:

—Fixed costs associated with nondisposables total $10,000 per year.

—Overhead, interest, and storage costs are either trivial or would remain the same for either disposable or nondisposable utensils.

—Each year you process 400,000 meal-equivalents in dietary.

A salesman representing a manufacturer and distributor of disposable utensils offers you disposables at $.11 per meal-equivalent. He claims a reduction in time associated with handling utensils and gives data in support of this claim from two hospitals in the area that adopted the disposable utensils. These data indicate a man-time cost of $.01 per meal-equivalent when using disposables.

a. Make the cases for both accepting and rejecting the salesman's offer. Include any factors that might not be self-evident from the numbers in your analysis.

b. If you think demand will increase 10 percent next year, would your decision be affected?

3.4 You currently buy individual disposables for the patient's bedside stand:

| | |
|---|---|
| toothbrush | $.15 |
| denture cup | .05 |
| wash basin | .20 |
| soap cake and holder | .07 |
| back rub | .25 |
| emesis basin | .15 |
| water glass | .05 |
| total | $.92 |

One set is used for each admission. Last year there were 10,000 admissions.

A salesman offers you a pre-packaged kit for $1.00 and claims that his kits reduce handling in room set-up by 4 man-minutes per admission. He backs this claim by micro-motion time studies which appear quite carefully done, and which your industrial engineer reviews favorably.

Your housekeeping personnel who perform the room set-up are paid $.03 per minute, and draw $.01 per minute in fringe benefits. The executive housekeeper recommends purchase of the kits, claiming that the product is more attractive and more convenient for nursing, and that speed in room cleaning is important to maintain high occupancy. No payroll reduction can be expected; the cleaning is done by full-time staff permanently assigned to individual floors. However, there are frequent delays when several patients leave at once, and these will be reduced.

The industrial engineer comments that similar kits could be prepared centrally by the hospital in unused available space in the housekeeping storeroom. This would also save 4 man-minutes per admission at the bedside and would be done by additional part-time personnel at $.03 per man-minute. Preparation would require 15,000 man-minutes. A plastic bag is necessary, and costs $.01. The executive housekeeper agrees but points out that the industrial engineer's method would be no more attractive or convenient for patient and nurse than the present method.

a. Assuming overhead, interest, storage, and capital costs to be trivial, estimate the marginal costs for adopting
   1. The salesman's proposal over the present method;
   2. The industrial engineer's proposal compared to the present method.
b. You decide in favor of the salesman's proposal. By rejecting the industrial engineer's proposal and the present method, what imputed prices (think carefully!) have you set upon
   1. The value of patient and nurse convenience?
   2. The value of reducing delay in making rooms available?

3.5 The daily demand for a certain item used by all patients is very stable and can be assumed constant at 200 units per day. It costs $50 to order any amount of the item from 1 to 50,000 units (the ordering cost does not include the price paid per item, but includes the cost of making the order, communicating with the supplier, arranging payment, taking delivery, etc.). It costs

$.02 per item per day to store the items (this includes cost of warehouse, utilities, warehouse personnel, insurance, etc.). In addition, there is the investment cost of the cash tied up in inventory of 10 percent per year, with a price of $17 per item.

a. What is the "optimal" number of units to order each time an order is placed?

b. Since "optimal" is relative, under what circumstances is this optimal?

3.6 Your hospital uses a disposable pack of personal items for the patient's bedside stand. This is provided in each room at the time the room is prepared for the next admission. The following data have been collected:

| | |
|---|---|
| Price: | $2.00 each. The price is set by annual contract and is constant unless more than twelve deliveries are made per year. |
| Cost of ordering: | $50.00 per order. |
| Storage cost: | $.25 per unit per year. |
| Interest rate: | 10 percent. |
| Usage: | 13,000 units per year. Usage is relatively constant and deliveries are prompt, requiring 5 days. |

a. Recommend the order quantity which the purchasing agent should use.

b. How sensitive is your recommendation to a 30 percent error in the cost of ordering?

c. State any additional assumptions necessary to your recommendations, other than those stated or implied above.

d. Indicate the minimum stock level at which the reorder should be placed, assuming stockout is to be avoided.

3.7 The following tasks are necessary to complete a small construction job.

| Task | Time in Weeks | Prede- cessors |
|---|---|---|
| 1 Excavation and footings | 6 | — |
| 2 Steel fabrication | 8 | — |
| 3 Steel erection, mechanical roughing, floor and exterior wall | 12 | 1,2 |
| 4 Boiler and mechanical delivery | 8 | — |

| Task | Time in Weeks | Prede-cessors |
|------|---------------|---------------|
| 5 Boiler and mechanical installation | 3 | 4 |
| 6 Glazing | 2 | 3 |
| 7 Interior wall | 15 | 3 |
| 8 Mechanical finishing and testing | 4 | 5,7 |
| 9 Finishes—floor and walls | 4 | 7 |
| 10 Clean-up and inspection | 2 | 9 |

a. Construct a PERT chart;

b. Calculate the minimum time for completion of the project;

c. Calculate the slack time for each task;

d. Identify the tasks on the critical path;

e. Construct a Gantt chart for the project.

3.8 Suppose in Problem 3.7 that it was worth $5,000 to accomplish the job one week ahead of schedule, $8,000 for two weeks ahead, and $10,000 for three weeks. Task 2 can be completed 3 weeks earlier if you pay overtime, amounting to $6,000. Task 4 can be decreased by one week if you pay $800 for special shipping. Task 1 can be reduced one week by paying overtime of $2,000. Which, if any, of these reductions should you purchase, and in what combination?

3.9 The Public Health Department took a kindergarten survey at a school near your hospital on two different occasions and found that approximately 33% of the children had been immunized against measles by the vaccine, 33% by the disease, 20% were definitely susceptible, and 14% had unknown but probably susceptible immunization status. The Public Health Officer asked if you would work with them to immunize 80% (300–400 children ages 1–9) of susceptible or probably susceptible children in the census tract around your hospital. The two of you worked out the following list of activities, the predecessors to each activity, and the expected time (working days) to complete each activity.

| Activities | Predecessor Activities | Expected Time (Days) |
|------------|------------------------|----------------------|
| 1. Gather demographic data | — | 1 |
| 2. Survey homes in area | — | 7 |
| 3. Estimate number of susceptible children 1–9 | 1, 2 | 5 |

| Activities | Predecessor Activities | Expected Time (Days) |
|---|---|---|
| 4. Review estimate and other details with each other | 3 | 2 |
| 5. Select clinic sites | 4 | 2 |
| 6. Schedule times at sites | 5 | 10 |
| 7. Arrange for manual injection guns and vials of vaccine | 6 | 3 |
| 8. Arrange for M.D. and nurse | 6 | 3 |
| 9. Arrange for two city cars and sound equipment | 4 | 1 |
| 10. Obtain volunteers' assistance | 6 | 3 |
| 11. Develop method to use car and sound equipment | 4 | 4 |
| 12. Develop educational material | 4 | 7 |
| 13. Print educational material | 12 | 10 |
| 14. Assemble educational material | 13 | 2 |
| 15. Distribute educational material | 14 | 4 |
| 16. Orient volunteers concerning procedures | 10 | 1 |
| 17. Notify households that clinic will open | 7, 8 | 1 |
| 18. Announce clinic will open on car loudspeakers | 6, 9, 11 | 5 |
| 19. Hold clinic | 15, 16, 17, 18 | 5 |

a. Draw a PERT network diagram.

b. Determine the minimum number of working days required to complete the project.

c. Identify the activities on the critical path.

d. Note the earliest starting time and latest starting time at each event node.

e. If you had to get the project done three days sooner than the minimum it would now take, how would you speed it up? Why?

(We thank Diane Hunter for the above exercise.)

## Additional Reading

Griffith, John R. "Measuring Service Areas and Forecasting Demand." In *Cost Control in Hospitals,* edited by John R. Griffith, Walton M. Hancock, and Fred C. Munson. Ann Arbor, Michigan: Health Administration Press, 1976.

# 4

# Simple Stochastic Analysis

## 4.1 INTRODUCTION

The analyses of the last chapter had an important characteristic in common: in each it was assumed that there was no uncertainty about what would occur. Demand was for exactly 400 visits a week, and each visit took exactly 20 minutes. We know that such decision environments do not exist "naturally" in the real world, but only to the extent that we assume them to be so for the analysis. In this chapter we will attempt to move closer to the "real world" by explicitly incorporating some of the stochastic elements in the preceding chapter's analysis which we assumed to be deterministic. To the extent that we do incorporate stochastic elements into the analysis, the more closely our analysis approaches the "real world," the more accurate our predictions and descriptions and the more useful the results for meeting objectives and maintaining control. Such increased sophistication is not without cost, and the analyses of this chapter and especially those of Chapter 5 will require both more data and greater analytical effort. Thus an important issue to keep in mind is a cost-benefit assessment of the analysis itself: Is the increase in accuracy from a more sophisticated analysis worth more than the increased cost of the analysis?

In every decision, there is uncertainty about what will happen no matter what we do (for example, what the demand for ICU beds will be next year); and uncertainty about what will happen if we perform a specific action (for example, how often will the ICU unit be full if we build only 16 ICU beds?). We will attempt to address the first type of uncertainty by forecasting, using both "point" and "distribution" forecasts (Chapter 7). In this chapter and in Chapter

5 we will attempt to treat the following two questions: *Given* that our best forecast of demand is $Y$ (or demand is normally distributed with mean $\bar{Y}$ and standard deviation $\sigma$), what is our best estimate of what will happen if we adopt Strategy A instead of Strategy B? And which strategy best meets the objectives of the organization? Recall that in terms of our decision-making framework, the first question is a Step 2 process (quantifying what will happen if we take a particular strategy), while the second question is a Step 3 process ("solving" for the best strategy).

What distinguishes a simple stochastic analysis from a complex one? All of our attempts to treat uncertainty involve *incorporating* the stochastic nature of the real world into the analysis. In a large sense, a complex stochastic analysis will include more of the stochastic phenomena *explicitly,* while the same decisions can be treated in a simple analysis by *implicitly* including such phenomena. For example, we can treat the decision of how many ICU beds to provide a community in a simple analysis by assuming the ICU census will be Poisson distributed with mean $\lambda$, and provide enough beds to meet demand 95 percent of the time by determining the 95th percentile of the distribution. By dealing only with the distribution of the census we include implicitly such stochastic phenomena as length of stay, variation of demand by day of week (if any), seasonal variation of admissions of ICU, and seasonal variations in length of stay, etc. A complex treatment would explicitly include many of these in the analysis, as we will see in the next chapter.

A second distinction between simple and complex treatment involves the number of measures of performance that are addressed. In the above example, simple analysis gives the percentage of days demand is met. A more complex treatment would yield the number of times patients were turned away, how long they waited on the medical floor until they could get a bed in ICU, how many surgical admissions were cancelled to avoid turning away ICU patients, etc. In essence, the complex treatment will provide greater *detail* in describing what will happen if we do A instead of B.

In this chapter, then, we begin our treatment of stochastic analyses by *explicitly* incorporating one (or at most two) of the stochastic elements of the real-world problem, and addressing only one (or at most two) measures of performance. In Chapter 5, using more sophisticated concepts and techniques, we will begin to include more stochastic elements and address multiple measures of performance.

## 4.2 RESOURCE-SIZE DECISIONS

Stochastic analysis of the resource-size decision brings up a new and interesting issue that a deterministic analysis avoids for the most part. Since in the stochastic environment the only way to guarantee that *all* demand will be met is to provide that level of resources that will meet the *most extreme* level of demand (the "busiest" day of the year, hour of the week, etc.), in essence we are now facing the issue of how much of total demand to meet; or more to the point, how much demand *not* to meet. Since the only reason that we do not meet all demand is that it is "too costly" to do so, the decision is actually one of balancing the cost of meeting the next increment of demand (i.e., providing the resources to meet it) versus the cost of not meeting the next increment of demand. Since the cost to meet the increment is usually expressed in terms of the cost of additional resources, it is typically easily measured. The main effort of the analysis, then, is determining the cost of *not* meeting demand.

> **Problem:** Returning to the Balham community's problem of planning for the pediatric primary care walk-in clinic of the last chapter, we will consider for the moment only the resource-size problem of *how many examining rooms* to provide.
>
> The first step in the modeling analysis is to formulate the model. The objective is to minimize total cost:
>
> $$TC(X) = C_1(X) + C_2(X)$$
>
> where $X$ is the number of examining rooms to provide (the decision variable), $C_1(X)$ is the annual cost of providing $X$ rooms, and $C_2(X)$ is the annual cost of providing *only* $X$ rooms—that is, the cost of turning away some patients or making them wait because we do not have enough rooms to meet all demand at all times.

We will expect that the two cost components will be related to $X$ as expressed generally in Figure 4.1. The cost of providing $X$ rooms will certainly increase with $X$, while the cost associated with unmet demand will decrease. The point where total cost $TC(X)$ is minimized gives the optimal number of rooms to provide.

It is useful to view the $C_2(X)$ as the product of two

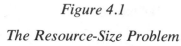

*Figure 4.1*

*The Resource-Size Problem*

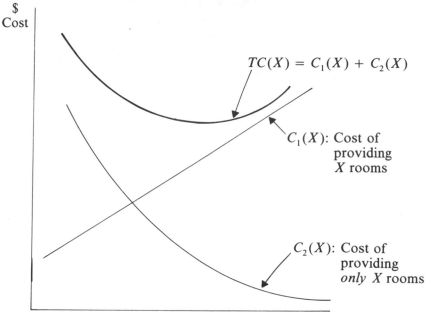

$$TC(X) = C_1(X) + C_2(X)$$

$C_1(X)$: Cost of
providing
$X$ rooms

$C_2(X)$: Cost of
providing
*only* $X$ rooms

$X$: Number of rooms

components: $f(X)$—the physical implications of providing
only $X$ rooms, and $u$—the *cost per unit* of such implications.*
This redefines the total cost objective as

$$TC(X) = C_1(X) + u \cdot f(X),$$

where, for our example, $f(X)$ is the number of patients
turned away per year, and $u$ is the cost of turning a patient
away.

We will expand this model when we treat the decision in a complex
stochastic analysis in Chapter 5 to include other implications such
as the costs of patients' waiting.

The second step in the analysis is to quantify the parameters
and the relationships of the model. The $C_1(X)$ is estimated by

---

*Recall that this was our approach in Chapter 2 with the OB merger problem, where we
divided cost of underserving into number underserved times cost per underserving.

accounting, engineering, and other techniques. It includes the cost to build and maintain the rooms (appropriately allocated over the life of the facility), equipment for the rooms, utilities, housekeeping, etc. (We might also include the necessary technical personnel as part of the room instead of as a separate resource-size problem, if they are indeed "tied" to the room. This is not likely the case in this example).

The $u$ must be measured subjectively for the most part. Because of the straightforwardness of this model and the fact that there is only one decision variable, we may wait and measure this cost *implicitly* in the next step of the analysis. (This will become a less satisfactory, but still possible, method of assessing $u$ when we use a more complex stochastic analysis.)

It is the estimation of the $f(X)$ that requires a new technique. What is the process that produces turnaways on a particular day, and how many interrelated stochastic phenomena make up that process? The process is as follows: (1) patients arrive; (2) they wait; (3) when a room becomes vacant, they are "served"; or (4) if the clinic closes while they wait, they are turned away (Figure 4.2). There are many stochastic elements to the process, the more important being

1. the number of patient arrivals that day, and the pattern of their arrival;

2. the average service time (in the examining rooms) that day, and the pattern of service time;

3. tardiness or absenteeism of physicians, nurses, and other personnel; their taking breaks, lunch, etc.;

## Figure 4.2

### Patient Flow in Clinic

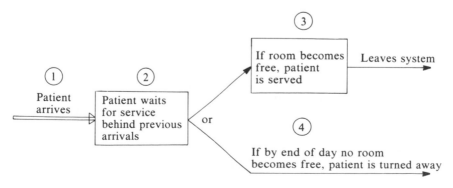

4. equipment breakdown in the examining rooms;

5. other instances of delay or of not being able to use rooms.

The simple analysis below will include all but the first of these *implicitly*, while a more complex analysis will begin to include the other elements explicitly. The simplest stochastic approach is to assume that the service time is fixed and that, for example, if we have $X$ rooms we can service $Y$ patients per day without turning any away according to the following table:

| $X$ | $Y$ |
| --- | --- |
| 1 | 30 |
| 2 | 58 |
| 3 | 82 |
| 4 | 100 |

Such data could conceivably be obtained by observing other clinics with similar characteristics and by making interpolations where necessary. An alternate method would be to attempt to measure service time and assume a utilization rate to determine $Y$. In either case, we will take the above data as fixed and deterministic in this analysis, leaving a more sophisticated approach to Chapter 5.

The only stochastic phenomenon we will treat *explicitly* here is demand, in terms of the number of patient arrivals per day. Suppose we have determined that demand in the busiest season of the year will follow the Poisson distribution, with means by day of the week as follows:

| Mon | Tue | Wed | Thu | Fri | Sat | Sun |
| --- | --- | --- | --- | --- | --- | --- |
| 70 | 75 | 80 | 75 | 70 | 30 | 0 |

(These estimates would rely heavily on both the projected number of patients per week, and the inferences from similar facilities in similar communities. The assumption that the number of visits is Poisson distributed at other clinics could be tested empirically. For additional discussion see Section 5.2.)

To calculate an $f(X)$ we need only to determine the *expected* number of patients who will be turned away each day for different $X$. For example, from the table showing number of rooms and number of patients serviced, if $X$(rooms) $= 3$, the clinic can serve 82 patients.

Now, consider the problem of determining how many patients will be turned away on Mondays, when the mean number of arrivals is 70, if we provide three rooms. As long as 82 or fewer patients arrive, there are no turnaways. The problems start when 83 or more patients arrive. Table 4.1 gives the analysis we need in order to calculate expected turnaways for Mondays if we provide three rooms. For each possible occurrence of column 1, column 2 gives the probability of the occurrence from the frequency distribution of a Poisson distributed random variable with mean 70 (these probabilities were calculated using the normal approximation to the Poisson, since most Poisson tables, like the one at the end of this text, do not cover Poisson means greater than 20). Column 3 gives the number of turnaways (column 1 minus 82) and column 4 the contribution of this occurrence to the expected number of turnaways. When we add this column, we get 0.305 (rounded to 0.31), which is the expected number of turnaways each Monday if we provide three rooms.

### Table 4.1

### Calculation of Expected Turnaway

| Arrivals $Y$ | Probability of $Y$ | Turnaways | Expected Turnaway |
|:---:|:---:|:---:|:---:|
| 83 | 0.0140 | 1 | 0.014 |
| 84 | 0.0115 | 2 | 0.023 |
| 85 | 0.0100 | 3 | 0.031 |
| 86 | 0.0078 | 4 | 0.031 |
| 87 | 0.0060 | 5 | 0.030 |
| 88 | 0.0047 | 6 | 0.028 |
| 89 | 0.0036 | 7 | 0.025 |
| 90 | 0.0026 | 8 | 0.021 |
| 91 | 0.0020 | 9 | 0.018 |
| 92 | 0.0015 | 10 | 0.015 |
| 93 | 0.0011 | 11 | 0.012 |
| 94 | 0.0008 | 12 | 0.010 |
| 95 | 0.0006 | 13 | 0.008 |
| 96 | 0.0004 | 14 | 0.006 |
| : | : | : | : |

Summation $\Sigma = 0.305$

The expected turnaway if we provide three and four rooms is displayed by day in Table 4.2 (assuming that $X = 1$ and $X = 2$ are not included, as they result in unacceptable turnaway rates at *any* reasonable value of $u$).

*Table 4.2*

*Expected Turnaway by Day of Week*

|                          | Mon | Tue  | Wed  | Thur | Fri | Sat | Weekly Total |
| ------------------------ | --- | ---- | ---- | ---- | --- | --- | ------------ |
| Average Demand           | 70  | 75   | 80   | 75   | 70  | 30  | 400          |
| Expected Turnaway if $X = 3$ | .31 | 1.06 | 2.65 | 1.06 | .31 | 0   | $5.39 = f(3)$ |
| Expected Turnaway if $X = 4$ | .00 | .01  | .04  | .01  | 0   | 0   | $.06 = f(4)$  |

To complete the second step of the analysis, assume that we have estimated that to build, equip, and maintain 3 rooms over the next 10 years (an arbitrary horizon) will cost $60,000 a year, while 4 rooms will cost $70,000 annually (the cost of building and equipping have been amortized appropriately over the 10 years). Thus the fourth room costs $10,000 a year or $193 a week.

The third step of the analysis is to solve for the optimal strategy. Recall that we did not establish a value for $u$ in Step 2. Since there are only two strategies to evaluate ($X = 3$ and $X = 4$) we may calculate what value we *imply* for $u$ if we take either strategy (and not the other). *If* we were to build 3 rooms, it would imply that the cost of the extra (fourth) room was greater than the cost of *not* providing the extra room:

$$\$193 > u \ (5.39 - .060)$$
$$\$193 > u \ (5.33)$$
$$u < \$193/5.33$$
$$u < \$36.$$

Thus, if we *were* to build the fourth, it would imply $u > \$36$. So instead of having to determine the value of $u$ in Step 2, we only have to decide if $u$ is less than or greater than $36. If there had been more than two possible strategies, the same method would have resulted in several *ranges* for the implied value of $u$, and the solution process is to determine into which range the actual $u$ falls. Note that it does not allow the decision maker to avoid dealing with $u$, nor does it make its evaluation less subjective. What it does allow is the avoidance of assigning a *point* evaluation to $u$, substituting a *range* evaluation instead.

The final step in the analysis is to assess the sensitivity of the model and its conclusions to changes or errors. In our case, we assess changes or errors in

1. the estimate of average demand,
2. the assumption of Poisson demand,
3. the cost of providing the rooms,
4. the value of $u$,
5. the number of patients which can be seen without turn-away if $X = 3$ and $X = 4$, and
6. the effect of making the simplifying (deterministic) assumptions.

Let's initially look at these individually, and then together (a much more complex task). The easiest is the value of $u$, since we know the effect of changes in $u$ from the analysis. The other elements can be assessed as to how changes in their values affect the implied breakpoint in $u$. For example, if the cost of providing the fourth room is actually $20,000 a year, the implied breakpoint for $u$ is $72. If this changes the decision of *which* $X$ is better ($X = 3$ or $X = 4$), then a more exact estimate of the cost of providing the fourth room should be obtained. Similarly, the sensitivity of the conclusion to points 1, 2, and 5 above can be assessed by repeating the analysis for possible values of these elements. The sensitivity of the model and its conclusions to point 6 is more complicated. The assessment may well involve us in performing a more sophisticated analysis (i.e., one which makes fewer simplifying assumptions). We will discuss more sophisticated analyses in Chapter 5.

Sensitivity to more than one element can be assessed *explicitly* by trying all combinations of changes. This quickly expands to unmanageable size, and some judgment must be used, such as analyzing only the most individually sensitive elements, and these only in pairs or in triplets.

To this point we have included explicitly only one stochastic element—demand—and considered only two measures of performance of the process—the number of patients turned away (ignoring, for example, the amount of time patients would have to wait for service), and, second, the cost to provide the rooms. To consider either more stochastic elements or more measures of performance moves us closer to complex analysis. Consider including the stochastic nature of service time explicitly in the analysis. One method of considering this element is to let the number of patients which can be serviced per day with $X$ rooms be a random variable $\bar{Z}$ following, for example, the Poisson distribution with $\lambda = 82$ for $X = 3$ and $\lambda = 100$ for $X = 4$. (How would these distributions be estimated?) The analysis involves the joint distribution of $\bar{Y}$ and $\bar{Z}$.

## 4.3 PROCEDURE DECISIONS

As in the resource-size problem, we may explicitly include some of the stochastic elements of procedure decisions in the analysis without making it complex. Again, however, we will need to make deterministic assumptions about many of the other real-world stochastic elements.

Reconsider the radiology problem of Section 3.3. Two of the major stochastic elements are

—demand (hourly, daily and monthly) and

—service times of the make option.


Let's consider the explicit inclusion of the stochastic nature of monthly demand into the analysis. (What are the implications of not treating demand hourly? Daily?) Suppose demand is expected to follow the following distribution:

| Demand/Month | $P$(Demand) |
|:---:|:---:|
| 800 | .1 |
| 900 | .2 |
| 1,000 | .2 |
| 1,100 | .2 |
| 1,200 | .1 |
| 1,300 | .1 |
| 1,400 | .1 |

The expected total cost of the make alternative is

$$\text{Exp}\,[FC(M) + VC(M)],$$

where Exp stands for expected. Since $FC$ does not change, but $VC(M)$ is a function of $D$, this reduces to

$$FC(M) + \text{Exp}\,[VC(M)].$$

Recall that the expected value of a *function* of a random variable is generally not equal to the value of the function at the expected value of the random variable:

$$\text{Exp } [f(\tilde{X})] \neq f(\text{Exp } [\tilde{X}]).$$

To calculate $\text{Exp } [f(\tilde{X})]$, we must sum overall possible values of $\tilde{X}$ the product

$$f(\tilde{X}) \cdot \text{prob}(\tilde{X}).$$

For our example,

| $\bar{D}$ | $VC(M)$ if $D = \bar{D}$ | $P(\bar{D})$ | $VC(M) \cdot P(\bar{D})$ |
|---|---|---|---|
| 800 | 8,000 | .1 | 800 |
| 900 | 9,000 | .2 | 1,800 |
| 1,000 | 10,000 | .2 | 2,000 |
| 1,100 | 11,000 | .2 | 2,200 |
| 1,200 | 12,000 | .1 | 1,200 |
| 1,300 | 13,000 | .1 | 1,300 |
| 1,400 | 14,000 | .1 | 1,400 |
| | | $\text{Exp } [VC(M)] =$ | 10,700 |

Thus the expected value of $TC$ is $10,700 + 11,000 = 21,700$. The expected value of $TC$ for the buy decision is calculated similarly:

| $\bar{D}$ | $VC(B)$ if $D = \bar{D}$ | $P(\bar{D})$ | $VC(B) \cdot P(\bar{D})$ |
|---|---|---|---|
| 800 | 17,600 | .1 | 1,760 |
| 900 | 19,800 | .2 | 3,960 |
| 1,000 | 22,000 | .2 | 4,400 |
| 1,100 | 24,200 | .2 | 4,840 |
| 1,200 | 26,400 | .1 | 2,640 |
| 1,300 | 28.600 | .1 | 2,860 |
| 1,400 | 30,800 | .1 | 3,080 |
| | | $\text{Exp } [VC(B)] =$ | 23,540 |

Thus we take alternative $M$.

Unfortunately, the concept of an indifference point is not manageable in the stochastic case. (Why not?) The extensions of this problem, described in Chapter 3, can be handled with stochastic demand in the same manner as above. The difference is that the fixed cost in some cases becomes "unfixed," and it is brought into the analysis under the expectation operation (Exp).

## 4.4 SCHEDULING DECISIONS: INVENTORY REVISITED

In the last chapter we formulated the inventory decision under several assumptions and then investigated the possibility of relaxing some of those assumptions, leaving the ones concerning stochastic demand and stochastic lead time to this chapter. It is suggested that the reader briefly review Section 3.4 before continuing.

The major implication of explicitly including stochastic demand and lead time in the analysis is that we thus introduce the cost of *stockout,* that is, of running out of an item before the next replenishment. Since demand is stochastic, it is possible to completely avoid stockout only by keeping enough inventory to meet the most extreme levels of demand. Unless the cost of stockout is extremely high (e.g., in the case of blood) and/or the cost of holding the item is extremely low, it will be likely that the optimal inventory strategy will allow some chance of stockout, when the cost of stockout has been balanced against the cost of avoiding stockout (holding extra inventory).

To make the analysis manageable, suppose that we *must* order only once a month. (The reader interested in more realistic and thus complex analyses is referred to Naddor.) Suppose further that lead time is zero, so that our strategy involves determining *to what level we should replenish stock for the coming month.* Redefine $Q$ as the level to which to replenish. Figure 4.3 gives the level of inventory over a typical six-month period when strategy $Q$ is employed. Note that during the third month, we experienced a stockout of $D_3 - Q$, where $D_3$ was the demand in Month 3. Generally, the amount of stockout $(S)$ will be

$$\bar{S} = \begin{cases} 0 \text{ if } \tilde{D} \le Q \\ \tilde{D} - Q \text{ if } \tilde{D} > Q. \end{cases}$$

Let $C_3$ be the cost *per item* of stocking out. Assume further that the monetary investment in the item is held for the whole month, so that we *always* have $pQ$ dollars invested in inventory, at interest rate $i/12$ per month. Finally, assume that we must always keep space for all $Q$ items, so that our warehousing cost is always $WQ/12$ (the division by 12 is to convert annual warehousing cost to monthly warehousing cost). Our *expected* cost *per month* if we use strategy $Q$ is

$$\text{Exp}\,[TC(Q)] = \text{Exp}\,[ipQ/12 + WQ/12 + C_3\bar{S}];$$

or since the only term involving a random variable is $C_3\,\bar{S}$,

## Figure 4.3

### Level of Inventory over Time

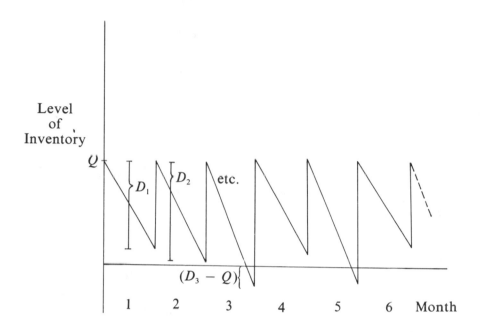

$$\text{Exp}\,[TC(Q)] = (ipQ + WQ)/12 + C_3\,\text{Exp}\,[\bar{S}].$$

Suppose demand has the following distribution.

| $\tilde{D}$ | $P(\tilde{D})$ |
| --- | --- |
| 200 | .1 |
| 300 | .3 |
| 400 | .3 |
| 500 | .2 |
| 600 | .1 |

What is expected stockout if we set $Q = 500$? If $\tilde{D}$ is 500 or less, there is no stockout. If $\tilde{D}$ is 600, we experience stockout of 100. The expected stockout is $100 \times .1 = 10$. For $Q = 400$, expected stockout $= 100 \times .2 + 200 \times .1 = 40$. For $Q = 300$, $\text{Exp}\,(\bar{S}) = .3 \times 100 + .2 \times 200 + .1 \times 300 = 100$ and for $Q = 200$, $\text{Exp}\,(\bar{S}) = .3 \times 100 + .3 \times 200 + .2 \times 300 + .1 \times 400 = 190$.

Like the resource-size problem, we may proceed either of two ways at this point. We may fix the cost of stockout $C_3$ and solve for optimal $Q$, or we may infer the range of $C_3$ implied by each of the five possible strategies. Following the second way, recall from the last chapter that $i = .1$, $W = 3.65$, and $p = \$6$. Thus $i/12 = .0085$, so that $ip/12 = .05$, and $W/12 = .30$. Table 4.3 gives the holding costs for each of the strategies and the related expected stockout.

### Table 4.3

### *Trial and Error Calculation of Optimal Q*

| $Q$ = | 200 | 300 | 400 | 500 | 600 |
|---|---|---|---|---|---|
| $ipQ/12$ = | 10 | 15 | 20 | 25 | 30 |
| $WQ/12$ = | 60 | 90 | 120 | 150 | 180 |
| Holding Costs | 70 | 105 | 140 | 175 | 210 |
| $\mathrm{Exp}(\tilde{S})$ | 190 | 100 | 40 | 10 | 0 |

*If* we choose $Q = 400$, what does it imply about $C_3$? First, it means that we did *not* choose $Q = 300$; thus the increase in cost of stocking out of $Q = 300$ over $Q = 400$ must be larger than the decrease in holding cost:

$$(100 - 40)\, C_3 \geq (140 - 105), \text{ or}$$

$$C_3 \geq .58.$$

But second, since we did *not* choose $Q = 500$,

$$(40 - 10)\, C_3 \leq (175 - 140), \text{ or}$$

$$C_3 \leq 1.17.$$

Thus, *if* we were to choose $Q = 400$ as optimal, we imply that

$$.58 \leq C_3 \leq 1.17.$$

Similarly, Table 4.4 gives the ranges of $C_3$ implied by choosing the other strategies.

To "solve" for optimal $Q$ means determining into which range $C_3$ actually falls, rather than having to determine a point value for $C_3$.

Sensitivity analysis for this problem is similar to the problems in the previous section.

## Table 4.4

### Implied Ranges for Cost of Stockout

| Strategy: $Q=$ | Implied Range $C$ |
|:---:|:---:|
| 200 | $C_3 \leq .40$ |
| 300 | $.40 < C_3 \leq .58$ |
| 400 | $.58 < C_3 \leq 1.17$ |
| 500 | $1.17 < C_3 \leq 3.50$ |
| 600 | $3.50 < C_3$ |

## 4.5 GRAPHICAL REPRESENTATION OF STOCHASTIC ANALYSIS: DECISION TREES

It is often easier to keep track of the decision-making framework for a stochastic analysis by using a decision tree. The alternatives, the measures of performance, the forecast of outcomes and their probabilities, and the calculations for the solution step are easily recorded in a decision tree format. To illustrate the use of the decision tree, we will reconsider the three examples from this chapter: the *make–buy* decision, the *inventory replenishment* decision, and the *number of examining rooms* decision. No additional information is required—we will simply draw the decision trees that underlie the decision framework for these examples.

The *make–buy* decision is the most straightforward. The decision tree is shown in Figure 4.4. A square represents a decision node—the decision maker must select one of the make–buy alternatives at this point on the tree. The circles represent chance nodes—the decision maker cannot select a specified demand for radiology examinations but rather must estimate the probability (chance) that a certain demand will occur. The outcome resulting from the decision maker's selecting one of the alternatives, and a certain demand's occurring, will be a cost to the institution. For the make alternative, this cost was given in Section 3.3 as

$$TC(M) = 11,000 + 10y,$$

and for the buy alternative as

$$TC(B) = 22y,$$

where $y$ = the number of examinations per month.

On the tree, then, the costs are placed at the tip of the last branches. For example, if the decision maker selected the make alternative, and the demand was 800 examinations per month, then

*Figure 4.4*

*Decision Tree for Make-Buy Decision*

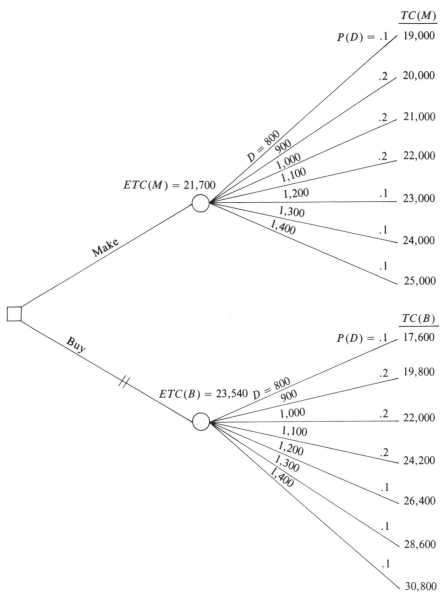

the total cost would be

$$TC(M) = 11,000 + 10(800)$$

$$= 19,000.$$

This is repeated for the tip of each branch.

The probability that 800 examinations will be demanded as given in Section 4.3 is recorded on the corresponding branch. This is repeated for each demand level. The possible outcomes (and corresponding demand) must be mutually exclusive and exhaustive for this analysis so that the probabilities add to 1.0. We now have all of the information from Sections 3.3 and 4.3 recorded on the decision tree. Next is the solution step.

The calculations in the solution step are also straightforward. We calculate the expected total cost ($ETC$) for each alternative, and, according to the analysis, select that alternative with the lowest $ETC$. The $ETC$ for an alternative is the sum of the total costs (branch tips) weighted by their probability. For example, the $ETC$ for the make alternative is

$$ETC\,(M) = .1(19,000) + .2(20,000) + .3(21,000) + .2(22,000)$$

$$+.1(23,000) + .1(23,000) + .1(24,000) + .1(25,000)$$

$$= 21,700.$$

Similarly, in the buy alternative the $ETC(B)$ is 23,540. $ETC$ is shown at the corresponding chance nodes at the end of each alternative. Note that these are the same values as given in Section 4.3. According to the analysis, the make alternative is preferred; therefore slashes are placed on the buy branch.

The extensions of Section 3.3, and any sensitivity analyses, can be incorporated in the analysis by replacing the appropriate total costs at the end of the branches and recalculating the $ETC$s. This is left as an exercise.

The decision tree for the *inventory replenishment* decision is shown in Figure 4.5. The added feature in the analysis of this decision compared to the make-buy decision is that instead of calculating the $ETC$, the expected stockout is calculated and ranges for $C_3$, the cost of running out of one item, are calculated. If instead we set $C_3$ at some value, this analysis and its tree would be identical to the make–buy analysis.

The alternatives shown at the decision node are replenishment levels set at $Q = 200, 300, 400, 500,$ and 600. Possible demand levels (mutually exclusive and exhaustive) are shown at the chance nodes with the probability of each level recorded on the branch. The difference between the demand level and $Q$, or the stockout, is the outcome and is recorded at the tip of each branch. The expected

*Figure 4.5*

*Decision Tree for Inventory Replenishment Decision*

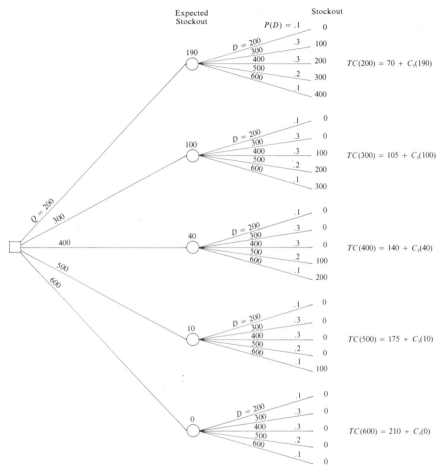

stockout is calculated by multiplying the probabilities for demand levels times the number of stockouts and summing at each chance node. The total cost for each alternative equals the holding cost for $Q$ plus $C_3$, the cost per stockout, times the expected number of stockouts for that alternative.

To obtain the ranges of $C_3$, the total cost equations for each pair of adjacent alternatives are set equal to each other and solved for $C_3$.

Finally, the tree for deciding the number of examining rooms is shown in Figure 4.6. The alternative number of rooms is shown at the decision node. For each day of the week, there is a different

## Figure 4.6

## Decision Tree for Number of Examining Rooms Decision

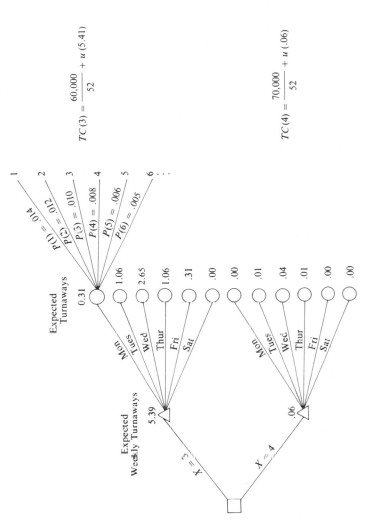

average number of arrivals. At the end of the Monday branch for $X = 3$ is the expected number of turnaways. The probability distribution for turnaways on Monday, calculated above from the normal distribution, is shown on the tree. To calculate the expected number of turnaways for Monday, the probability times the number of turnaways is summed for the chance node at the tip of the Monday branch. This process would need to be repeated for each day of the week and each alternative. (This is not shown on the tree.)

To get the expected number of turnaways per week, the daily expected numbers are summed. This step is shown by the triangle on the tree—a composite evaluation node. There is no choice at this point, and there is no chance—every day will occur for certain. Therefore, we cannot use the square or circle to denote this point. The expected number of turnaways at each triangle is recorded. The expected total weekly cost for each alternative is calculated, using the expected total cost equation

$$ETC(X) = C_1(X) + u \cdot f(X),$$

where $X$ = number of examining rooms and $u$ = cost of one turnaway. To obtain the range of $u$, the same steps are followed as for the inventory replenishment decision.

There are three important extensions to the above analysis that should be considered when using the decision tree: *sequential decisions, utility,* and *subjective probability.*

The idea of sequential decisions can be seen in operation by realizing that running out of an item in the replenishment decision or turning away a patient in the number of examining rooms decision are also decisions—even though we treated them as outcomes in the above analysis. Rather than simply turning away a patient when there are not enough examining rooms, we could decide to use another room; one that is less well-equipped, more cramped, or less private. Or, we could send the patient to another clinic, or ask him to return on another day.

Rather than run out of stock and do without, we could purchase the items from a local retail store, or make do with a less preferred item, or request a special delivery. Sequential decisions are being made—first about the replenishment level, then about the method for quick delivery or substitution if we run out.

The sequential decision for turnaways is diagrammed in the decision tree in Figure 4.7. The possible outcomes are cure, disability, death, or some other characteristic of patient health. In order to

Figure 4.7

Decision Tree for Sequential Decisions

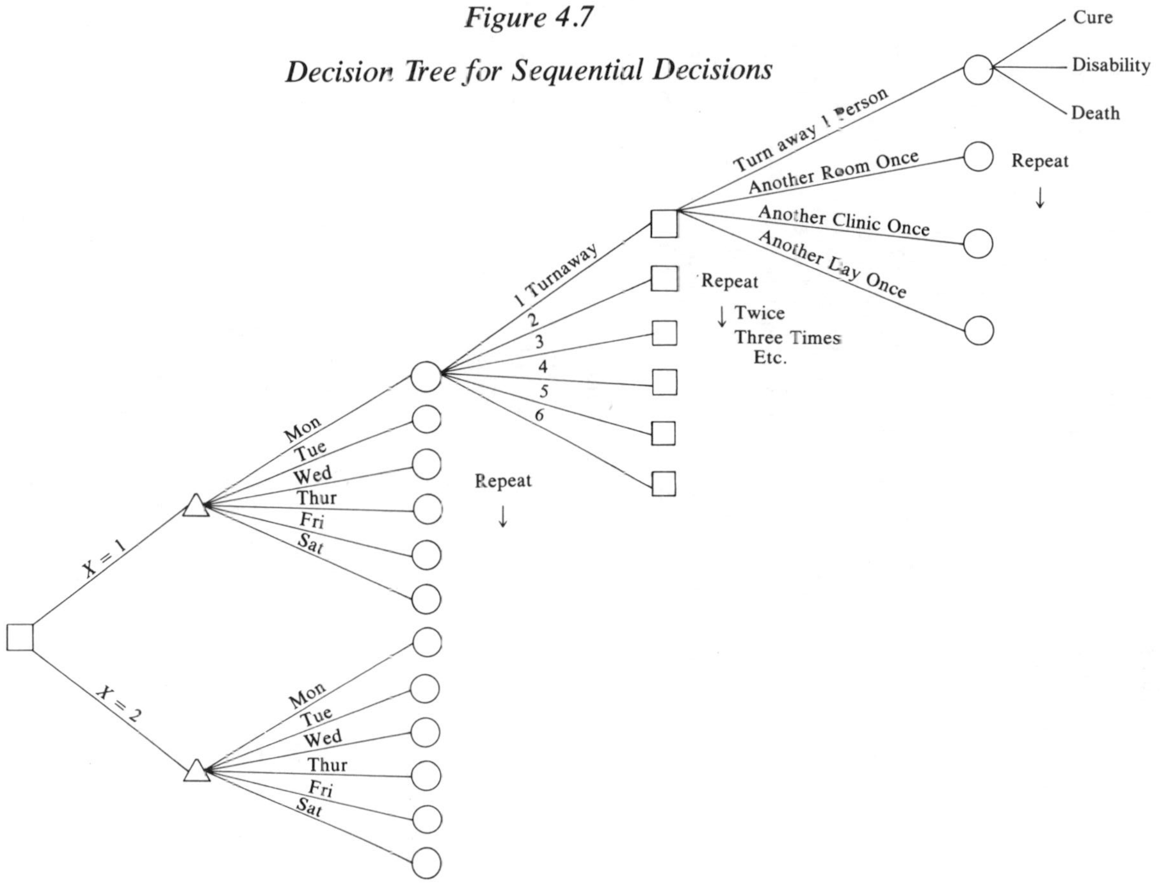

perform the analysis, a preference for being cured, disabled, or dead must be quantified. The general term for quantifying preference is utility—the value we place on an outcome. (The preference measurement for various states of health are beyond this book, and the interested reader is referred to Blishke, et al.) We will further discuss measuring preference or utility in Chapter 9 and illustrate several methods for doing it.)

We also need probabilities of a patient's becoming cured, disabled, or deceased, given the selection of one of the alternatives: turnaway, another room, another clinic, or another day. In the analysis, the probabilities would be multiplied times the utilities to obtain expected utility at the end of each decision branch. We select the alternative with the highest expected utility, assign that value to the decision node, and use it in calculating the expected utility at the next chance node. Finally, there would be an expected utility at the end of the two alternatives we were originally deciding between, and we would select that alternative with the highest expected utility.

The probabilities of a patient's becoming cured, disabled, or deceased would be difficult to obtain by conducting a study and observing the frequency with which these states occur—as we could have done for the probability of turnaways. However, we could ask physicians to make *estimates* of the probabilities, called *subjective* probabilities. We will return to this topic in Chapter 9.

### Exercises

4.1 You are the administrator of a relatively large rural hospital (250 beds) that has a high occupancy rate (MED/SURG units are at 94 percent occupancy). An emergency patient that must be admitted is normally admitted to the MED/SURG unit. However, if it is full, as it often is with an occupancy rate of .94, the emergency patient is turned away. You are considering remodeling the Emergency Room (ER) so that there would be a holding area. Emergency patients could spend one night in the holding area if the MED/SURG unit was filled, and then be transferred to the first open MED/SURG bed the following day.

Your quantitative staff specialist provides you with the following information and recommendations.

—Since census drops off on Friday and Saturday nights, the average number of "overflow" emergency patients requiring a place in the holding area is 0 for these two nights.

—The heaviest demand for MED/SURG beds is Monday, Tuesday, and Wednesday nights, when the average number of overflow ER patients is 2 per night.

—On Sunday and Thursday nights, the average number of overflow patients is 1 per night.

—Assume the distribution of overflow patients follows a Poisson distribution with the averages given above (round probabilities off to nearest hundredth).

—If you open an ER holding area, one RN per bed ($12,000 per year each, including fringe benefits) will have to be added on the night shift.

—To provide these beds, the ER will have to be remodeled with costs estimated at $6,000 per year spread over the useful life of the ER for the first bed, and an *additional* $4,000 per year for each additional bed.

a. Following carefully the four steps of analyzing decisions, decide how many beds you would provide. What cost or range of costs are you willing to incur to avoid turning away an emergency patient when the MED/SURG unit is full?

b. Suggest the most likely sensitivity analyses you would want your quantitative specialist to perform. Why these?

4.2 You are the administrator of a large (600 bed) hospital in the suburbs of a large (1 million) city. There are presently 3 treatment rooms in your emergency facility (ER), and last year about 5,000 patients were treated in the treatment rooms. The head nurse says that 3 rooms seems about right, since they are seldom all used at the same time, and she can remember only two times last year when a fourth was needed. A large nearby hospital, however, is closing its ER service, and since your hospital is the only other one in the vicinity, you expect that beginning about one year from now you'll get most of its ER business; it also treated about 5,000 patients in its treatment rooms last year. The chief MD in ER suggests that you double the number of treatment rooms, since business will double.

You consult your quantitative staff specialist (your employee with a Master's in Industrial Engineering). He happens to have the following data gathered last year. He observed the arrival of patients between 4 P.M. and 1 A.M.—by far the busiest time of the day, when 60 percent of the ER patients are treated—and found the following:

| Number of rooms being used when patient arrived | Number of patients observed (total = 100) |
|:---:|:---:|
| 0 | 42 |
| 1 | 36 |
| 2 | 21 |
| 3 | 1 |

Your quantitative staff specialist points out that the distribution is very close to the Poisson, with mean equal to 1. He suggests that when business doubles, the distribution of the number of rooms being used when a patient arrives will be Poisson, with mean equal to 2, as follows:

| Number of rooms being used when patient arrived, if 6 rooms were provided | Probability (total = 1.0) |
|:---:|:---:|
| 0 | .14 |
| 1 | .27 |
| 2 | .27 |
| 3 | .18 |
| 4 | .09 |
| 5 | .04 |
| 6 | .01 |

You look into the cost of providing a fourth, fifth, and sixth treatment room in the ER. Your hospital architect estimates that the fourth room would cost about $20,000 in remodeling and about $20,000 in equipment. Since it will have a useful life of about 10 years, you figure it will cost about $4,000 a year. The fifth would cost *another* $60,000 remodeling and *another* $20,000 to equip. The sixth would cost another $40,000 and $20,000 to remodel and equip respectively. The current number of personnel could serve the fourth, but another nurse would have to be hired to serve the fifth (she could also serve the sixth, if there were a sixth), and she would cost about $12,000 a year, including fringe benefits.

    a. Following carefully the four steps of analyzing decisions, determine the appropriate number of rooms to provide. State all assumptions you use, but *make them reasonable*. Subjective costs should be "priced out" by the analysis, but use your own values and recommend the appropriate number of rooms to provide, pointing out exactly what your decision implies about the subjective costs. Show how sensitive your results arc to errors in measurement of the different costs in the model you build.

b. Evaluate your analysis above. Discuss how, if you had more time and money, you might gather more data, use a different approach, etc.

c. Discuss the roles of the Health Administrator (yourself in the above problem) and quantitative specialists (including the industrial engineer, your accountants, or others you used or might use) in the above analysis.

4.3 a. In Chapter 3 Exercises, Question 3.1, how would your decision change if your analysis took into account the stochastic nature of monthly demand? Assume demand is expected to follow the following distribution. (Also assume demand will not be anything but these five amounts.)

| Exams/Month | Probability (Demand) |
|---|---|
| 840 | .07 |
| 870 | .24 |
| 900 | .38 |
| 930 | .24 |
| 960 | .07 |

b. How can you perform a sensitivity analysis now? Do it for variable cost; assume radiologist's salary will be $8,000.

4.4 For the radiology problem of Section 4.3 (see text), suppose it is not clear exactly what salary would be negotiated with the radiologist, but it is likely to be no less than $5000/month and no more than $9000/month. Is the decision to make or buy sensitive to the radiologist's salary in the stochastic case where demand is expected to follow the distribution (as in Section 4.3)? Interpret the results of your analysis.

4.5 In Section 3.3, two extensions of the above problem were considered. The first was: suppose that for up to 750 additional radiology exams per month, the make alternative would require one additional radiologist, two technologists, and two rooms. For between 750 and 1250 exams per month, the make alternative would require still another technologist and one more room. For between 1,250 and 1,750 exams per month, there would need to be still another room and technologist plus a half-time additional radiologist at $4,000 per month. Assume the first radiologist would cost $7,000 per month (i.e., do not do the sensitivity analysis).

Suppose further that for the buy alternative, it would be necessary to hire two carriers to transport patients, reports, etc., and one secretary; and that there would be other fixed costs amounting to $4,000 a month. With the hospital supporting $4,000 of the buy alternative in this way, the charge per exam from the private group would be $20 per exam. Should you make or buy? Why?

4.6 A second extension in Section 3.3 to the above problem was to suppose the private group now offers you rates as follows:

| | | |
|---|---|---|
| 0–499 | exams/month | $25/exam |
| 500–999 | exams/month | 20/exam |
| 1,000–1,499 | exams/month | 18/exam |
| 1,500+ | exams/month | 16/exam |

Assume the other facts described in Exercise 4.5 still hold. Should you make or buy? Why?

4.7 Reconsider Problem 3.2. The butcher cuts meat on the day before it is to be served and must finish all cutting before he leaves, even if he must work overtime. He is able to cut exactly 25 lbs. of servable meat per hour. Depending on the menu and the number of patients on particular diets, the amount of meat he must cut varies per day according to the following distribution:

| lbs/day | Probability |
|---|---|
| 150 | .1 |
| 175 | .2 |
| 200 | .3 |
| 225 | .2 |
| 250 | .2 |

The butcher is paid $3.50/hr. (including fringe benefits) for regular time and $5.00 overtime (including fringe benefits). He works 5 days a week, and a part-time butcher fills in for his weekends and vacations, etc., at the same pay rate. The butcher is paid for 8 hrs./day even if he works less than 8.

Assuming the meat prices are those in Problem 3.2, build a case for either keeping the butcher(s) or going to portion-ready cuts.

4.8 Reconsider Problem 3.6. Assume now that usage is stochastic with a mean of 36 units per day and a standard deviation of 6 units per day. Assume this mean and standard deviation hold for every day of the year. In addition, assume the following:

—You must order once a month (30 days).

—The lead time to receiving the order is zero (rather than the 5 days as in Problem 3.6).

—The disposable packs of personal items come in cartons of 33 and you cannot order partial cartons (and you are short entire cartons, not partial cartons).

—The monetary investment in the packs is held for the whole month.

—You must always keep space for the maximum number of packs stored.

a.  To what level should you replenish stock for the coming month? (Since you can only order cartons, how many cartons should be ordered?)

b.  Calculate the cost of stockout you implied by the levels you set.

c.  Which level would you select and why?

Recall from statistics that the distribution resulting from summing normal distributions (over 30 days, for example) is a normal distribution with the mean equal to the sum of the means and the variance equal to the sum of the variances. The standard deviation is *not* the sum of the standard deviations, but the square root of the summed variance.

4.9 Reconsider Problem 3.6. Assume now that usage is stochastic with a mean of 36 units per day and a standard deviation of 6 units per day. Assume this mean and standard deviation hold for every day of the year. In addition, assume the following facts.

—You may order at any time and therefore plan to order $Q$ from Problem 3.6.

—The lead time for deliveries is 5 days.

—The disposable packs of personal items come in cartons of 13 and you cannot order partial cartons (and you are short entire cartons, not partial cartons).

—The monetary investment in the packs is held for the whole month.

—You must always keep space for the maximum number of packs stored.

a.  At what point (number of cartons) should you set the minimum stock level for reorder?

b. Calculate the cost of stockout implied by the levels you set.

c. Which level would you select and why?

4.10 Return to the Physician Assistant "inventory" problem at the end of Section 3.4. Suppose the distribution of PAs staying with the clinic is as follows:

| Stay | Probability |
|------|-------------|
| exactly 1 yr. | .2 |
| exactly 2 yrs. | .3 |
| exactly 3 yrs. | .5 |

Suppose that training sessions will be held only once every 3 years. If the clinic has too many (i.e., more than 120), the extra ones perform as nurses (which could have been hired for $3000 a year less than a PA). If the clinic has too few PAs, however, it must hire physicians that cost $10,000 more than a PA per year. How many PAs should be trained each three years?

4.11 The daily number of visits to your Physical Therapy (PT) department follows the distribution

| Visits | $P$(visits) |
|--------|-------------|
| 20 | .6 |
| 25 | .2 |
| 30 | .2 |

Although it is known by 7 A.M. each day how many *visits* will occur that day, the number of *hours* of PT that will be required that day is stochastic as follows: given that the number of visits is

| 20 | | 25 | | 30 | |
|------|------------|------|------------|------|------------|
| hours | $P$(hours) | hours | $P$(hours) | hours | $P$(hours) |
| 24 | .5 | 24 | .2 | 24 | 0 |
| 28 | .4 | 28 | .3 | 28 | .1 |
| 32 | .1 | 32 | .3 | 32 | .4 |
| 36 | 0 | 36 | .2 | 36 | .5 |

The staffing decision for the PT department is made in two stages.

1) You must provide a "core" staff, which does not change for 6 months, of either 3 PTs (or $3 \times 8 = 24$ hours) at $400 a day, or 3-1/2 PTs (or 28 hours) at $450 a day.

2) Then at 7 A.M., after the number of visits for that day is known, you either

a) rely on overtime (at $20 an hour) to cover any hours of demand over the "core" hours available, or

b) call in a complete extra PT shift of 8 hours, which costs you $100. If these 8 extra hours still do not cover demand, you must use overtime ($20 an hour) for the excess.

(*Example:* you have staffed the core at 3 PTs, or 24 hours. At 7 A.M. today you find that there will be 30 visits. You decide to call in the extra shift, giving you 32 hours. The demand from the 30 visits happens to take 36 hours today, so you also must use 4 hours overtime.)

Draw a two stage decision tree for the two stages of staffing decision, deciding which core size (3 or 3-1/2) to use, and how you will react to the 7 A.M. decision.

## Additional Reading

Blishke, W. R., Bush, J. W., and Kaplan, R. M. "Successive Internal Analysis of Preference Measures in a Health Status Index." *Health Services Research,* Summer 1975, p. 181.

Hillier, F. S. and Lieberman, G. J. *Introduction to Operations Research.* San Francisco: Holden-Day, 1974.

Naddor, E. *Inventory Systems.* New York: John Wiley and Sons, 1966.

Wagner, H. M. *Principles of Operations Research With Applications to Managerial Decisions.* Englewood Cliffs, N.J.: Prentice-Hall, 1969.

# 5

# Complex Stochastic Analysis

## 5.1 INTRODUCTION

In the last chapter we framed our pediatric clinic resource-size decision in terms of balancing the cost of providing a certain level of resources (examining rooms) against the cost of that level of resources' not being able to meet all demands. We measured the unmet demand in terms of expected average turnaway per year. But does "average turnaway" completely describe the implications of providing only $X$ examining rooms? Turnaway might be too coarse a measure. What will be the average amount of time patients have to wait for service? How many will be waiting at any given time? Will they wait for the receptionist, then wait for an examination, then wait for the doctor's report? What will happen when a patient returns on a scheduled visit? How should return patients be scheduled? How often will the last examining room be used? The next to last room? How often will the clinic have to be operated on an overtime basis?

Our analysis in the last chapter also made several important simplifying assumptions. What if service time is now considered to be stochastic? What if physicians (or nurses, receptionists, etc.) arrive late? What if scheduled return patients arrive late (or not at all)? What is the effect of day of week (or time of day) on patient arrival patterns?

Complex stochastic analysis can be differentiated from simple stochastic analysis in these two important ways: (1) the measures of performance addressed in the objective function represent a finer measurement of the implications of choosing each alternative; and (2) many of the simplifying assumptions necessary for a simple analysis are relaxed, making possible a closer representation of the real-world process. Complex analysis also allows analysis of some processes that are so complex by nature that a simple stochastic analysis is not meaningful, such as the scheduling of inpatient admissions to hospitals.

We will use the same decision framework for complex analyses that we used in the previous chapters. The differences will be in an objective function in Step 1 with more terms and more (and more complex) decision variables, and, in Step 2, more sophisticated techniques for quantifying the relationships of the objective function. We will spend much of our time on two closely related techniques of such quantification: *queueing* and *simulation.* Both are rather complex, and a significant amount of both mathematical and computer sophistication is required to carry out a full-scale analysis. Thus we will focus on what the administrator must know in order to manage the quantitative specialist on the staff who is carrying out a complex analysis. This will begin with an understanding of the *queueing flow process* (Section 5.2), then move into investigating which of the simpler models can be solved by mathematics, to the limitations of mathematically solvable queueing models, and finally to the assumptions that must be made to use them. The importance of queueing models, however, lies in their role as the basic framework for most simulation models; we discuss this further in Section 5.3. The most effective way to gain insight into the manager's role in analyzing complex phenomena and the role of queueing and simulation in decision making is to present successful applications of simulation in health administration decision making in some detail. Two such examples are the resource-size problem of how many obstetric beds are appropriate to meet demand (Section 5.4), and scheduling inpatient admissions to hospitals (Section 5.5).

## 5.2 THE QUEUEING FLOW PROCESS

**Problem:** Returning to our resource-size decision of the preceding chapters, how many examining rooms ($X$) should we provide to meet the demand for pediatric walk-in patients in our proposed new clinic? Assume now that "average number of turnaways" is too coarse a measure of the costs of not meeting all demand. We now want measures of how long patients will have to wait and of how many will be waiting on the average. Also, we feel uncomfortable about the assumption that the service (examination) time is deterministic, and we want to incorporate its true stochastic nature into the analysis.

Our first step is to formulate the objective function for the resource-size decision. Our objective is still to minimize total cost. The formulation is

$$TC(X) = C_1(X) + C_2(X)$$

where $C_1(X)$ is the annual cost of providing and maintaining $X$ examining rooms and $C_2(X)$ is the cost associated with providing *only* $X$ rooms. We now expand $C_2(X)$ to reflect our new measures of performance:

$$TC(X) = C_1(X) + u \cdot W(X) + v \cdot L(X)$$

where
  $u$ = the cost per minute of average patient wait,
  $W(X)$ = the average patient wait (in minutes),
  $v$ = cost per patient waiting, and
  $L(X)$ = average number of patients waiting.
(At this stage we will examine only these two wait measures. With the simulation examples we will expand the objective to include other measures.)

The quantification (decision-making framework, Step 2) of $C_1(X)$, $u$, and $v$ in the objective function are the same as in previous chapters: we find values for $C_1(X)$ by using accounting methods, expert opinion, etc., and for $u$ and $v$ by subjective means (or, more likely, by leaving the quantification of $u$ and $v$ to Step 3). It is the quantification of the $W(X)$ and $L(X)$ that requires new techniques.

In order to quantify $W(X)$ and $L(X)$, we regard the arrival, service (examination and treatment), and discharge of patients as a queueing flow process (see Figure 5.1). Patients arrive randomly for service and wait in a *queue* to be served. If one of the $X$ rooms is free and there is no one in line before him, the patient waits zero minutes, and immediately occupies an empty exam room. If all rooms are full, he waits until one is free; if there are other patients also waiting, he waits his turn. After service is performed, the patient leaves the room, freeing it immediately for the next waiting patient. If no patient is waiting, the room(s) becomes idle.

Notice that there are only two independent stochastic elements in the flow process: the *arrival process* and the *service process*. (These of course may not be independent of one another. For the time

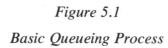

*Figure 5.1*

*Basic Queueing Process*

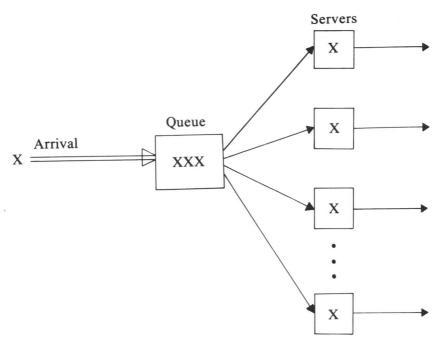

being, however, we will assume they are.) Although the amount of time a patient waits, how many wait with him, and when he is discharged are also stochastic, we will see that they depend on (and can be derived from) the arrival and service process. In addition to these two independent stochastic processes we must also consider the *queue discipline*, defined as the manner in which the patients will be called from the queue (for example, first come, first served; last come, first served; random; shortest expected service time first; most ill first), and the *number of servers* (the number of examining rooms *X* in our example). These four elements—the arrival process, the service process, the queue discipline, and the number of servers— will be said to completely define the queueing system. (There are some other descriptors that are beyond the scope of our use here; see Wagner, for example, in Additional Reading.)

**The Arrival Process**

Since the arrival process is a stochastic process, in many cases we can describe it with a probability distribution. There are two options. We could specify the distribution of times between arrivals,

*Figure 5.2*

*Interarrival Distribution*

| Time Between Arrivals (Hours) | Observed Frequency (100 Patients) |
|---|---|
| .1 | 60 |
| .2 | 21 |
| .3 | 8 |
| .4 | 4 |
| .5 | 4 |
| .6 | 1 |
| .7 | 0 |
| .8 | 1 |
| .9 | 1 |

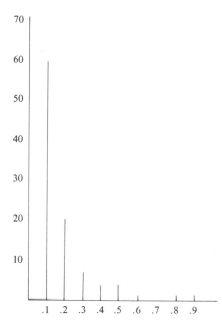

known as the *interarrival time* (see Figure 5.2), or we could specify the distribution of the number of arrivals per minute, per hour, or per day, called the *arrival rate* (see Figure 5.3). One may generally be derived from the other.

Suppose, for instance, we observe the distribution of the arrival rate of a nearby pediatric clinic which seems to have a level of demand similar to what we expect for our pediatric clinic. By observing the process on twelve consecutive Wednesdays from approximately 8:00 A.M. to 4:00 P.M. (100 hours), we find the *empirical arrival rate distribution* of Figure 5.3, which has a mean of 8 per hour. If we

*Figure 5.3*

*Arrival Rate Distribution*

| Observed Arrivals (Per Hour) | Observed Frequency (100 Hours) |
|:---:|:---:|
| 0 | 1 |
| 1 | 1 |
| 2 | 1 |
| 3 | 3 |
| 4 | 6 |
| 5 | 8 |
| 6 | 13 |
| 7 | 13 |
| 8 | 15 |
| 9 | 9 |
| 10 | 10 |
| 11 | 8 |
| 12 | 3 |
| 13 | 4 |
| 14 | 2 |
| 15 | 1 |
| 16 | 0 |
| 17 | 1 |
| 18 | 1 |

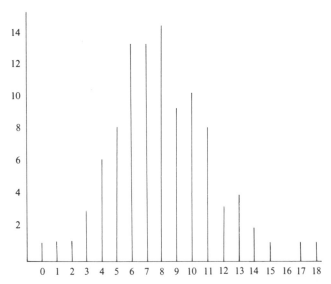

believe that the observed clinic's arrival experience is very similar
to what will happen at our proposed pediatric clinic, we might use
this empirical distribution for our analysis. There are two problems
with doing this, however. First, we may be uneasy with the assumption
that our arrival process, both in magnitude (the average rate) and

## Figure 5.4

### The Poisson Distribution

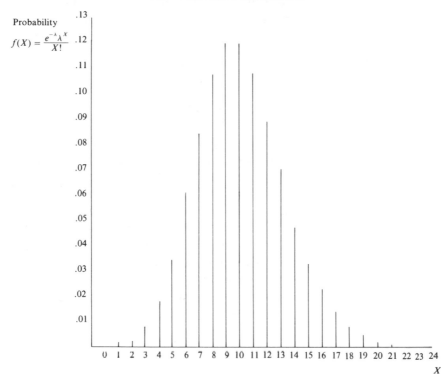

Arrivals per Hour (Mean = λ = 10)

in pattern (the shape of the distribution) will be the same as that of the observed pediatric clinic. Second, it is more difficult (but not impossible) to use empirical distributions in a queueing analysis, although they are easily used in simulation. Thus, the actual arrival process is often approximated by a theoretical distribution—one that can be easily described mathematically and which can be easily altered to fit our situation.

If arrivals are (1) independent of one another and are (2) independent of the time of day (of week, of year, etc.), it can be shown that the arrival rate can be described with the *Poisson distribution* (see Figure 5.4) with its mean λ (lambda) equal to the average number of arrivals per unit of time.* We would feel more confident with the assumption that the arrival process at the proposed

---

*The Poisson distribution is given by $f(X) = e^{-\lambda} \lambda^X / X!$ Table IV in the Appendix gives $f(X)$ for $\lambda = .1$ to $\lambda = 20$.

clinic will follow the Poisson distribution if we knew that the arrival process was Poisson at the *existing* clinic. (We would of course only feel more comfortable; it would not guarantee that the new clinic will have the same arrival process as the existing clinic, only suggest it.) We test the hypothesis that the arrival process at the existing clinic is Poisson with the $\chi^2$ (chi-square) goodness of fit test. This test is a comparison of the *actual* distribution of arrivals with the arrival distribution that would have been found if the process had been exactly Poisson, called the *expected* distribution. The actual distribution is given in Figure 5.3. If the arrival process had been *exactly* Poisson, we would have expected the distribution to be that of Column 4 of Table 5.1. (Column 4 is obtained by multiplying column 3 by 100—the sample size of the actual distribution.)

Of course we would not expect to have observed the distribution of Column 4 exactly because of the random deviation of the process, even if it were Poisson, and because we only observed 100 hours. The question is, then, whether the difference between the actual distribution and the expected distribution is due to random sampling error, or whether the actual distribution represents a distribution other than a Poisson. We test the hypothesis that the actual distribution is Poisson by using the $\chi^2$ goodness of fit statistic:

$$\chi^2 = \sum_i \frac{(A_i - E_i)^2}{E_i},$$

where $i$ indexes the categories (rows of Table 5.1) of arrivals per hour. (The $\chi^2$ test requires that the $E_i$ must be greater than or equal to 5, and so we must combine some of the categories as shown in Table 5.1, column 4.)

If the hypothesis is true, then the $\chi^2$ statistic follows the $\chi^2$ distribution (see Table III in Appendix) with $n - k - 1$ degrees of freedom, where $n$ is the number of categories (rows) *after* combining, and $k$ is the number of parameters being estimated (e.g., only one for the exponential or Poisson, but two for the normal). For our case $n = 9$ and $k = 1$. The last column of Table 5.1 gives the calculation of the $\chi^2$ statistic. From Table III, if the hypothesis *is* true, we would find this large a difference about 90 percent of the time (that is, the $\chi^2$ distribution with $n - k - 1 = 9 - 1 - 1 = 7$ degrees of freedom has 90 percent of its tail to the right of 2.83). Thus we might accept the hypothesis, and conclude that the arrival process at the existing clinic is indeed Poisson.

Note that in this test we are trying to *accept* the null hypothesis

## Table 5.1

### $\chi^2$ Goodness of Fit Test for Arrival Rate Distribution

| (1) Arrivals Per Hour | (2) $A_i$ Actual Frequency Observed | (3) Expected Probability ($\lambda = 8$) | (4) $E_i$ Expected Frequency ((3) × 100) | (5) Actual Minus Expected | (6) Actual Minus Expected Squared | (7) $\chi^2$ ((6) ÷ (4)) |
|---|---|---|---|---|---|---|
| 0 | 1 ⎫ | .0003 | .03 ⎫ | | | |
| 1 | 1 ⎪ | .0027 | .27 ⎪ | | | |
| 2 | 1 ⎬ 12 | .0107 | 1.07 ⎬ 9.96 | 2.04 | 4.16 | .42 |
| 3 | 3 ⎪ | .0286 | 2.86 ⎪ | | | |
| 4 | 6 ⎭ | .0573 | 5.73 ⎭ | | | |
| 5 | 8 | .0916 | 9.16 | −1.16 | 1.35 | .15 |
| 6 | 13 | .1221 | 12.21 | .79 | .62 | .05 |
| 7 | 13 | .1396 | 13.96 | −.96 | .92 | .07 |
| 8 | 15 | .1396 | 13.96 | 1.04 | 1.08 | .08 |
| 9 | 9 | .1241 | 12.41 | −3.41 | 11.63 | .94 |
| 10 | 10 | .0993 | 9.93 | .07 | .00 | .00 |
| 11 | 8 ⎫ 11 | .0722 | 7.22 ⎫ 12.03 | −1.03 | 1.06 | .09 |
| 12 | 3 ⎭ | .0481 | 4.81 ⎭ | | | |
| 13 | 4 ⎫ | .0296 | 2.96 ⎫ | | | |
| 14 | 2 ⎪ 9 | .0169 | 1.69 ⎪ | | | |
| 15 | 1 ⎬ | .0090 | .90 ⎬ 6.30 | 2.70 | 7.29 | 1.16 |
| 16 | 0 ⎪ | .0045 | .45 ⎪ | | | |
| 17 | 1 ⎪ | .0021 | .21 ⎪ | | | |
| 18 | 1 ⎭ | .0009 | .09 ⎭ | | | |
| | 100 | 1.0000 | 100.00 | | | $\chi^2 = \overline{2.94}$ |

and are thus put in a statistically weak position. This requires that we offer a sufficient sample size to make the test fair, and that we also try to fit other distributions to the data as well. In other hypothesis testing where we are trying to obtain a *rejection* of the null hypothesis, a smaller sample may be less likely to find significant evidence to reject, so that the analysis requires us to look for enough evidence to reject, using larger samples if necessary. In the goodness of fit case, the shoe is on the other foot, and we want to obtain the *best* evidence possible, to be sure *it* is not good enough to reject the null hypothesis. Of course, another difference is that while we were happier in prior tests to obtain statistics far out in the $\chi^2$ distribution (the 99th, the 95th, etc.), in this test we are happier to find statistics in the *lower* percentiles (the 5th, 10th, 20th, etc.), since these give *less* evidence against the null hypothesis that we want to *accept*.

Having established that the arrival process of the existing clinic is Poisson, we might then assume that the arrival process at the proposed clinic will be Poisson (still a tentative assumption, but perhaps the best we can do). Recall that on Wednesdays we expect an average of 80 patients a day. If the clinic is open eight hours, this implies an average of 10 patients an hour. Thus we might tentatively assume that the arrival process will be Poisson with $\lambda = 10$, as in Figure 5.4. (We might note here that if the distribution of the arrival *rate* is Poisson with mean $\lambda$, then the distribution of the *interarrival time* is exponential* with mean equal to $1/\lambda$—see Wagner for derivation.)

## The Service Process

As with the arrival process, we can either observe an empirical distribution of the time of service at the nearby clinic or assume that time of service follows a theoretical distribution. For example, suppose that from the same observations we used to derive the arrival distributions, we observe the service (examination) distribution of Figure 5.5, which has a mean of $1/3$ hour. A commonly used theoretical distribution for service time is the exponential distribution (see Figure 5.6). Other distributions, including the normal distribution, are also sometimes used. Note, however, that there is always some probability that a service time will be negative with a normal distribution, which becomes a serious misrepresentation when the ratio of the mean

---

*The exponential distribution is given by $f(X) = \mu e^{-\mu X}$. The cumulative is given by $F(X) = 1 - e^{-\mu X}$.

## Figure 5.5

## Distribution of Service Time

| Observed Time | | Observed Frequency |
|---|---|---|
| Minutes | Hours | (100 Patients) |
| 5 | .083 | 26 |
| 10 | .167 | 18 |
| 15 | .250 | 13 |
| 20 | .333 | 11 |
| 25 | .417 | 6 |
| 30 | .500 | 5 |
| 35 | .583 | 4 |
| 40 | .667 | 4 |
| 45 | .750 | 2 |
| 50 | .833 | 2 |
| 55 | .917 | 2 |
| 60 | 1.000 | 2 |
| 65 | 1.083 | 1 |
| 70 | 1.167 | 1 |
| 75 | 1.250 | 0 |
| 80+ | 1.333+ | 3 |

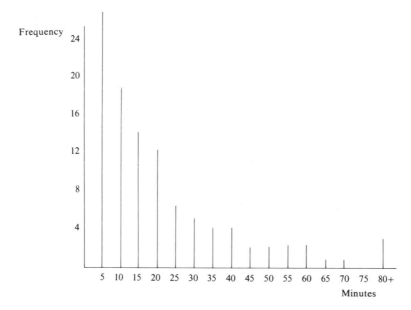

to the standard deviation is less than 2 or 3, for example. We will examine another commonly used distribution, the Gamma distribution, below.

As with the arrival process, it is common to observe an empirical distribution first from an actual service process similar to the one of interest, and then to try to "fit" it to several theoretical distributions.

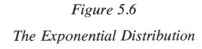

*Figure 5.6*

*The Exponential Distribution*

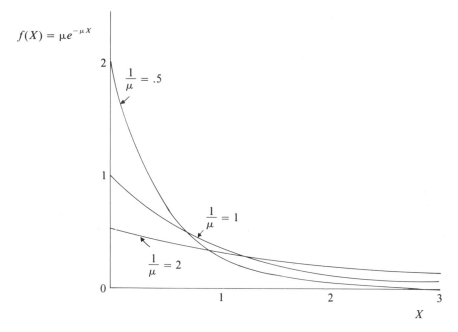

Let us suppose that we have used the $\chi^2$ goodness of fit test to test the empirical distribution of Figure 5.5 against the exponential distribution with mean = 1/3 hour (Table 5.2) and are satisfied that the latter sufficiently represents our pediatric service process. (We will call the mean service time $1/\mu$, meaning $\mu$ is the mean service *rate*: the average number of patients that can be served per physician per hour. If the service *time* is distributed exponentially with mean of $1/\mu$, then service *rate* is distributed Poisson with mean $\mu$.)

The other two characteristics needed to specify a queueing system are the queue discipline and the number of servers. The queue discipline of our pediatric clinic example is actually very complex. Some arrivals will have been scheduled from earlier visits, while others will be first-time walk-ins. Also, some will be emergent, requiring faster service. Finally, if there is more than one physician, some arrivals may be designated to a particular physician while others may take the first available. We will deal with these complexities later, but for the moment we will assume that the queue discipline is on a first-come-first-served (FCFS) basis.

We have already made several important simplifying assumptions:

## Table 5.2

## $\chi^2$ *Goodness of Fit Test for Service Time Distribution*

| Interval (Minutes) | $A_i$ Observed Frequency (100 Patients) | $E_i$ Expected Frequency (100 Patients) | $\dfrac{(A_i - E_i)^2}{E_i}$ |
|---|---|---|---|
| 0 – 7.5 | 26 | 31.3 | .90 |
| 7.5–12.5 | 18 | 15.2 | .52 |
| 12.5–17.5 | 13 | 11.8 | .12 |
| 17.5–22.5 | 11 | 9.2 | .35 |
| 22.5–27.5 | 6 | 7.2 | .20 |
| 27.5–32.5 | 5 | 5.6 | .06 |
| 32.5 37.5 | 4 ⎫ 8 | 4.4 ⎫ 7.8 | .01 |
| 37.5–42.5 | 4 ⎭ | 3.4 ⎭ | |
| 42.5–47.5 | 2 ⎫ | 2.6 ⎫ | |
| 47.5–52.5 | 2 ⎬ 6 | 2.1 ⎬ 6.3 | .01 |
| 52.5–57.5 | 2 ⎭ | 1.6 ⎭ | |
| 57.5–62.5 | 2 ⎫ | 1.2 ⎫ | |
| 62.5 67.5 | 1 | 1.0 | |
| 67.5–72.5 | 1 ⎬ 7 | .8 ⎬ 5.7 | .30 |
| 72.5–77.5 | 0 | .6 | |
| 77.5–∞ | 3 ⎭ | 2.1 ⎭ | |

$$\chi^2 = 2.47$$
with 7 degrees of freedom
$$(n-k-1=9-1-1=7)$$

arrivals are Poisson, service is exponential, and queue discipline is FCFS. We have purposely chosen these conditions, in order to structure the queueing model so that it can be solved mathematically. Solving mathematically means that, by using mathematical techniques, we can derive the average waiting time and the average queue length in terms of only three parameters: the mean arrival rate, the mean service time, and the number of servers. The process is complex, and the derivation of the solution of even the simplest example is beyond the scope of this text. (The interested reader is referred to Wagner.) We can state the solution of the queueing model with *one* server for the *steady state* of the process (see discussion of steady state below) as follows. If the arrival rate is Poisson with mean $\lambda$ and the service time is exponential with mean $1/\mu$, then the expected steady state waiting line length $[L(1)]$ is

$$L(1) = \frac{\lambda^2}{\mu(\mu - \lambda)}$$

and the average waiting time $[W(1)]$ is

$$W(1) = \frac{L(1)}{\lambda}.$$

Further, it can be shown that the *distribution* of waiting time for a particular patient is exponential with mean equal to $W(1)$. Since the cumulative density function for the exponential with mean $1/\mu$ is

$$F(X) = 1 - e^{-\mu x},$$

the probability that a particular patient will have to wait $X$ time units (e.g., hours) or less is

$$F(X) = 1 - e^{-x/W(1)},$$

and the probability he will have to wait more than $X$ time units is $1 - F(X)$. The probability that there will be exactly $n$ patients in the system (being served or waiting) at any time is $(1 - \lambda/\mu)(\lambda/\mu)^n$. These results assume that the average time between arrivals $(1/\lambda)$ is *strictly greater* than the average service time $1/\mu$; otherwise both the waiting time and the waiting line go to infinity.

For our process, where we expect an average of 10 arrivals per hour ($\lambda = 10$) and service averages $1/3$ of an hour ($\mu = 3$), the waiting line and waiting time for one server (examining room) in the long run go to infinity: $1/\lambda < 1/\mu$. Thus we will not be able to evaluate the case where there is only one examining room (see Exercise 5.2 for a single server example).

For more than one server, if we define $\rho$ (rho) as $\rho = \lambda/\mu$ (called the traffic intensity) and define $X$ as the number of servers (examining rooms), the expected waiting time $[W(X)]$ is given by

$$W(X) = \frac{\dfrac{\rho^x}{X!(1 - \rho/x)} \cdot \dfrac{1}{\displaystyle\sum_{j=0}^{x-1} \rho^j/j! + \dfrac{\rho^x}{X!(1 - \rho/x)}}}{\mu X - \lambda}$$

and

$$L(X) = W(X) \cdot \lambda.$$

As awkward as the equation looks, with a calculator it takes relatively little time to substitute values from our problem to find $W(X)$ and $L(X)$ for several values of $X$. Table 5.3 gives the calculated values

## Table 5.3

### Expected Wait Time and Queue Length

| Exam Rooms | Expected Wait (Hours) | Expected Queue Length |
|---|---|---|
| 4 | .33 | 3.3 |
| 5 | .07 | 0.7 |
| 6 | .02 | 0.2 |
| 7 | .006 | 0.06 |
| 8 | .002 | 0.02 |

for $\lambda = 10$, $\mu = 3$, and thus $\rho = 10/3$ or 3.33. (The interested student is again referred to Wagner for the derivation of the equation for $W(X)$.) As in the case of a single server, the distribution of wait time is exponential.

Our decision now becomes one of returning to the objective function and balancing the $C_1(X)$ against the $W(X)$ and $L(X)$, where the values of $u$ and $v$ must be subjectively assessed as in the examples of previous chapters.

We present the solution to the Poisson arrival/exponential service model only for demonstration. Results for queueing models using other distributions of arrival and service have also been derived, the results being available either as equations or in tables. The important point is that the mathematical "solution" to *certain* queueing situations is available without the expense of simulation. There are several limitations of mathematically-solved queueing analyses. Some of the more important are listed below.

1. Stationarity of the arrival and service process is assumed. For example, it would be difficult to include the fact that arrivals are heavier in the earlier hours, peaking after lunch, or that they are generally heavier early in the hour than they are late in the hour, or that the physician speeds up the examinations near the end of the day, etc.

2. Independence of arrival and service is assumed. For example, it would be difficult to model a physician speeding up an examination because many other patients are waiting.

3. The number of servers is assumed fixed. For example, it is difficult to model a clinic situation in which there is one physician on duty from 8:00 A.M. to about 9:00 A.M., two

more arriving randomly between 9:00 and 10:00, two going to lunch from 12:00 P.M. to 1:00 P.M., etc.

4. There is very little ability to incorporate important exceptions to the general flow. For example, it is difficult to model an examination's being temporarily delayed while a patient leaves to get an X-ray, and the physician begins to examine another patient.

5. It is difficult to model any but very simple processes. For example, it may be that for some situations a nurse is required (are they all busy at this moment?), or that the examination would go faster if a nurse were available, etc.

6. Most results of mathematically solved queueing models address "steady state" results. The steady state of a process refers to the process's having reached a point at which it is independent of its starting conditions. For example, assume that the arrival rate of our clinic *is* stationary during the day (from 8 A.M. to 4 P.M.). Since the clinic is empty at 8 A.M. we would expect patients who arrive the first hour (or the first few hours) to be subject to less waiting time than patients who arrived later, because the earlier patients had the benefit of the starting condition of empty facilities. Later in the afternoon, we would expect this effect to have worn off, so that we would say that sometime during the day, when the starting conditions are no longer influential, the process had reached steady state. Note that if the arrival rate or service rate is not stationary or if the number of servers is not fixed, the process *never* reaches steady state, since just as it is about to "recover" from the last change in one of the rates, a new rate change occurs. Thus by using only steady state results, much of the actual process may be ignored for those processes which are not continuous (and stationary) around the clock.

If queueing models are so limited, why have we included them here? There are three reasons. First, the queueing flow framework is basic to simulation modeling, which does not have the above limitations. Second, the results from a queueing model are often useful as starting points for a simulation analysis. Third, since mathematically solved queueing models are relatively cheap and fast to solve (we'll see why when we examine simulation), a decision maker may be willing to base his decision on such approximate results rather than incur the expense and time of simulation. The issue is whether the gain in information from a more sophisticated analysis is worth the additional cost in time and money.

## A Queueing Example: Obstetrics

Before leaving mathematically solvable queueing models, we will look at the most reasonable application of such an analysis for a patient flow process: obstetrics. The reader should review the obstetrics problem developed in Chapter 2. We will treat the same analysis in Section 5.4 with simulation, going through the complete decision-making framework: here we will look only at modeling the process.

The patient flow in OB is diagrammed in Figure 5.7. Patients arrive randomly at the hospital and wait for one of $L$ beds in the labor facility. The patient then goes to one of $D$ delivery beds, then to one of $R$ recovery beds, and finally to one of $P$ postpartum beds. Before each of these moves, the patient may have to wait until a bed is free. We will be concerned with how long patients will have to wait on the average before entering each facility (labor, delivery, recovery, and postpartum) as a function of how many beds are provided in each facility.

For one such study, data from the records of 588 OB patients over a four-month period were gathered, giving the distribution of interarrival times for the patients shown in Figure 5.8. Under the assumption that arrivals were stationary throughout the day, week, and year, several of the theoretical distributions for which queueing results have been mathematically derived were fitted (testing with the $\chi^2$ goodness of fit test) to the distribution of Figure 5.8, and the exponential distribution with mean $1/\mu = 3.81$ hours provided the best fit. We will examine this assumption and fit more closely when we again analyze the OB decision with simulation in Section 5.4. Thus arrivals are assumed to be Poisson with $\lambda = 1 \div 3.81 = .26$ per hour.

The same patient records gave the service time distribution in labor shown in Figure 5.9. It too was fitted to the exponential distribution with $1/\mu = 4.5$ hours. (Although it is not a very close fit by the $\chi^2$ test, it was the best fit of all distributions tried. Again in Section 5.4 we will re-examine this fit with the greater latitude of simulation.)

We are now in a position to analyze the labor process—the initial queueing system in the OB patient flow. From the equation for waiting time above we obtain the expected waiting time for the

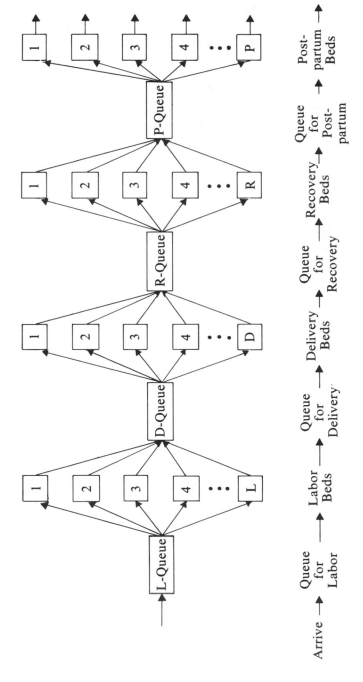

*Figure 5.7*

*Multi-Server, Multi-Stage Queueing Process*

## Figure 5.8

## *Interarrival Distribution for OB Patients*

| MEAN=3.810 | SUM=588 | EXPONENTIAL | | | | |
| --- | --- | --- | --- | --- | --- | --- |
| INTERARRIVAL TIME | ACTUAL FREQ | ACTUAL PROB | ACTUAL CDF | EXPO FREQ | EXPO PROB | EXPO CDF | CHI SQR |
| 0.50 | 112 | 0.190 | 0.190 | 105.1 | 0.179 | 0.179 | 0.46 |
| 1.00 | 60 | 0.102 | 0.293 | 59.4 | 0.101 | 0.280 | 0.01 |
| 1.50 | 56 | 0.095 | 0.388 | 52.1 | 0.089 | 0.368 | 0.29 |
| 2.00 | 54 | 0.092 | 0.480 | 45.7 | 0.078 | 0.446 | 1.51 |
| 2.50 | 41 | 0.070 | 0.549 | 40.1 | 0.068 | 0.514 | 0.02 |
| 3.00 | 40 | 0.068 | 0.617 | 35.1 | 0.060 | 0.574 | 0.67 |
| 3.50 | 34 | 0.058 | 0.675 | 30.8 | 0.052 | 0.626 | 0.33 |
| 4.00 | 28 | 0.048 | 0.723 | 27.0 | 0.046 | 0.672 | 0.04 |
| 4.50 | 25 | 0.043 | 0.765 | 23.7 | 0.040 | 0.713 | 0.07 |
| 5.00 | 19 | 0.032 | 0.798 | 20.8 | 0.035 | 0.748 | 0.15 |
| 5.50 | 14 | 0.024 | 0.821 | 18.2 | 0.031 | 0.779 | 0.98 |
| 6.00 | 11 | 0.019 | 0.840 | 16.0 | 0.027 | 0.806 | 1.56 |
| 6.50 | 10 | 0.017 | 0.857 | 14.0 | 0.024 | 0.830 | 1.15 |
| 7.00 | 13 | 0.022 | 0.879 | 12.3 | 0.021 | 0.851 | 0.04 |
| 7.50 | 10 | 0.017 | 0.896 | 10.8 | 0.018 | 0.869 | 0.06 |
| 8.00 | 9 | 0.015 | 0.912 | 9.5 | 0.016 | 0.885 | 0.02 |
| 8.50 | 5 | 0.009 | 0.920 | 8.3 | 0.014 | 0.899 | 1.31 |
| 9.00 | 6 | 0.010 | 0.930 | 7.3 | 0.012 | 0.912 | 0.22 |
| 9.50 | 6 | 0.010 | 0.940 | 6.4 | 0.011 | 0.923 } | 0.02 |
| 10.00 | 5 | 0.009 | 0.949 | 5.6 | 0.010 | 0.932 } | 0.21 |
| 10.50 | 7 | 0.012 | 0.961 | 4.9 | 0.008 | 0.940 } | |
| 11.00+ | 23 | 0.039 | 1.000 | 35.0 | 0.060 | 1.000 | 4.11 |

CHI SQUARE (19) = 13.25           13.25

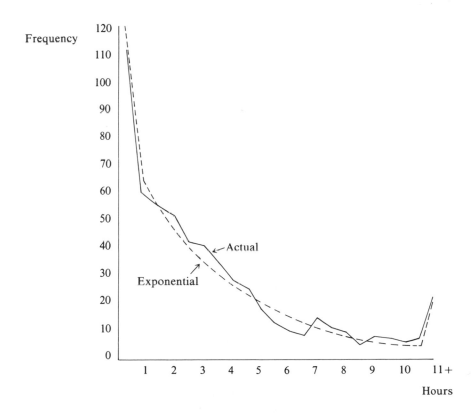

## Figure 5.9

### Service Time Distribution in Labor

MEAN=4.497          SUM=588          EXPONENTIAL

| SERVICE TIME | ACTUAL FREQ | ACTUAL PROB | ACTUAL CDF | EXPO FREQ | EXPO PROB | EXPO CDF | CHI SQR |
|---|---|---|---|---|---|---|---|
| 0.50 | 76 | 0.129 | 0.129 | 90.3 | 0.154 | 0.154 | 2.27 |
| 1.00 | 57 | 0.097 | 0.226 | 52.4 | 0.089 | 0.243 | 0.41 |
| 1.50 | 35 | 0.060 | 0.286 | 46.9 | 0.080 | 0.322 | 3.00 |
| 2.00 | 25 | 0.043 | 0.328 | 41.9 | 0.071 | 0.394 | 6.83 |
| 2.50 | 34 | 0.058 | 0.386 | 37.5 | 0.064 | 0.457 | 0.33 |
| 3.00 | 31 | 0.053 | 0.439 | 33.6 | 0.057 | 0.515 | 0.20 |
| 3.50 | 33 | 0.056 | 0.495 | 30.0 | 0.051 | 0.566 | 0.29 |
| 4.00 | 28 | 0.048 | 0.543 | 26.9 | 0.046 | 0.611 | 0.05 |
| 4.50 | 24 | 0.041 | 0.583 | 24.0 | 0.041 | 0.652 | 0.00 |
| 5.00 | 30 | 0.051 | 0.634 | 21.5 | 0.037 | 0.689 | 3.34 |
| 5.50 | 25 | 0.043 | 0.677 | 19.3 | 0.033 | 0.722 | 1.72 |
| 6.00 | 29 | 0.049 | 0.726 | 17.2 | 0.029 | 0.751 | 8.05 |
| 6.50 | 22 | 0.037 | 0.764 | 15.4 | 0.026 | 0.777 | 2.81 |
| 7.00 | 17 | 0.029 | 0.793 | 13.8 | 0.023 | 0.801 | 0.75 |
| 7.50 | 17 | 0.029 | 0.821 | 12.3 | 0.021 | 0.822 | 1.76 |
| 8.00 | 12 | 0.020 | 0.842 | 11.0 | 0.019 | 0.840 | 0.08 |
| 8.50 | 11 | 0.019 | 0.861 | 9.9 | 0.017 | 0.857 | 0.13 |
| 9.00 | 15 | 0.026 | 0.886 | 8.8 | 0.015 | 0.872 | 4.29 |
| 9.50 | 10 | 0.017 | 0.903 | 7.9 | 0.013 | 0.886 | 0.55 |
| 10.00 | 8 | 0.014 | 0.917 | 7.1 | 0.012 | 0.898 | 0.12 |
| 10.50 | 8 | 0.014 | 0.930 | 6.3 | 0.011 | 0.908 | 0.44 |
| 11.00 | 11 | 0.019 | 0.949 | 5.7 | 0.010 | 0.918 | 5.02 |
| 11.50 | 6 | 0.010 | 0.959 | 5.1 | 0.009 | 0.927 | 0.17 |
| 12.00 | 6 | 0.010 | 0.969 | 4.5 | 0.008 | 0.934 | 2.25 |
| 12.50 | 7 | 0.012 | 0.981 | 4.1 | 0.007 | 0.941 | |
| 13.00 | 3 | 0.005 | 0.986 | 3.6 | 0.006 | 0.947 | 0.12 |
| 13.50 | 3 | 0.005 | 0.991 | 3.3 | 0.006 | 0.953 | |
| 14.00 | 5 | 0.009 | 1.000 | 27.6 | 0.047 | 1.000 | 18.55 |

CHI SQUARE (24) = 63.52                                                              63.52

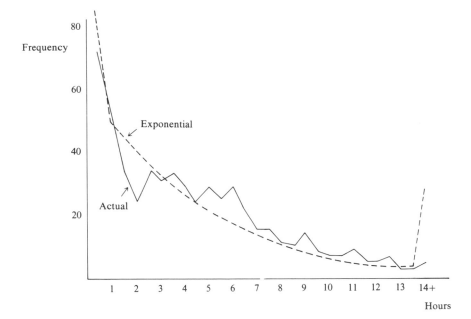

labor facility as a function of the number of beds shown in Table 5.4.

A fortunate characteristic of queueing systems with Poisson arrival is that the distribution of *departures* is often also Poisson with the same mean. That is, patients leave the labor room (and

## Table 5.4

### Expected Waiting Time for Labor Beds

| Number of Labor Beds L | Average Wait (Hours) W(L) | Average Wait (Minutes) |
|---|---|---|
| 2 | 2.410 | 140.5 |
| 3 | .327 | 19.6 |
| 4 | .054 | 3.3 |
| 5 | .009 | .5 |

arrive for delivery) according to the same distribution (and mean) that they arrive for labor. Thus our arrival process for the second queueing system—delivery—is also Poisson with $\lambda = .26$. The patient records yielded delivery service times shown in Figure 5.10. The delivery service is clearly not exponential. This time the best fit came from a member of the Gamma* distribution, although again the fit is not very close—check the $\chi^2$ value. (Note that we estimate two parameters of the Gamma distribution, so that the $k$ of $n - k - 1$ is 2 for calculating the degrees of freedom for the $\chi^2$ test.) Results have been derived for queueing systems with Poisson arrival and Gamma service, and are available in tables (see Warner reference at end of chapter). These are given in Table 5.5.

At the time of the analysis, there was no recovery facility at the existing hospitals, but the OB physicians wanted to implement such a phase at the proposed merged OB facility. Thus the recovery service distribution had to be obtained by asking OB physicians what percentage of patients would stay 0 hours, 1/2 hour, 1 hour, etc., in recovery (the technique is discussed in Chapter 9). The resulting distribution is shown in Figure 5.12. It was also fitted to a Gamma

---

*The Gamma distribution is given by

$$g(y) = \frac{a(ay)^{b-1} e^{-ay}}{(b-1)!},$$

and its cumulative distribution as

$$G(y) = 1 - \sum_{j=0}^{b-1} \frac{(ay)^j e^{-ay}}{j!}$$

where $a$ and $b$ are the two parameters defining the shape of the distribution. The mean of the Gamma is equal to $b/a$. The Gamma can take on many shapes, as shown in Figure 5.11 where $a$ is fixed at 1 and $b$ takes on different values. The Gamma is fitted to an empirical distribution by trying different values of $b$ (and $a = b/\text{mean}$) and choosing the one that best fits the empirical distribution. Gamma with $a = 10.371$ and $b = 8$ is shown in Figure 5.10.

## Figure 5.10

### Service Time Distribution for Delivery

MEAN = .771          SUM = 588          GAMMA WITH A = 10.371 AND B = 8

| SERVICE TIME | ACTUAL FREQ | ACTUAL PROB | ACTUAL CDF | GAMMA FREQ | GAMMA PROB | GAMMA CDF | CHI SQR |
|---|---|---|---|---|---|---|---|
| 0.17 | 28 | 0.048 | 0.048 | 3.1 | 0.005 | 0.005 | 0.00 |
| 0.33 | 43 | 0.073 | 0.121 | 38.9 | 0.066 | 0.071 | 0.44 |
| 0.50 | 130 | 0.221 | 0.342 | 114.1 | 0.194 | 0.265 | 2.23 |
| 0.67 | 148 | 0.252 | 0.594 | 147.2 | 0.250 | 0.516 | 0.00 |
| 0.83 | 124 | 0.211 | 0.804 | 126.2 | 0.215 | 0.730 | 0.04 |
| 1.00 | 44 | 0.075 | 0.879 | 83.6 | 0.142 | 0.872 | 18.74 |
| 1.17 | 24 | 0.041 | 0.920 | 42.7 | 0.073 | 0.945 | 8.17 |
| 1.33 | 13 | 0.022 | 0.942 | 19.6 | 0.033 | 0.978 | 2.24 |
| 1.50 | 6 | 0.010 | 0.952 | 8.2 | 0.014 | 0.992 | |
| 1.67 | 2 | 0.003 | 0.956 | 3.0 | 0.005 | 0.997 | |
| 1.83 | 3 | 0.005 | 0.961 | 1.0 | 0.002 | 0.999 | |
| 2.00 | 4 | 0.007 | 0.968 | 0.4 | 0.001 | 1.000 | |
| 2.17 | 3 | 0.005 | 0.973 | 0.1 | 0.000 | 1.000 | |
| 2.33 | 3 | 0.005 | 0.978 | 0.0 | 0.000 | 1.000 | |
| 2.50 | 2 | 0.003 | 0.981 | 0.0 | 0.000 | 1.000 | 35.72 |
| 2.67 | 3 | 0.005 | 0.986 | 0.0 | 0.000 | 1.000 | |
| 2.83 | 0 | 0.000 | 0.986 | 0.0 | 0.000 | 1.000 | |
| 3.00 | 3 | 0.005 | 0.991 | 0.0 | 0.000 | 1.000 | |
| 3.17 | 1 | 0.002 | 0.993 | 0.0 | 0.000 | 1.000 | |
| 3.33 | 2 | 0.003 | 0.997 | 0.0 | 0.000 | 1.000 | |
| 3.50 | 2 | 0.003 | 1.000 | 0.0 | 0.000 | 1.000 | |

CHI SQUARE $(n-k-1=9-2-1=6)=67.58$                                              67.58

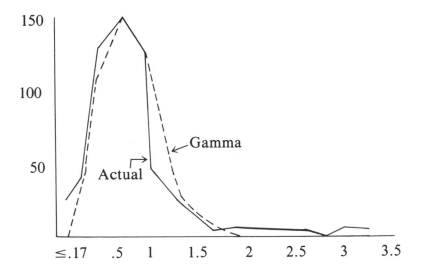

## Table 5.5

### Expected Waiting Time for Delivery Beds

| Number of Delivery Beds D | Average Wait (Hours) W(D) |
|---|---|
| 1 | .112 |
| 2 | .007 |
| 3 | .0004 |

*Figure 5.11*

*The Gamma Distribution*

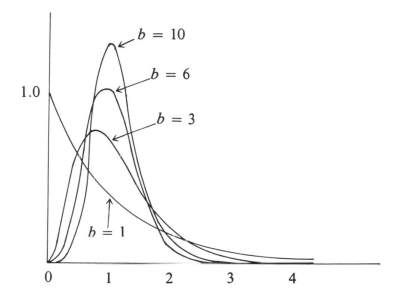

distribution, with $a = 2.623$ and $b = 18$. Table 5.6 gives expected waiting times for recovery as a function of the number of recovery beds provided. Finally, the observed length of stay in postpartum displayed in Figure 5.13 was fitted to the Gamma with $a = 4.6$ and $b = 18$, and expected waiting times are given in Table 5.7.

It should be pointed out that the result of the queueing analysis— waiting times—serves as a quantification for only one of the terms of the objective function of the decision-making framework: after quantification of the other (cost) terms, the trade-off between providing too many versus too few beds is addressed in the solution step of the framework. The reader should also carefully review the implications of the assumptions that were made in the OB process that allowed the above queueing analysis, especially a stationary arrival rate throughout the day and independence of service time from occupancy. Are there other patient flow processes that are as close as the OB process in meeting the requirements of mathematically solvable queueing models? What about patient flow through X-ray? Through the emergency room? What explicit assumptions would one have to make about these two processes to allow a similar analysis?

*Figure 5.12*

*Service Time Distribution for Recovery*

MEAN=3.050          SUM=100          GAMMA WITH A=2.623 AND B=8

| SERVICE TIME | ACTUAL FREQ | ACTUAL PROB | ACTUAL CDF | GAMMA FREQ | GAMMA PROB | GAMMA CDF | CHI SQR |
|---|---|---|---|---|---|---|---|
| 1.00 | 2 | 0.020 | 0.020 | 4.7 | 0.047 | 0.047 | 0.00 |
| 2.00 | 35 | 0.350 | 0.370 | 28.8 | 0.288 | 0.336 | 1.32 |
| 3.00 | 35 | 0.350 | 0.720 | 36.1 | 0.361 | 0.697 | 0.03 |
| 4.00 | 18 | 0.180 | 0.900 | 20.5 | 0.205 | 0.902 | 0.30 |
| 5.00 | 6 | 0.060 | 0.960 | 7.4 | 0.074 | 0.975 |  |
| 6.00 | 2 | 0.020 | 0.980 | 2.0 | 0.020 | 0.995 | 0.00 |
| 7.00 | 2 | 0.020 | 1.000 | 0.5 | 0.005 | 1.000 |  |

CHI SQUARE (2)=1.38                                                          1.38

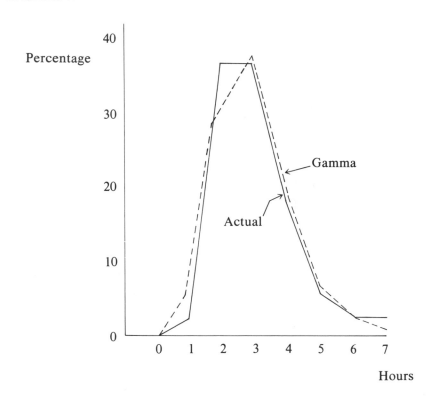

*Table 5.6*

*Expected Waiting Time for Recovery Beds*

| Number of Recovery Beds R | Average Wait (Hours) W(R) |
|---|---|
| 1 | 3.03 |
| 2 | .38 |
| 3 | .05 |
| 4 | .01 |

## Table 5.7

## Expected Waiting Time for Postpartum Beds

| Number of Postpartum Beds P | Average Wait (Hours) W(P) |
|---|---|
| 30 | 2.47 |
| 31 | 1.12 |
| 32 | .68 |
| 33 | .31 |
| 34 | .10 |

## Figure 5.13

## Service Time Distribution for Postpartum Stay

MEAN=3.912        SUM=588        GAMMA WITH A=4.602 AND B=18

| SERVICE TIME | ACTUAL FREQ | ACTUAL PROB | ACTUAL CDF | GAMMA FREQ | GAMMA PROB | GAMMA CDF | CHI SQR |
|---|---|---|---|---|---|---|---|
| 1.00 | 0 | 0.000 | 0.000 | 0.2 | 0.000 | 0.000 | 0.00 |
| 2.00 | 24 | 0.041 | 0.041 | 26.8 | 0.046 | 0.046 | 0.29 |
| 3.00 | 232 | 0.395 | 0.435 | 179.2 | 0.305 | 0.351 | 15.58 |
| 4.00 | 224 | 0.381 | 0.816 | 237.1 | 0.403 | 0.754 | 0.72 |
| 5.00 | 70 | 0.119 | 0.935 | 113.1 | 0.192 | 0.946 | 16.45 |
| 6.00 | 18 | 0.031 | 0.966 | 27.2 | 0.046 | 0.992 | |
| 7.00 | 10 | 0.017 | 0.983 | 4.0 | 0.007 | 0.999 | |
| 8.00 | 0 | 0.000 | 0.983 | 0.4 | 0.001 | 1.000 | |
| 9.00 | 0 | 0.000 | 0.983 | 0.0 | 0.000 | 1.000 | |
| 10.00 | 4 | 0.007 | 0.990 | 0.0 | 0.000 | 1.000 | |
| 11.00 | 0 | 0.000 | 0.990 | 0.0 | 0.000 | 1.000 | 1.30 |
| 12.00 | 0 | 0.000 | 0.990 | 0.0 | 0.000 | 1.000 | |
| 13.00 | 0 | 0.000 | 0.990 | 0.0 | 0.000 | 1.000 | |
| 14.00 | 1 | 0.002 | 0.991 | 0.0 | 0.000 | 1.000 | |
| 15.00 | 2 | 0.003 | 0.995 | 0.0 | 0.000 | 1.000 | |
| 16.00 | 3 | 0.005 | 1.000 | 0.0 | 0.000 | 1.000 | |

CHI SQUARE (3)=34.34                                                     34.34

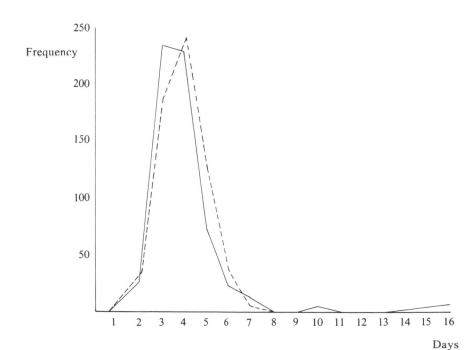

## 5.3 SIMULATION

In the last section we saw that the major shortcoming of mathematically solvable queueing models is that they must be relatively noncomplex, and this limits their ability to mimic the real-world process of interest. Although there are many instances in industrial situations in which such models are applicable, it is usually difficult to be comfortable with the simplifying assumptions when analyzing health planning and operations problems.

Simulation is a method to solve virtually any model of a queueing nature. It is conceptually different from the mathematical solution in that the model is actually operated through simulated time and the results of the operation are observed. Thus instead of *deducing* the results through mathematics, we *generate* them. The most important drawback of simulation is cost in money and time. While a mathematical queueing solution can involve from several days' to several weeks' work, an initial simulation study can involve from several man-months to several man-years plus a significant amount of computer usage; subsequent studies using the same model, however, take relatively little time. We will thus want to keep in mind a cost-benefit view of simulation: will the benefit associated with more information outweigh the increased cost of the analysis?

We will begin with a very simple process. Suppose patients arrive at the office of a family physician who has a solo practice; they wait until the physician is free, are seen by the physician one at a time, and are then released. Figure 5.14 shows this process. Suppose patients arrive according to the following distribution. Each hour there is a 50 percent chance that no patients will arrive and a 50 percent chance that exactly one patient will arrive. Finally suppose that the physician will spend one hour with 50 percent of the patients and two hours with the other 50 percent.

As in the previous section, it is useful to view the arrival and service processes as independent stochastic elements. To simulate the physician's office process, we simply simulate the independent elements, keep track of time and where patients are, and accumulate statistics (results) of interest.

How can we simulate the arrival of patients? We need a device that randomly generates one event (no arrivals) half the time and another event (one arrival) the other half. Flipping a "fair" coin does this. Associate heads with the event "zero patients arrive this hour" and tails with "one patient arrives this hour." Now, to simulate the first hour's arrivals, flip the coin. Suppose we get "tails." There is no one in the waiting room (we've just begun), so the arriving

## Figure 5.14

### Patient Flow in Physician's Office

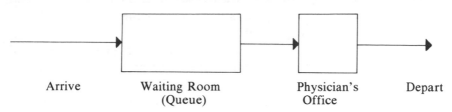

| Arrive | Waiting Room (Queue) | Physician's Office | Depart |

patient goes directly to the physician. How long will he remain with the physician? We can simulate his stay with the physician by flipping the coin again: heads—he stays one hour, tails—two hours. By keeping track of the flow of patients, how many are waiting, how busy the physician is, etc., we simulate the whole process. Figure 5.15 details the results of one day's (eight hours') simulation.

How well do the statistics "average wait = .5" and "average utilization = .89" represent the actual, long-run results of the model (not the real-world process, but the model)? If we were to run the simulation again, would we get the same results? A simulation run

## Figure 5.15

### Simulation of Patient Flow Process

| Hour | Arrival Coin Flip | Service Coin Flip | Waiting Room | Physician Office |
|------|-------------------|-------------------|--------------|------------------|
| 1 | Tails (#1) | Tails | — | Patient #1 ↓ |
| 2 | Tails (#2) | Heads | Patient #2 | Patient #1 → |
| 3 | Tails (#3) | Heads | Patient #3 | Patient #2 → |
| 4 | Heads | — | — | Patient #3 → |
| 5 | Tails (#4) | Heads | — | Patient #4 → |
| 6 | Heads | — | — | — |
| 7 | Tails (#5) | Tails | — | Patient #5 ↓ |
| 8 | Tails (#6) | Heads | Patient #6 | Patient #5 → |
| | | | | Patient #6 → |

(Physician works one hour overtime)
Number of simulated patients = 6.
Average wait = $3/6$ = .5 hour.
Average utilization of physician = $8/9$ or 89%
Average queue length = $3/8$

is referred to as part of an "experiment," in that the results from several simulation runs are viewed as a sample (in the statistical sense) from the population of (in our case) daily results of a solo practice physician's office. Thus if we repeat the above simulation run twenty times, we generate a sample of size twenty for both average daily wait and average daily utilization. Using statistical concepts, we can make inferences from our sample to the "true" population statistics, complete with confidence intervals on our estimates of population statistics. We will examine this procedure more closely below. First, we will look at the simulation of a slightly more complex process.

Most arrival and service distributions are much more complex than the 50–50 of the last example. Suppose the rate of arrivals is Poisson, with mean of .5 per hour. Table 5.8 gives the Poisson frequency and cumulative distribution for $\lambda = .5$. We should recognize the assumptions that we are implying by using the Poisson—arrivals are independent of one another; and the assumption of using the same Poisson distribution throughout the eight-hour day implies that the arrival rate does not change throughout the day. We will deal below with the case in which these assumptions cannot be made.

Note that what we mean by a Poisson arrival process with $\lambda = .5$ is that in 61 percent of the hours there will be zero arrivals, and in 30 percent of the hours there will be one arrival, and in 7.6 percent of the hours there will be two arrivals, and so on. To simulate this process, we need a scheme that randomly generates zero, one, two, etc. arrivals in such a way that in the long run, the proportion of hours with zero arrivals will be .61, hours with one arrival will be .3, and so on.

Suppose that we have a mechanism that generates random numbers of three digits in a way that each of the one thousand

*Table 5.8*

*Frequency and Cumulative Distributions*
*of Poisson with $\lambda = .5$*

| $X$ | $f(X)$ | $F(X)$ |
|---|---|---|
| 0 | .607 | .607 |
| 1 | .303 | .910 |
| 2 | .076 | .986 |
| 3 | .013 | .998 |
| 4 | .002 | 1.000 |

possible numbers has an equal chance of being generated next. Now, if we associate exactly 607 of these numbers (say 0 through 606) with the event "zero arrivals," and exactly 303 of them (say 607 through 909) with the event "one arrival," and so on, then by generating a random number between 0 and 999 and observing into which range it falls we would generate arrivals according to the Poisson distribution with $\lambda = .5$. Note that what we are doing is mapping the uniform distribution from 0 to 1 into the cumulative distribution of the Poisson arrival process (see Figure 5.16). This is the procedure used to simulate any distribution (including empirical), for any process, arrival, or service.

Random numbers can be obtained from two sources. One source is a random number table such as Table 5.9 which has been carefully generated such that each number is independent of previous numbers in the table, and each number has an equal chance of occurring each time. The second source usually used in computer simulations is a subroutine that generates random numbers. (An alternative would be to store the table in the computer, but it is easier to generate them.)

## Figure 5.16

### Cumulative Distribution Mapped on Uniform Distribution

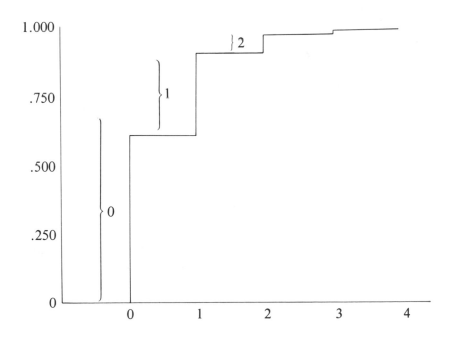

## Table 5.9

### Table of Random Numbers

| | | | | | | | | | | | | | |
|---|---|---|---|---|---|---|---|---|---|---|---|---|---|
| 5822 | 4931 | 7192 | 8765 | 7866 | 8305 | 9035 | 9467 | 5482 | 7693 | 6815 | 1649 | 8559 | 6508 |
| 2013 | 3508 | 2929 | 5999 | 9633 | 3805 | 6130 | 2531 | 0014 | 7306 | 3707 | 6487 | 5561 | 4978 |
| 9813 | 4079 | 6154 | 0207 | 5858 | 3282 | 6970 | 2280 | 0949 | 5172 | 2488 | 8380 | 7887 | 1898 |
| 0405 | 5350 | 8450 | 2547 | 9232 | 2471 | 1731 | 8148 | 3307 | 6506 | 9270 | 7069 | 8980 | 0259 |
| 0730 | 2050 | 5726 | 5902 | 3876 | 0134 | 5921 | 4314 | 2594 | 6732 | 7046 | 1688 | 6712 | 5079 |
| 0061 | 4653 | 7369 | 2337 | 7699 | 5161 | 1672 | 3582 | 6438 | 6393 | 0412 | 4933 | 5887 | 0924 |
| 2566 | 7074 | 9346 | 2412 | 0355 | 0415 | 9297 | 2044 | 8590 | 3143 | 1549 | 1003 | 2074 | 3416 |
| 1824 | 0202 | 4794 | 6942 | 8501 | 8529 | 4662 | 1208 | 5288 | 0858 | 7553 | 7590 | 7566 | 7081 |
| 4391 | 2612 | 6152 | 3400 | 5031 | 9586 | 2236 | 7135 | 2687 | 1904 | 7240 | 6303 | 2656 | 9209 |
| 1348 | 5205 | 9094 | 7718 | 4459 | 7286 | 3583 | 5927 | 3308 | 6503 | 9248 | 6958 | 8515 | 8467 |
| 4167 | 8802 | 5302 | 2592 | 7838 | 3697 | 1632 | 6519 | 4429 | 7898 | 7521 | 4046 | 6584 | 3089 |
| 9272 | 7830 | 3526 | 0686 | 2379 | 8102 | 7199 | 0275 | 6854 | 8651 | 0219 | 3450 | 8728 | 1319 |
| 9359 | 4284 | 1470 | 0262 | 8342 | 7694 | 1080 | 7233 | 3674 | 6946 | 8606 | 9121 | 7274 | 1549 |
| 3826 | 9015 | 9655 | 6793 | 3861 | 2025 | 7400 | 6176 | 0452 | 7125 | 8683 | 7969 | 9664 | 6261 |
| 0589 | 7177 | 7760 | 1970 | 1978 | 4134 | 6996 | 4770 | 5654 | 0996 | 5087 | 1560 | 3568 | 7369 |
| 2103 | 6293 | 8829 | 6331 | 8523 | 4161 | 8256 | 2088 | 8222 | 0539 | 9230 | 0534 | 0127 | 5957 |
| 4592 | 3937 | 2294 | 8329 | 9332 | 1024 | 2153 | 3702 | 2838 | 3704 | 6684 | 6765 | 0428 | 1686 |
| 6259 | 2379 | 7940 | 6227 | 5903 | 9373 | 3107 | 4284 | 7735 | 7852 | 7495 | 4296 | 8323 | 1271 |
| 2718 | 4863 | 4716 | 4528 | 4719 | 7562 | 2897 | 9318 | 9837 | 5156 | 2403 | 8008 | 6420 | 6443 |
| 0877 | 7273 | 5741 | 8992 | 2280 | 2747 | 5960 | 1029 | 2535 | 5949 | 2874 | 3700 | 6336 | 4709 |
| 1228 | 4990 | 8881 | 8373 | 0313 | 6517 | 6279 | 9021 | 7611 | 4480 | 8378 | 9941 | 4243 | 5991 |
| 7760 | 2633 | 5957 | 2047 | 8666 | 3569 | 3420 | 8394 | 9587 | 1972 | 5547 | 5535 | 3279 | 9859 |
| 9642 | 9121 | 7948 | 5600 | 2065 | 1991 | 3361 | 2245 | 3218 | 9099 | 5626 | 1866 | 0562 | 6576 |
| 4391 | 7159 | 3438 | 6195 | 6220 | 1570 | 3432 | 6464 | 7893 | 9179 | 4039 | 1620 | 3364 | 5609 |
| 3373 | 9754 | 8162 | 1190 | 3674 | 1336 | 4944 | 7644 | 1361 | 9373 | 3982 | 9538 | 1384 | 2462 |
| 2318 | 1747 | 9618 | 1983 | 5340 | 4187 | 7062 | 4682 | 4533 | 5063 | 9577 | 1891 | 5149 | 3878 |
| 6926 | 6647 | 7548 | 5466 | 4856 | 9946 | 5966 | 6280 | 3985 | 7386 | 8448 | 4210 | 9225 | 7456 |
| 1710 | 3150 | 3511 | 2711 | 4665 | 3593 | 9572 | 5088 | 4380 | 0488 | 3502 | 6619 | 8197 | 9608 |
| 3874 | 6774 | 5777 | 3692 | 0156 | 7705 | 4824 | 9598 | 4168 | 8621 | 4219 | 7719 | 8339 | 0564 |
| 8333 | 4918 | 4514 | 2815 | 6261 | 2234 | 7051 | 2198 | 9728 | 8588 | 3970 | 6524 | 3416 | 1773 |
| 9897 | 3422 | 1458 | 7947 | 4556 | 5813 | 3869 | 0896 | 0556 | 5272 | 6628 | 2313 | 4226 | 4540 |
| 9200 | 4342 | 3248 | 0410 | 3221 | 5637 | 4835 | 8270 | 6103 | 2189 | 8205 | 9527 | 3318 | 4162 |
| 5107 | 3177 | 3100 | 0007 | 2136 | 2758 | 7316 | 9075 | 8605 | 9953 | 2265 | 4015 | 3702 | 6077 |
| 3144 | 4167 | 6702 | 2710 | 5939 | 1239 | 3977 | 2714 | 0486 | 8486 | 6545 | 2894 | 8452 | 4666 |
| 1924 | 9552 | 9995 | 3998 | 4027 | 8181 | 2838 | 3401 | 4859 | 8541 | 7518 | 8237 | 1754 | 6391 |
| 2558 | 7824 | 3920 | 3098 | 3309 | 1967 | 2016 | 4394 | 8215 | 9746 | 4540 | 9518 | 6250 | 1834 |
| 4753 | 2009 | 9275 | 7564 | 1910 | 3377 | 3070 | 8026 | 0526 | 0921 | 0784 | 6419 | 1452 | 0939 |
| 2563 | 6926 | 8485 | 8577 | 5090 | 3350 | 4286 | 5564 | 4808 | 8769 | 9337 | 7099 | 8558 | 7453 |
| 7699 | 9113 | 5387 | 0300 | 3315 | 7188 | 3289 | 5036 | 0613 | 8354 | 4603 | 2429 | 3149 | 7031 |
| 3843 | 9774 | 4056 | 6367 | 1698 | 2886 | 2031 | 6205 | 8953 | 7867 | 6627 | 8953 | 4077 | 3880 |
| 6585 | 4586 | 8246 | 8197 | 4969 | 6041 | 1520 | 4754 | 4840 | 6253 | 3960 | 7480 | 9235 | 8087 |
| 5404 | 9638 | 9190 | 8397 | 7668 | 0428 | 3558 | 7491 | 2922 | 0112 | 4373 | 5225 | 1988 | 4901 |
| 1518 | 4994 | 6301 | 2858 | 0431 | 6865 | 7308 | 2065 | 6613 | 1091 | 7022 | 2314 | 0683 | 3277 |
| 3506 | 1548 | 7727 | 2430 | 5035 | 8335 | 4695 | 3154 | 6663 | 1595 | 9598 | 3227 | 2983 | 8848 |
| 6245 | 7832 | 0786 | 4228 | 8286 | 1665 | 5416 | 7507 | 6294 | 0195 | 6254 | 5396 | 1646 | 1305 |
| 3015 | 6349 | 0954 | 8580 | 2894 | 0139 | 4790 | 7487 | 1805 | 3451 | 4458 | 5685 | 3984 | 2737 |
| 0563 | 8742 | 7378 | 5588 | 7128 | 2475 | 0691 | 1872 | 5007 | 3195 | 4108 | 5886 | 8343 | 7086 |
| 7426 | 0778 | 7829 | 9974 | 9374 | 6479 | 4509 | 8736 | 1839 | 2405 | 7876 | 5610 | 2776 | 6169 |
| 2025 | 6626 | 1535 | 9568 | 3594 | 5450 | 0355 | 3076 | 5256 | 3850 | 5794 | 0109 | 8507 | 0063 |
| 3811 | 2300 | 9500 | 6299 | 2290 | 7048 | 1679 | 6639 | 4720 | 8573 | 8955 | 6567 | 8809 | 3744 |

To be sure that you understand the procedure of simulating a process by its cumulative distribution, try using Table 5.8 and Table 5.9 to generate five hours of arrivals according to the Poisson distribution with $\lambda = .5$. You may begin choosing consecutive numbers at any point in the random number table, and move either across the table or down the table.

Now suppose service time for the solo-practice physician is exponential with mean $1/\mu = 1.5$ hours. The frequency distribution for the exponential is

$$f(X) = \mu e^{-\mu X},$$

and the cumulative distribution is given by

$$F(X) = 1 - e^{-\mu X}.$$

Thus

$$1 - F(X) = e^{-\mu X}$$

and

$$\ln (1 - F(X)) = - \mu X,$$

or

$$X = - \frac{\ln (1 - F(X))}{\mu}.$$

We have thus defined the exponentially distributed random variable $X$ in terms of $F(X)$, where $F(X)$ varies from 0 to 1, and is a term we can generate with our uniformly distributed random numbers. Recall that $1/\mu = 1.5$. Now suppose our first random number is 3,284 (which we convert to .328). Our first exponentially distributed service time is

$$X = \frac{-\ln (1 - .328)}{.667} = \frac{-\ln (.672)}{.667} = \frac{.397}{.667} = .595 \text{ hours.}$$

Generating functions, which allow generation of random variables with random numbers, can be derived for any continuous or discrete distribution—theoretical or empirical.

Now that we can generate arrivals and service times, we can resimulate the eight-hour day of the physician's office as before with the new arrival and service distributions (see Exercises 5.3 through 5.6).

Suppose that we separate patients into two types: Type 1 which generally needs less time (say service is exponential with $1/\mu = .5$) and Type 2 which needs more time ($1/\mu = 2$). Further, suppose Type 1 patients arrive (independently of the Type 2 patients) at a Poisson rate with $\lambda = 1.7$ and Type 2 patients arrive with Poisson rate as follows:

between 8 A.M. and 10 A.M.    $\lambda = 1.3,$
between 10 A.M. and noon      $\lambda = 1.5,$
between noon and 4 P.M.       $\lambda = 1.2.$

Finally, suppose there are now three physicians.

This does not add new conceptual difficulties to the simulation, only more "housekeeping"—keeping track of when to use which generating table or function, which patients are of which type, with which physician, etc. (Physicians who may go to lunch, take breaks, etc., create additional items to keep track of.) Moreover, in order to obtain simulation results which we believe actually represent the process, we would have to simulate many eight-hour days. (Do patients arrive at the same rate on Mondays as on Tuesdays? If not, we may need different arrival generating functions for each day of the week.)

All this leads to the conclusion that anything but the simplest simulation must be done on a computer. Using a computer does not add anything conceptually but it provides the "housekeeping" and the speed. The computer is carefully programmed to simulate the processes in the hospital—how Type 1 patients are treated differently from Type 2 or 3, etc., what happens at the end of each day, how patients are to be scheduled for return visits, etc. The program includes an overall clock to keep track of time and appropriate accumulators to accumulate waiting time, idle time, service failures, etc., as they occur during simulation.

Writing such a simulation program for a computer can be a time-consuming task if the general-purpose programming languages (FORTRAN, BASIC, PL/I, etc.) are used. Fortunately, special-purpose simulation languages have been developed which reduce programming time by as much as a factor of 100. Currently the most popular are GPSS and SIMSCRIPT, although there are many others, and new ones are under development. We will briefly investigate GPSS (General Purpose Simulation System) in the obstetrics example of the next section.

Before looking at a complete application, four more considerations are necessary. Recall that the output of one simulation run is actually one observation in a sample (or one point in a sample space). We are collecting a sample from which to make inferences about the true nature of the physician's office model if it were run indefinitely, just as we would choose a sample of people's heights to make inferences about the height of the total population. Thus a complete simulation analysis involves several runs, each run being a sample point (observation). Just as with any statistical inference analysis, we then estimate means and variances from our sample runs. For example, suppose we make ten independent simulation runs and find the average waiting times to be those of Table 5.10.

From the central limit theorem, we know that an unbiased estimate of the population is $\bar{X}$ and an estimate of the $\sigma$ of the distribution of sample means is $S/\sqrt{n}$. Using these inferences from the central limit theorem, confidence intervals can be constructed for the population to indicate estimates of what the results would be if we simulated the model indefinitely.

Notice, however, that the central limit theorem requires *independence* between sample points. For a continuous process such as obstetrics—the pediatric clinic is not continuous since it shuts down every day—there is a danger of the sample points not being independent. If one long run is made and simply divided into 10 segments for a sample of 10, the ending condition of sample point 3 is the beginning condition of sample point 4. This is usually remedied either by making the runs relatively long ("washing out" the effect) or by running a short time between sample segments and throwing out the results of such short runs.

Why should we make one long run and divide it up rather than make *n* short runs, beginning with a new place in the random number table each time? Consider a continuous process like the postpartum obstetrics unit. When we begin our simulation, there is no one in the unit. This is a non-normal situation. Thus the first few weeks of the simulation run is necessary to build up the census to its "normal"

*Table 5.10*

*Results of Ten Independent Simulation Runs*

| Run | Average Wait |
|:---:|:---:|
| 1 | 14.8 |
| 2 | 22.7 |
| 3 | 16.3 |
| 4 | 14.9 |
| 5 | 18.3 |
| 6 | 17.6 |
| 7 | 20.1 |
| 8 | 20.9 |
| 9 | 17.4 |
| 10 | 17.1 |

$$\bar{X} = 18.01$$
$$S = 2.55$$
$$S/\sqrt{10} = .81$$

range: this is called a start-up run. The process is said to be in its steady state once it begins operating in its normal range. Steady state does not mean stationary—it means that the process is independent of its starting conditions. Thus to make $n$ small runs, we would also need to run $n$ start-up times before each run to make sure each run began in its steady state. Note that this is no problem for the non-continuous process, as we are interested in the non-steady state results as well as the steady state (if it in fact ever reaches steady state).

The final consideration is the length of the run and the number of runs. The two cannot be considered separately, since a sample of $n$ very long runs is likely to have much smaller sample variance than $n$ short runs. The longer the runs, the smaller the sample can be, and vice versa. The estimate of needed sample size / run length is made as in any sampling experiment. First some estimate of sample variance is needed, perhaps from a set of small pilot runs of varying lengths. With this estimate, working backwards from a desired confidence range will yield the necessary sample size.

## 5.4 A RESOURCE-SIZE EXAMPLE: OBSTETRICS MERGER

In Chapter 2 we developed the obstetrics (OB) merger decision in the decision-making framework, leaving the details of quantification, solution, and sensitivity analysis steps to later chapters. In Section 5.2 we analyzed the quantification step with queueing. It would be helpful for the reader to review the OB merger problem as outlined in Chapter 2 and analyzed in Section 5.2 before proceeding.

Recall that the last two alternatives were actually each a set of options, with each member of the set specifying a number of labor, delivery, recovery, and postpartum beds to be provided at the merged site. The quantification problem was to predict how many patients would be expected to have to wait for service if $L$ labor beds, $D$ delivery beds, $R$ recovery beds, and $P$ postpartum beds were provided, for different values of $L$, $D$, $R$, and $P$.

Recall the OB process (Figure 5.7). The first step of the analysis was to estimate the distribution of the arrival process to the proposed merged unit. This included combining into a single process the patients who would have come to the two separate units if no merger took place.

To estimate the magnitude of annual OB usage, linear regression (see Chapter 7) was used to extend past trends into a ten-year horizon. The fertility rate (number of live births per thousand women 15 to 44 years old) was projected independently of the population of

15 to 44–year old women, the latter estimate being obtained from population experts. The fertility rate showed a downward trend, while population showed an upward trend. The combination was a slight downward trend. The current annual births for the two units combined was 2,300 and the forecasted estimate yielded 2,200 a year in ten years. The distribution of interarrival time in ten years was assumed to be the same as the present distribution but with proportionately larger mean and variance.

The present distribution was measured by obtaining arrival times of all OB patients in January, April, July, and October of the current year: 588 patients in all. (About 20 man-days were required to gather and analyze the data for all arrival and service distributions.) The interarrival distribution is shown in Figure 5.8. The distribution showed a close fit to the exponential distribution. Upon closer inspection, however, it was found that approximately 57 percent of the patients arrived during the A.M. hours and 43 percent during the P.M. hours. (Why? The best guess is that the arrivals are coordinated with physicians' schedules, although this is not verified.) The empirical interarrival distribution of patients arriving in the A.M. was tested against the exponential distribution with equal mean, $(1/\lambda = 3.3)$, and arrivals in the P.M. against the exponential distribution with equal mean, $1/\lambda = 4.42$ (see Figure 5.17). Since the actual arrival pattern was not stationary, to represent arrivals accurately the arrival pattern of the simulation would have to be unstationary as well. Increasing the current interarrival means by 2,300/2,200 gave $(23/22) \times 3.31 = 3.46$ for the A.M. and $(23/22) \times 4.42 = 4.62$ for the P.M.; these results define the exponential interarrival distributions of Figure 5.18 for the simulation. (The computer program that was used required the discrete approximation.)

The service time in the labor room was examined next, using the same patient records. It was found that the time of *delivery* was distributed evenly over the time of day, and that the difference between unstationary arrival in the labor facility and stationary delivery was an unstationary labor room service time: patients arriving in the A.M. tended to stay longer than those arriving in the P.M. The overall average for labor stay was 4.5 hours (Figure 5.9), but the distribution of stay in the A.M. and P.M. had means of 5.0 hours and 3.84 hours, respectively. Thus the labor stay was also assumed to be unstable, and separate labor service times were used for the A.M. and P.M.—the empirical distributions of Figure 5.19.

Service times in the delivery room (Figure 5.10) and in the postpartum area (Figure 5.13) appeared to be stationary, and the

*Analysis for Decision Making*

## *Figure 5.17*

## *Empirical Interarrival Distributions for OB Patients*

A.M. ARRIVALS

MEAN= 3.310          SUM= 350          EXPONENTIAL

| | ACTUAL FREQ | ACTUAL PROB | ACTUAL CDF | EXPO FREQ | EXPO PROB | EXPO CDF | CHI SQR |
|---|---|---|---|---|---|---|---|
| 0.50 | 78 | 0.223 | 0.223 | 71.0 | 0.203 | 0.203 | 0.70 |
| 1.00 | 40 | 0.114 | 0.337 | 39.1 | 0.112 | 0.315 | 0.02 |
| 1.50 | 36 | 0.103 | 0.440 | 33.6 | 0.096 | 0.411 | 0.17 |
| 2.00 | 28 | 0.080 | 0.520 | 28.9 | 0.083 | 0.493 | 0.03 |
| 2.50 | 28 | 0.080 | 0.600 | 24.9 | 0.071 | 0.564 | 0.40 |
| 3.00 | 23 | 0.066 | 0.666 | 21.4 | 0.061 | 0.625 | 0.12 |
| 3.50 | 20 | 0.057 | 0.723 | 18.4 | 0.053 | 0.678 | 0.14 |
| 4.00 | 14 | 0.040 | 0.763 | 15.8 | 0.045 | 0.723 | 0.21 |
| 4.50 | 15 | 0.043 | 0.806 | 13.6 | 0.039 | 0.762 | 0.15 |
| 5.00 | 9 | 0.026 | 0.831 | 11.7 | 0.033 | 0.795 | 0.62 |
| 5.50 | 8 | 0.023 | 0.854 | 10.0 | 0.029 | 0.824 | 0.42 |
| 6.00 | 6 | 0.017 | 0.871 | 8.6 | 0.025 | 0.849 | 0.81 |
| 6.50 | 5 | 0.014 | 0.886 | 7.4 | 0.021 | 0.870 | 0.79 |
| 7.00 | 5 | 0.014 | 0.900 | 6.4 | 0.018 | 0.888 | 0.30 |
| 7.50 | 7 | 0.020 | 0.920 | 5.5 | 0.016 | 0.904 | 0.42 |
| 8.00 | 4 | 0.011 | 0.931 | 4.7 | 0.013 | 0.917 ⎫ | |
| 8.50 | 3 | 0.009 | 0.940 | 4.1 | 0.012 | 0.929 ⎬ 0.19 | |
| 9.00 | 3 | 0.009 | 0.949 | 3.5 | 0.010 | 0.939 ⎭ | |
| 9.50 | 2 | 0.006 | 0.954 | 3.0 | 0.009 | 0.947 ⎫ | |
| 10.00 | 1 | 0.003 | 0.957 | 2.6 | 0.007 | 0.955 ⎬ 0.08 | |
| 10.50 | 4 | 0.011 | 0.969 | 2.2 | 0.006 | 0.961 ⎭ | |
| 11.00+ | 11 | 0.031 | 1.000 | 13.6 | 0.039 | 1.000 | 0.50 |

CHI SQUARE (16) = 6.04                                                              6.04

P.M. ARRIVALS

MEAN= 4.420          SUM= 238          EXPONENTIAL

| | ACTUAL FREQ | ACTUAL PROB | ACTUAL CDF | EXPO FREQ | EXPO PROB | EXPO CDF | CHI SQR |
|---|---|---|---|---|---|---|---|
| 0.50 | 34 | 0.143 | 0.143 | 37.1 | 0.156 | 0.156 | 0.27 |
| 1.00 | 20 | 0.084 | 0.227 | 21.5 | 0.090 | 0.246 | 0.10 |
| 1.50 | 20 | 0.084 | 0.311 | 19.2 | 0.081 | 0.327 | 0.03 |
| 2.00 | 26 | 0.109 | 0.420 | 17.1 | 0.072 | 0.399 | 4.59 |
| 2.50 | 13 | 0.055 | 0.475 | 15.3 | 0.064 | 0.463 | 0.35 |
| 3.00 | 17 | 0.071 | 0.546 | 13.7 | 0.057 | 0.521 | 0.81 |
| 3.50 | 14 | 0.059 | 0.605 | 12.2 | 0.051 | 0.572 | 0.26 |
| 4.00 | 14 | 0.059 | 0.664 | 10.9 | 0.046 | 0.618 | 0.88 |
| 4.50 | 10 | 0.042 | 0.706 | 9.7 | 0.041 | 0.659 | 0.01 |
| 5.00 | 10 | 0.042 | 0.748 | 8.7 | 0.037 | 0.695 | 0.20 |
| 5.50 | 6 | 0.025 | 0.773 | 7.8 | 0.033 | 0.728 | 0.40 |
| 6.00 | 5 | 0.021 | 0.794 | 6.9 | 0.029 | 0.757 | 0.54 |
| 6.50 | 5 | 0.021 | 0.815 | 6.2 | 0.026 | 0.783 | 0.23 |
| 7.00 | 8 | 0.034 | 0.849 | 5.5 | 0.023 | 0.806 ⎫ | |
| 7.50 | 3 | 0.013 | 0.861 | 4.9 | 0.021 | 0.827 ⎭ 0.03 | |
| 8.00 | 5 | 0.021 | 0.882 | 4.4 | 0.019 | 0.845 ⎫ | |
| 8.50 | 2 | 0.008 | 0.891 | 3.9 | 0.017 | 0.862 ⎭ 0.20 | |
| 9.00 | 3 | 0.013 | 0.903 | 3.5 | 0.015 | 0.877 ⎫ | |
| 9.50 | 4 | 0.017 | 0.920 | 3.1 | 0.013 | 0.890 ⎭ 0.02 | |
| 10.00 | 4 | 0.017 | 0.937 | 2.8 | 0.012 | 0.902 ⎫ | |
| 10.50 | 3 | 0.013 | 0.950 | 2.5 | 0.011 | 0.912 ⎬ 1.98 | |
| 11.00+ | 12 | 0.050 | 1.000 | 20.9 | 0.088 | 1.000 ⎭ | |

CHI SQUARE (15) = 12.0                                                              12.00

## Figure 5.18

### Exponential Interarrival Distributions

| | A.M. | | P.M. | |
|---|---|---|---|---|
| | MEAN = 3.460 | | MEAN = 4.620 | |
| | EXPO PROB | EXPO CDF | EXPO PROB | EXPO CDF |
| 0.50 | 0.195 | 0.195 | 0.150 | 0.150 |
| 1.00 | 0.108 | 0.303 | 0.087 | 0.237 |
| 1.50 | 0.094 | 0.397 | 0.078 | 0.315 |
| 2.00 | 0.081 | 0.478 | 0.070 | 0.386 |
| 2.50 | 0.070 | 0.548 | 0.063 | 0.449 |
| 3.00 | 0.061 | 0.609 | 0.057 | 0.505 |
| 3.50 | 0.053 | 0.662 | 0.051 | 0.556 |
| 4.00 | 0.046 | 0.707 | 0.046 | 0.601 |
| 4.50 | 0.039 | 0.747 | 0.041 | 0.642 |
| 5.00 | 0.034 | 0.781 | 0.037 | 0.679 |
| 5.50 | 0.030 | 0.810 | 0.033 | 0.712 |
| 6.00 | 0.026 | 0.836 | 0.030 | 0.741 |
| 6.50 | 0.022 | 0.858 | 0.027 | 0.768 |
| 7.00 | 0.019 | 0.877 | 0.024 | 0.792 |
| 7.50 | 0.017 | 0.894 | 0.021 | 0.813 |
| 8.00 | 0.014 | 0.908 | 0.019 | 0.832 |
| 8.50 | 0.012 | 0.920 | 0.017 | 0.850 |
| 9.00 | 0.011 | 0.931 | 0.015 | 0.865 |
| 9.50 | 0.009 | 0.940 | 0.014 | 0.879 |
| 10.00 | 0.008 | 0.948 | 0.012 | 0.891 |
| 10.50 | 0.007 | 0.955 | 0.011 | 0.902 |
| 11.00 | 0.006 | 0.961 | 0.010 | 0.912 |
| 11.50 | 0.005 | 0.966 | 0.009 | 0.921 |
| 12.00 | 0.005 | 0.971 | 0.008 | 0.929 |
| 12.50 | 0.004 | 0.975 | 0.007 | 0.937 |
| 13.00 | 0.003 | 0.978 | 0.006 | 0.943 |
| 13.50 | 0.003 | 0.981 | 0.006 | 0.949 |
| 14.00 | 0.003 | 0.984 | 0.005 | 0.954 |
| 14.50 | 0.002 | 0.986 | 0.005 | 0.959 |
| 15.00 | 0.002 | 0.988 | 0.004 | 0.963 |
| 15.50 | 0.002 | 0.989 | 0.004 | 0.967 |
| 16.00 | 0.001 | 0.991 | 0.003 | 0.970 |
| 16.50 | 0.001 | 0.992 | 0.003 | 0.973 |
| 17.00 | 0.001 | 0.993 | 0.003 | 0.976 |
| 17.50 | 0.001 | 0.994 | 0.002 | 0.979 |
| 18.00 | 0.001 | 0.995 | 0.002 | 0.981 |
| 18.50 | 0.001 | 0.996 | 0.002 | 0.983 |
| 19.00 | 0.004 | 1.000 | 0.017 | 1.000 |

empirical distributions were used for the simulation. The estimated distribution of recovery service time (Figure 5.12) was also used.

A simulation program was written in General Purpose Simulation System (GPSS) language (about three man-days to write and debug) (see Figure 5.20). Patients were allowed to leave the postpartum only between the hours of 10 A.M. and 4 P.M. A sample of one year's run evaluating $L = 4$, $D = 2$, $R = 3$, and $P = 34$ appears in Figure 5.21: Figure 5.22 interprets the output. A "sample" of five runs using different random numbers gave the results shown in Figure 5.23, from which rather narrow confidence intervals were calculated.

## Figure 5.19

### Empirical Service Time Distribution for Labor

| Length of Stay (Hours) | Frequency All Day (588 Patients) | Frequency A.M. (346 Patients) | Probability A.M. | CDF A.M. | Frequency P.M. (242 Patients) | Probability P.M. | CDF P.M. |
|---|---|---|---|---|---|---|---|
| ≤.5 | 76 | 36 | .104 | .104 | 40 | .165 | .165 |
| 1.0 | 57 | 30 | .087 | .191 | 27 | .112 | .277 |
| 1.5 | 35 | 22 | .064 | .254 | 13 | .054 | .331 |
| 2.0 | 25 | 13 | .038 | .292 | 12 | .050 | .380 |
| 2.5 | 34 | 20 | .058 | .350 | 14 | .058 | .438 |
| 3.0 | 31 | 17 | .049 | .399 | 14 | .058 | .496 |
| 3.5 | 33 | 17 | .049 | .448 | 16 | .066 | .562 |
| 4.0 | 28 | 18 | .052 | .500 | 10 | .041 | .603 |
| 4.5 | 24 | 14 | .040 | .540 | 10 | .041 | .645 |
| 5.0 | 30 | 15 | .043 | .584 | 15 | .062 | .707 |
| 5.5 | 25 | 15 | .043 | .627 | 10 | .041 | .748 |
| 6.0 | 29 | 16 | .046 | .673 | 13 | .054 | .802 |
| 6.5 | 22 | 11 | .032 | .705 | 11 | .045 | .847 |
| 7.0 | 17 | 12 | .035 | .740 | 5 | .021 | .868 |
| 7.5 | 17 | 10 | .029 | .769 | 7 | .029 | .897 |
| 8.0 | 12 | 8 | .023 | .792 | 4 | .017 | .913 |
| 8.5 | 11 | 7 | .020 | .812 | 4 | .017 | .930 |
| 9.0 | 15 | 13 | .038 | .850 | 2 | .008 | .938 |
| 9.5 | 10 | 6 | .017 | .867 | 4 | .017 | .955 |
| 10.0 | 8 | 8 | .023 | .890 | 0 | .000 | .955 |
| 10.5 | 8 | 7 | .020 | .910 | 1 | .004 | .959 |
| 11.0 | 11 | 7 | .020 | .931 | 4 | .017 | .975 |
| 11.5 | 6 | 5 | .014 | .945 | 1 | .004 | .979 |
| 12.0 | 6 | 5 | .014 | .960 | 1 | .004 | .983 |
| 12.5 | 7 | 6 | .017 | .977 | 1 | .004 | .987 |
| 13.0 | 3 | 1 | .003 | .980 | 2 | .008 | .996 |
| 13.5 | 3 | 3 | .009 | .989 | 0 | .000 | .996 |
| 14+ | 5 | 4 | .011 | 1.000 | 1 | .004 | 1.000 |
| Mean | 4.5 | 5.0 | | | 3.84 | | |

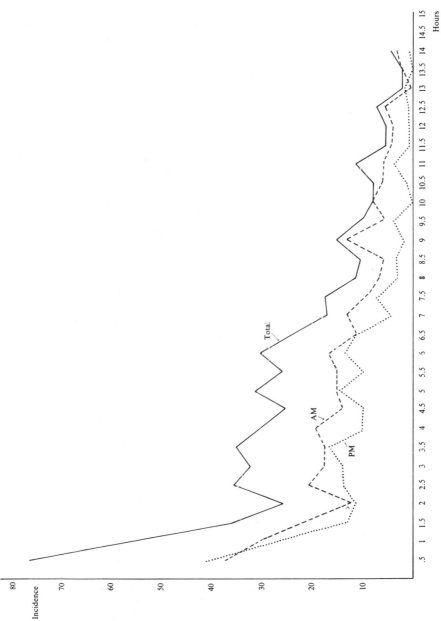

*Figure 5.20*

*GPSS Simulation Program*

```
                 STORAGE        S$LABOR,4/S$DELIV,2/S$RECOV,3/S$POSTP,34
        *
        EXPON    FUNCTION       RN1,C24
        0,0/.1,.104/.2,.222/.3,.355/.4,.509/.5,.69/.6,.915/.7,1.2
        .75,1.38/.8,1.6/.84,1.83/.88,2.12/.9,2.3/.92,2.52/.94,2.81/.95,2.99
        .96,3.2/.97,3.5/.98,3.9/.99,4.6/.998,5.3/.999,7/.9997,8
        1.0,9
        DUSE     FUNCTION       RN2,C17
        0,0/.0001,5.2/.048,15.2/.121,24.4/.342,35.6/.594,44.8
        .804,55/.879,66/.920,75.4/.942,84.2/.952,95.8/.956,104.6
        .961,115/.968,125/.981,175/.991,195/1.0,225
        RUSE     FUNCTION       RN3,C9
        0,0/.0001,30/.02,90/.37,150/.72,210/.9,270/.96,330/.98,390/1.0,450
        OBUSE    FUNCTION       RN4,C10
        0,0/.0001,2160/.041,3600/.435,5040/.816,6480/.935,7820
        .966,9260/.983,10800/.99,20800/1.0,30800
        *
        LABOR    TABLE          S$LABOR,0,1,12
        QLABO    QTABLE         LABOR,0,10,30
        DELIV    TABLE          S$DELIV,0,1,5
        QDELI    QTABLE         DELIV,0,10,30
        RECOV    TABLE          S$RECOV,0,1,10
        QRECO    QTABLE         RECOV,0,10,30
        POSTP    TABLE          S$POSTP,25,1,50
        QPOST    QTABLE         POSTP,0,30,30
        *
                 INITIAL        X1,208                 SET ARRIVAL MEAN TO AM VALUE
                 INITIAL        X2,300                 SET LABOR STAY TO AM VALUE
                 GENERATE       1440,,720              GENERATE TRANS EACH NOOR
                 SAVEVALUE      1,277                  RESET ARRIVAL MEAN TO PM VALUE
                 SAVEVALUE      2,228                  RESET LABOR STAY TO PM VALUE
                 TERMINATE
                 GENERATE       1440                   GENERATE TRANS EACH MIDNIGHT
                 SAVEVALUE      1,208                  RESET ARRIVAL MEAN TO AM VALUE
                 SAVEVALUE      2,300                  RESET LABOR STAY TO AM VALUE
                 TERMINATE
        *
        CLOXS    GENERATE       1440,,600              GENERATE TRANS EACH 10AM
                 LOGICS         FLAG                   OPEN DISCHARGE GATE
                 TERMINATE      0
        CLOXR    GENERATE       1440,,1260             GENERATE TRANS EACH 9PM
                 LOGICR         FLAG                   CLOSE DISCHARGE GATE
                 TERMINATE      0
        IATG     GENERATE       X1,FN$EXPON            GENERATE PATIENT ARRIVALS
                 ASSIGN         1,X2,I                 ASSIGN LABOR STAY TO PARAMETER 1
        QLABO    QUEUE          LABOR                  PATIENT QUEUES LABOR ROOM
                 TABULATE       LABOR                  TABULATE # ALREADY IN LABOR
                 ENTER          LABOR                  ENTER LABOR ROOM
                 DEPART         LABOR                  DEPART LABOR QUEUE
                 ADVANCE        P1                     LABOR STAY AS IN PARAMETER 1
                 LEAVE          LABOR                  LEAVE LABOR BED
        QDELV    QUEUE          DELIV                  PATIENT QUEUES FOR DELIVERY
                 TABULATE       DELIV                  TABULATE # ALREADY IN DELIVERY
        BACK     ENTER          DELIV                  ENTER DELIVERY ROOM
                 DEPART         DELIV                  LEAVE DELIVERY QUEUE
                 ADVANCE        FN$DUSE                DELIVERY STAY
                 LEAVE          DELIV                  LEAVE DELIVERY ROOM
        QRECO    QUEUE          RECOV                  PATIENT QUEUES RECOVERY
                 TABULATE       RECOV                  TABULATE # ALREADY IN RECOVERY
                 ENTER          RECOV                  ENTER RECOVERY ROOM
                 DEPART         RECOV                  LEAVE RECOVERY QUEUE
                 ADVANCE        FN$RUSE                RECOVERY STAY
                 LEAVE          RECOV                  LEAVE RECOVERY ROOM
        QPOST    QUEUE          POSTP                  PATIENT QUEUES FOR POSTPARTUM
                 TABULATE       POSTP                  TABULATE # ALREADY IN POSTP
                 ENTER          POSTP                  ENTER POSTP WARD
                 DEPART         POSTP                  LEAVE POSTP QUEUE
                 ADVANCE        FN$OBUSE               POSTP STAY
                 GATE LS        FLAG                   DELAY DISCHARGE IF GATE IS CLOSED
                 LEAVE          POSTP                  PATIENT IS DISCHARGED
        HIMAI    TERMINATE                             *
        *
        KNTRL    GENERATE       87433                  START-UP PERIOD
                 TERMINATE      1
                 START          1
                 RESET                                 CLEAR ALL TABULATIONS
        KNTRL    GENERATE       525600                 ONE YEAR SIMULATION
                 TERMINATE      1
                 START          1
                 END
```

*Figure 5.21*

## Output of GPSS Simulation Program

| STORAGE | CAPACITY | ENTRIES | AVERAGE CONTENTS | AVERAGE TIME/UNIT | CURRENT CONTENTS | MAXIMUM CONTENTS |
|---|---|---|---|---|---|---|
| LABOR | 4 | 2220 | 1.127 | 266.786 | 2 | 4 |
| DELIV | 2 | 2218 | .193 | 45.815 | | 2 |
| RECOV | 3 | 2219 | .770 | 182.271 | 1 | 3 |
| POSTP | 34 | 2239 | 24.403 | 5728.578 | 27 | 34 |

| QUEUE | MAXIMUM CONTENTS | AVERAGE CONTENTS | TOTAL ENTRIES | ZERO ENTRIES | PERCENT ZERO | AVERAGE TIME/TRANS | $AVERAGE TIME/TRANS |
|---|---|---|---|---|---|---|---|
| LABOR | 3 | .010 | 2219 | 2155 | 97.1 | 2.585 | 89.656 |
| DELIV | 2 | .000 | 2218 | 2193 | 98.8 | .170 | 15.159 |
| RECOV | 4 | .010 | 2218 | 2122 | 95.6 | 2.551 | 58.958 |
| POSTP | 7 | .056 | 2218 | 2121 | 95.6 | 13.323 | 304.649 |

$AVERAGE TIME/TRANS = AVERAGE TIME/TRANS EXCLUDING ZERO ENTRIES

TABLE LABOR
ENTRIES IN TALBE 2219

| UPPER LIMIT | OBSERVED FREQUENCY | PER CENT OF TOTAL | CUMULATIVE PERCENTAGE |
|---|---|---|---|
| 0 | 687 | 30.95 | 30.9 |
| 1 | 838 | 37.76 | 68.7 |
| 2 | 465 | 20.95 | 89.6 |
| 3 | 165 | 7.43 | 97.1 |
| 4 | 64 | 2.88 | 100.0 |

TABLE QLABO
ENTRIES IN TABLE 2219

| UPPER LIMIT | OBSERVED FREQUENCY | PER CENT OF TOTAL | CUMULATIVE PERCENTAGE |
|---|---|---|---|
| 0 | 2155 | 97.11 | 97.1 |
| 10 | 4 | .18 | 97.2 |
| 20 | 12 | .54 | 97.8 |
| 30 | 1 | .04 | 97.8 |
| 40 | 1 | .04 | 97.9 |
| 50 | 3 | .13 | 98.0 |
| 60 | 6 | .27 | 98.3 |
| 70 | 5 | .22 | 98.5 |
| 80 | 5 | .22 | 98.7 |
| 90 | 3 | .13 | 98.9 |
| 100 | 2 | .09 | 99.0 |

*Figure 5.21 (Continued)*

*Output of GPSS Simulation Program*

| UPPER LIMIT | OBSERVED FREQUENCY | PER CENT OF TOTAL | CUMULATIVE PERCENTAGE |
|---|---|---|---|
| 110 | 2 | .09 | 99.0 |
| 120 | 3 | .13 | 99.2 |
| 130 | 2 | .09 | 99.3 |
| 140 | 3 | .13 | 99.4 |
| 150 | 2 | .09 | 99.5 |
| 160 | 2 | .09 | 99.6 |
| 170 | 1 | .04 | 99.6 |
| 180 | 0 | .00 | 99.6 |
| 190 | 0 | .00 | 99.6 |
| 200 | 0 | .00 | 99.6 |
| 210 | 1 | .04 | 99.7 |
| 220 | 2 | .09 | 99.8 |
| 230 | 1 | .04 | 99.8 |
| 240 | 0 | .00 | 99.8 |
| 250 | 1 | .04 | 99.9 |
| 260 | 0 | .00 | 99.9 |
| 270 | 1 | .04 | 99.9 |
| 280 | 0 | .00 | 99.9 |
| OVERFLOW | 1 | .04 | 100.0 |

AVERAGE VALUE OF OVERFLOW 395.00

TABLE DELIV
ENTRIES IN TABLE 2218

| UPPER LIMIT | OBSERVED FREQUENCY | PER CENT OF TOTAL | CUMULATIVE PERCENTAGE |
|---|---|---|---|
| 0 | 1848 | 83.31 | 83.3 |
| 1 | 343 | 15.46 | 98.7 |
| 2 | 27 | 1.21 | 100.0 |

TABLE QDELI
ENTRIES IN TABLE 2218

| UPPER LIMIT | OBSERVED FREQUENCY | PER CENT OF TOTAL | CUMULATIVE PERCENTAGE |
|---|---|---|---|
| 0 | 2193 | 98.87 | 98.8 |
| 10 | 11 | .49 | 99.3 |
| 20 | 9 | .40 | 99.7 |
| 30 | 1 | .04 | 99.8 |
| 40 | 2 | .09 | 99.9 |
| 50 | 2 | .09 | 100.0 |

**TABLE RECOV**
**ENTRIES IN TABLE** 2218

| UPPER LIMIT | OBSERVED FREQUENCY | PER CENT OF TOTAL | CUMULATIVE PERCENTAGE |
|---|---|---|---|
| 0 | 1019 | 45.94 | 45.9 |
| 1 | 818 | 36.88 | 82.8 |
| 2 | 285 | 12.84 | 95.6 |
| 3 | 96 | 4.32 | 100.0 |

**TABLE QRECO**
**ENTRIES IN TABLE** 2218

| UPPER LIMIT | OBSERVED FREQUENCY | PER CENT OF TOTAL | CUMULATIVE PERCENTAGE |
|---|---|---|---|
| 0 | 2122 | 95.67 | 95.6 |
| 10 | 15 | .67 | 96.3 |
| 20 | 15 | .67 | 97.0 |
| 30 | 7 | .31 | 97.3 |
| 40 | 9 | .40 | 97.7 |
| 50 | 4 | .18 | 97.9 |
| 60 | 5 | .22 | 98.1 |
| 70 | 8 | .36 | 98.5 |
| 80 | 5 | .22 | 98.7 |
| 90 | 4 | .18 | 98.9 |
| 100 | 8 | .36 | 99.2 |
| 110 | 2 | .09 | 99.3 |
| 120 | 2 | .09 | 99.4 |
| 130 | 1 | .04 | 99.5 |
| 140 | 3 | .13 | 99.6 |
| 150 | 1 | .04 | 99.6 |
| 160 | 1 | .04 | 99.7 |
| 170 | 0 | .00 | 99.7 |
| 180 | 1 | .04 | 99.7 |
| 190 | 2 | .09 | 99.8 |
| 200 | 2 | .09 | 99.9 |
| 210 | 0 | .00 | 99.9 |
| 220 | 0 | .00 | 99.9 |
| 230 | 0 | .00 | 99.9 |
| 240 | 1 | .04 | 100.0 |

**TABLE POSTP**
**ENTRIES IN TABLE** 2218

| UPPER LIMIT | OBSERVED FREQUENCY | PER CENT OF TOTAL | CUMULATIVE PERCENTAGE |
|---|---|---|---|
| 25 | 1338 | 60.32 | 60.3 |
| 26 | 163 | 7.34 | 67.6 |
| 27 | 134 | 6.04 | 73.7 |
| 28 | 128 | 5.77 | 79.4 |

# Figure 5.21 (Continued)

## Output of GPSS Simulation Program

| UPPER LIMIT | OBSERVED FREQUENCY | PER CENT OF TOTAL | CUMULATIVE PERCENTAGE |
|---|---|---|---|
| 29 | 106 | 4.77 | 84.2 |
| 30 | 97 | 4.37 | 88.6 |
| 31 | 63 | 2.84 | 91.4 |
| 32 | 49 | 2.20 | 93.6 |
| 33 | 43 | 1.93 | 95.6 |
| 34 | 97 | 4.37 | 100.0 |

TABLE QPOST
ENTRIES IN TABLE 2218

| UPPER LIMIT | OBSERVED FREQUENCY | PER CENT OF TOTAL | CUMULATIVE PERCENTAGE |
|---|---|---|---|
| 0 | 2121 | 95.62 | 95.6 |
| 30 | 7 | .31 | 95.9 |
| 60 | 8 | .36 | 96.3 |
| 90 | 6 | .27 | 96.5 |
| 120 | 4 | .18 | 96.7 |
| 150 | 8 | .36 | 97.1 |
| 180 | 7 | .31 | 97.4 |
| 210 | 7 | .31 | 97.7 |
| 240 | 2 | .09 | 97.8 |
| 270 | 7 | .31 | 98.1 |
| 300 | 4 | .18 | 98.3 |
| 330 | 4 | .18 | 98.5 |
| 360 | 5 | .22 | 98.7 |
| 390 | 1 | .04 | 98.7 |
| 420 | 3 | .13 | 98.9 |
| 450 | 1 | .04 | 98.9 |
| 480 | 2 | .09 | 99.0 |
| 510 | 2 | .09 | 99.1 |
| 540 | 2 | .09 | 99.2 |
| 570 | 1 | .04 | 99.2 |
| 600 | 1 | .04 | 99.3 |
| 630 | 2 | .09 | 99.4 |
| 660 | 3 | .13 | 99.5 |
| 690 | 1 | .04 | 99.5 |
| 720 | 0 | .00 | 99.5 |
| 750 | 0 | .00 | 99.5 |
| 780 | 1 | .04 | 99.6 |
| 810 | 1 | .04 | 99.6 |
| 840 | 1 | .04 | 99.7 |
| OVERFLOW | 6 | .27 | 100.0 |

AVERAGE VALUE OF OVERFLOW 990.50

## Figure 5.22

## Explanation of GPSS Output

The first block of results shows the CAPACITY of each facility for this run (the L, D, R, and P), the AVERAGE CONTENTS (occupancy = average contents/capacity), the number of patients who ENTERED each facility, and the AVERAGE length of stay (in minutes). The CURRENT CONTENTS was the number of patients left when the simulation stopped, and MAXIMUM CONTENTS was the maximum census observed during the simulation.

The second block of results summarizes activity in each of the four queues preceding each facility. MAXIMUM CONTENTS is maximum waiting line length and AVERAGE CONTENTS is average length. TOTAL ENTRIES is the number of patients passing through the queue, with ZERO ENTRIES of them having no wait. AVERAGE TIME/TRANS is average wait for all patients passing through, where $AVERAGE is the average just for those who waited a positive amount of time.

The last 4 blocks of results give more detail for each facility and queue. TABLE LABOR is interpreted as follows. Let X = UPPER LIMIT and Y = OBSERVED FREQUENCY. There were Y patients who arrived to find X labor beds already occupied. For example, there were 64 patients who arrived to find all four beds full—thus these 64 patients had to wait in the queue. There were 165 patients who arrived to find exactly three beds already occupied, and they immediately occupied the fourth bed. Thus the fourth bed was used by 64 + 165 = 229 patients, or by 229/2,219 = 10.3% of the patients who went through the labor facility.

TABLE QLABO gives the distribution of waiting times for all patients who went through the labor facility. Most (2,155) had zero wait, four waited 0 to 10 minutes, twelve waited 10 to 20 minutes, etc.

## Figure 5.23

## Results of Five Runs with Three Labor Beds

|  | Number of Patients with Non-Zero Wait | $ Average Wait (Minutes) | Number of Patients Using Third Bed |
|---|---|---|---|
| Run #1 | 266 | 131 | 719 |
| Run #2 | 258 | 131 | 694 |
| Run #3 | 218 | 121 | 680 |
| Run #4 | 248 | 128 | 698 |
| Run #5 | 273 | 134 | 736 |
| Average | 252 | 129 | 705 |
| $\sqrt{S^2}$ | 21.5 | 5 | 22.3 |
| $\sqrt{S^2/N}$ | 9.6 | 2.2 | 10 |
| 95% Confidence Interval | 277 to 227 | 135 to 123 | 723 to 679 |

(Similar intervals for all relevant results are easily calculated.) The narrowness of the confidence intervals most likely comes from the length of the runs and the overall stability of the process. Table 5.11 summarizes results for different *L, D, R,* and *P.* These were the quantifications that then became the focus of the solution step of the decision-making framework as outlined in Chapter 2.

The final step was sensitivity analysis, which first involved increasing and decreasing the interarrival rate to test the sensitivity to errors in the forecast of future demand and the sensitivity to possible reductions in service times. For example, arrival rates that generated 2,200 + 10 percent were simulated, giving changes in most measures of about 4 percent. Two interesting additional sensitivities were measured. First, it was found that significantly fewer labor beds were needed if arrivals were stationary (i.e., one interarrival distribution for both A.M. and P.M.): why? Second, a significant reduction in postpartum beds could be obtained by allowing a wider discharge range (say, from 8 A.M. to 9 P.M.). Other operations policies could easily have been tested by the model with very little effort.

The cost of the simulation analysis was approximately 20 mandays (including data gathering) and approximately $200 in computer time. This did not include the estimation of construction costs to build or modify existing facilities.

## 5.5 A SCHEDULING EXAMPLE: ADMISSIONS SCHEDULING

One of the major operational controls on the use of the resources of the hospital comes at the time of a patient's admission. The admissions process, for most hospitals, can be viewed as that of Figure 5.24. On the left side are the different types of patients who are seeking admission to the hospital. On the right are the separate units of the hospital. Intensive care unit (ICU) and cardiac care unit (CCU) patients go directly to the ICU/CCU, where they remain several days before being transferred to the medical or surgical unit (MED/SURG unit). If the ICU/CCU is full, they may be temporarily held in the MED/SURG unit, or if that is full, in a temporary emergency room (ER) holding area if one exists. If that is full, they must be *turned away*. (Turnaway may actually mean inappropriate treatment in the hall, etc. The point is that an inappropriate situation arises when there is no room.) It may be possible to transfer an existing ICU/CCU patient to the MED/SURG unit before he would normally have been transferred, to make room for the new ICU/CCU patient. We will call this a *forced transfer*.

The emergency (ER) patient normally is admitted to the

## Table 5.11

### Summary of Results from Simulation Analysis
#### (Of 2,210 Patients)

| | Number of Beds Provided | Number (%) of Patients with Non-Zero Wait | Average Wait (All Patients) (Minutes) | $ Average Wait (Patients with Non-Zero Wait) | Number of Patients Using Last Bed |
|---|---|---|---|---|---|
| Labor | 3 | 266 (12%) | 15.7 | 131.0 | 719 |
| | 4 | 64 ( 3%) | 2.6 | 89.7 | 229 |
| | 5 | 9 ( 1%) | .3 | 72.3 | 53 |
| | 6 | 0 ( 0%) | .0 | .0 | 13 |
| Delivery | 2 | 25 ( 1%) | .2 | 15.2 | 370 |
| | 3 | 0 ( 0%) | .0 | .0 | 33 |
| Recovery | 2 | 438 (20%) | 17.9 | 90.6 | 1,242 |
| | 3 | 96 ( 4%) | 2.6 | 59.0 | 381 |
| | 4 | 28 ( 1%) | .6 | 47.4 | 103 |
| | 5 | 3 ( 1%) | .0 | 16.0 | 20 |
| Postpartum | 30 | 405 (18%) | 107.3 | 587.4 | 515 |
| | 32 | 173 ( 8%) | 38.4 | 483.4 | 241 |
| | 34 | 97 ( 4%) | 13.3 | 304.6 | 140 |
| | 36 | 65 ( 3%) | 7.3 | 247.4 | 54 |
| | 38 | 7 ( 1%) | .7 | 216.3 | 13 |
| | 40 | 2 ( 1%) | .0 | 48.0 | 8 |

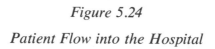

*Figure 5.24*

*Patient Flow into the Hospital*

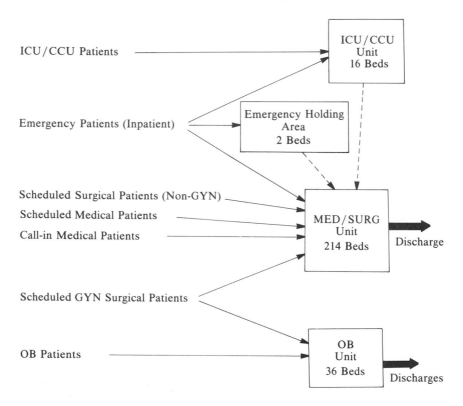

MED/SURG unit. If it is full, he may be held in an ER holding area (if there is one) or held on the ICU/CCU until there is a bed free. Otherwise, he is turned away.

Non-ER surgical patients are usually given a definite future date of admission, determined by when a bed will be free and by the patient's and physician's convenience. Obtaining such a firm date is called being *scheduled.* If the hospital is one which has high occupancy on the MED/SURG units, the scheduled date may be several weeks to several months in the future. We will call the time between when a scheduled patient asks for admission and when he is actually scheduled for admission the *surgical delay.* If a scheduled patient's firm date arrives and there is no room for him on the MED/SURG units, he is *cancelled.* (Thus ER and ICU/CCU patients are turned away and scheduled patients are cancelled.)

Most non-ER medical patients are "urgent," requiring admission as soon as possible. For hospitals with high MED/SURG occupancy, it is typical for these patients to form a *waiting line* for free beds. We will call these patients *call-in* patients, as they are generally called in for admission on the same day they are to be admitted. Call-in patients are not turned away or cancelled, since they are not called until it is certain a bed is free. (Call-in patients who wait too long on the waiting line may be declared ER patients by their physicians so that they can obtain immediate admission.) With the scheduling system designed below, it will be possible to *schedule* some urgent medical patients, if their firm date is not too far distant. Such scheduled patients may also maintain a place on the waiting line in case a bed becomes available before their firm date. As we did with surgical patients, we will call the time between a medical patient's request for admission and his actual admission the *medical delay*.

Non-ER gynecology (GYN) patients fall into the same categories as surgery patients, except some of them may be given beds on the obstetrics (OB) unit if there is room and if hospital policy permits. Thus GYN patients are scheduled and are subject to cancellation. Finally, OB patients are essentially ER patients who go to a special unit—OB. OB patients are thus subject to turnaway.

Like the other decisions we have examined, there are two "competing" sets of factors affected by how patients are admitted. The first set of factors is the use of the resources, which we can measure by the average occupancies on the separate units, and in some cases by the variance of the census. Unnecessarily low occupancies (or high variance) on these units means wasted resources. The second set of factors affected by the admissions process concerns the patient (and his physician). The key elements of this set of factors are

—the probability of *turnaway* for ER, OB and ICU/CCU patients;

—the probability of *cancellation* for scheduled patients;

—the *delay* for both medical and surgical patients, and the balance between these two delays;

—the possibility of scheduling urgent medical patients so that they may have a *firm date* rather than being subjected to call-in;

—the probability that an ICU/CCU patient will have to remain on the ICU/CCU unit after he should have been transferred to the MED/SURG because the latter is full (we will call this a *failed transfer*);

—the probability that an ICU/CCU patient will be *force transferred* to make room for another ICU/CCU patient.

The scheduling decision is thus the determination of a *scheduling system* that provides the correct balance between the two factors and among the separate elements of the second set of factors. We call this a scheduling decision because all of the resources (number of beds) are fixed. To some extent demand is also fixed, since we assume that we cannot increase or decrease its magnitude. We will, of course, manipulate the pattern of admissions.

It is important to begin by distinguishing between a hospital that is *overbedded* and one that is not. Overbedding means that the census on the MED/SURG units is in the 80 percent or below range. Thus patients seldom have to wait for admission because there are always beds free (i.e., no waiting line, and scheduling delay is determined by patient and physician convenience), and there is very little chance of ER or ICU/CCU turnaway, again because the hospital seldom reaches capacity.

When a hospital is overbedded the first of the two factors listed above (resource use) becomes the focus, since the second set of factors is not, by the definition of overbedding, presenting problems. Typically the census of the MED/SURG units of the overbedded hospital is subject to large fluctuations, essentially reflecting the random requests for admission and random length of stay. Figure 5.25 represents such a census. The resource use problem emerges because personnel staffing levels must be based on maintaining adequate care to the current census a certain percentage (say 90 percent) of the time (see Figure 5.25), allowing understaffing to occur only 10 percent of the time. If the variance of Figure 5.25 could somehow be "damped," the same 90 percent staffing policy would result in lower staffing levels (see Figure 5.26).

An attempt to damp this variance is reported by Briggs (see Additional Reading). Briggs evaluated scheduling policies which would delay admission of those patients at the "peaks" of Figure 5.25 until the next "valley." The trade-off is thus between variation (and improving resource use) and delaying patients.

Using a large simulation model of the admissions process of the hospital, Briggs simulated the effect of policies which would subject different percentages of patients to a short (one- to five-day)

Figure 5.25

Census Level over Time

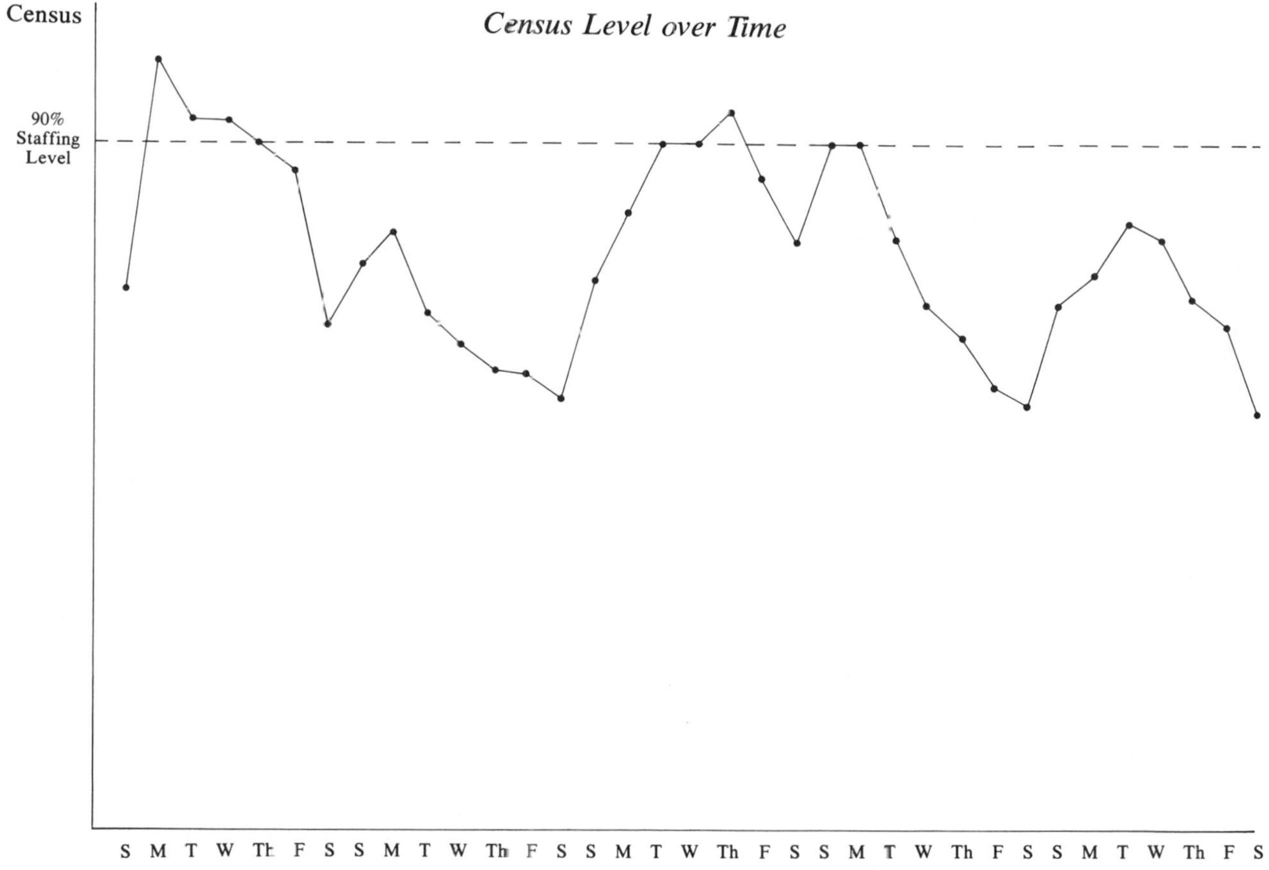

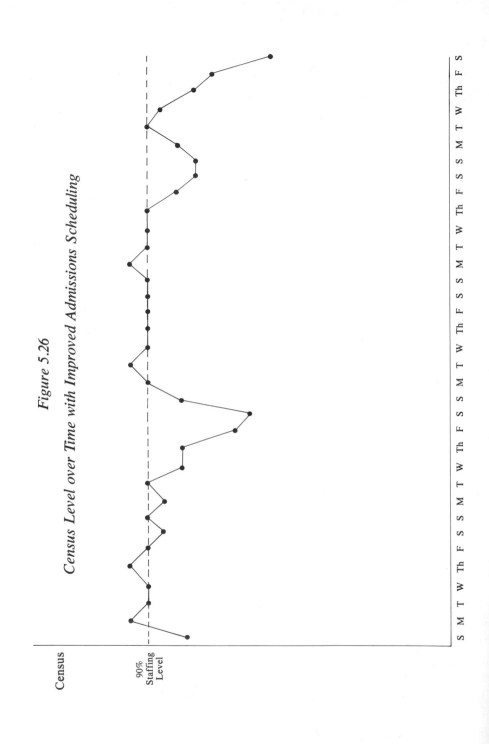

Figure 5.26

Census Level over Time with Improved Admissions Scheduling

delay. The simulation indicated that variance could be reduced by 19 percent if 5 percent of the patients were delayed, by 50 percent if 15 percent of the patients were delayed, and by 63 percent if 22 percent of the patients were delayed. The analysis indicated that if the staffing policy of a hospital dictated understaffing only 10 percent of the time (i.e., providing a level of staff to meet demand 90 percent of the time) at the 300 bed hospital where the study was conducted, annual nursing staff savings (in 1971) of about $1,000 for every percentage point (up to 22 percent) of patients delayed could be achieved. The decision thus becomes one of evaluating the cost of delaying patients. Briggs specified the set of rules that would achieve any level of variance reduction (and associated proportion of patients delayed) and let the hospital decide how it would make the trade-off.

The hospital which is not overbedded is characterized by high (90 to 95 percent or higher) occupancy on the MED/SURG units, a waiting line of urgent medical patients, surgical scheduling delay of from several weeks to several months, and positive probabilities of cancellations, turnaways, and failed transfers. Balancing latter elements of the objective for hospitals that are short of beds becomes much more delicate than in the case of an overbedded hospital.

Before we continue with our examination of the non-overbedded situation, it is important that we again keep in mind the decison framework of the analysis. So far we have described the process and specified the objectives (and hinted at their measure of performance). To be more specific, our objectives are the following:

1. maximize occupancy on the MED/SURG (designated OCM), occupancy on the ICU/CCU (OCI), and occupancy on the OB (OCO) units;
2. minimize the number of
   —ICU/CCU turnaways (TUI) per week
   —ER turnaways (TUE) per week
   —OB turnaways (TUO) per week
   —cancellations (CAN) per week
   —failed transfers (FAL) per week
   —forced transfers (FOR) per week;
3. maximize the number of scheduled urgent medical patients (SCM) per week; and
4. maintain the ratio of average surgical delay to the average medical delay at some desired ratio; let RAT be the *actual* ratio.

Our decision variable will be the scheduling system we adopt: $S$. This will be a set of rules which governs the flow of all patients to all units. The above measures of performance are thus all *functions* of $S$ (e.g., OCM $(S)$, CAN $(S)$, etc.).

Our objective function can thus be stated:

$$\text{Minimize } TC(S) = C_1[100 - OCM(S)] + C_2[100 - OCI(S)]$$

$$+ C_3[100 - OCO(S)]$$

$$+ C_4TUI(S) + C_5TUE(S) + C_6TUO(S)$$

$$+ C_7CAN(S) + C_8FAL(S) + C_9FOR(S)$$

$$+ C_{10}DIF(S) - C_{11}SCM(S),$$

where $TC(S)$ is the total cost of adopting scheduling scheme $S$; $C_1$ to $C_{10}$ are the cost per incident of each element (the opportunity cost of "lost" occupancy for the first three); $C_{11}$ stands for the benefit of scheduling a medical patient who would otherwise be on call-in status; and DIF is the difference between RAT and the desired ratio of delay to wait.

Because of the anticipated difficulty of measuring the $C_i$, we will find it more manageable to adopt the following model:

$$\text{Maximize } OCM(S) + C_1'OCI(S) + C_2'OCO(S) + C_3'SCM(S)$$

subject to

$$TUI(S) \leq A_1,$$
$$TUE(S) \leq A_2,$$
$$TUO(S) \leq A_3,$$
$$CAN(S) \leq A_4,$$
$$FAL(S) \leq A_5,$$
$$FOR(S) \leq A_6, \text{ and}$$
$$A_7 \leq RAT(S) \leq A_8,$$

where

$C_1'$ is the *ratio* of the benefit of an extra point of occupancy in the ICU/CCU to an extra point of occupancy in the MED/SURG for a week,

$C_2'$ is the same ratio for OB and MED/SURG,

$C_3'$ is the ratio of the benefit of a scheduled medical patient to an extra point of occupancy on MED/SURG for a week,

and the $A_i$ are appropriate "minimum allowable values."

This approach allows a "satisficing" rather than optimal solution, where the trade-off among turnaways, transfers, and occupancy can be examined in the sensitivity analysis step of the decision-making framework.

The final task in the first step of the decision-making framework is to define the decision variable $S$. A scheduling system is a set of rules that defines how each of the patient types is to be scheduled and/or admitted into each unit. The following general system or set of rules from Hancock, Warner, Heda and Fuhs (see Additional Reading) will provide the framework for such systems.

1. *The Surgical Allowance:* the maximum number of surgical patients to be scheduled for admission by day of week.

   *Example:*

   | Sun | Mon | Tue | Wed | Thurs | Fri | Sat |
   |-----|-----|-----|-----|-------|-----|-----|
   | 16  | 14  | 14  | 12  | 12    | 0   | 0   |

2. *The Medical Allowance:* the maximum number of urgent medical patients to schedule by day of week.

   *Example:*

   | Sun | Mon | Tue | Wed | Thurs | Fri | Sat |
   |-----|-----|-----|-----|-------|-----|-----|
   | 2   | 2   | 1   | 1   | 1     | 7   | 7   |

3. *The Census Reduction Allowance:* the number of beds that *should* be left empty each day on the MED/SURG units.

   *Example:*

   | Sun | Mon | Tue | Wed | Thurs | Fri | Sat |
   |-----|-----|-----|-----|-------|-----|-----|
   | 13  | 9   | 6   | 6   | 6     | 6   | 18  |

(The census reduction allowance is actually the combination of two allowances. First, there is a need to allow empty beds to meet ER and ICU/CCU arrivals who will come in the late afternoon and at night: the ER allowance. Second, since admissions are typically much higher than discharges on Sundays, Mondays, and often Tuesdays, there is a need to keep some beds empty over the weekend to meet such a net inflow: the weekend allowance.)

4. *The Cancellation Allowance:* the number of beds that *must* be kept empty even if some patients have to be cancelled. (Thus, we will not cancel patients to meet the census reduction allowance.)

   *Example:*

   | Sun | Mon | Tue | Wed | Thurs | Fri | Sat |
   |-----|-----|-----|-----|-------|-----|-----|
   | 4   | 4   | 4   | 4   | 4     | 4   | 4   |

5. *The Call-in Allowance:* the maximum number of patients per day to be called in.

| *Example:* | Sun | Mon | Tue | Wed | Thurs | Fri | Sat |
|---|---|---|---|---|---|---|---|
|  | 10 | 8 | 8 | 8 | 8 | 10 | 10 |

6. *The OB Allowance:* the number of beds that must be left open for OB patients (i.e., we may put GYN patients on the OB floor until there are these many beds left empty).

| *Example:* | Sun | Mon | Tue | Wed | Thurs | Fri | Sat |
|---|---|---|---|---|---|---|---|
|  | 8 | 8 | 8 | 8 | 8 | 8 | 8 |

7. *Priorities:*

   a) are forced transfers (of ICU/CCU) allowed?

   b) if there are only, say, three non-OB beds free in the hospital, and there is an ICU/CCU, an ER, a scheduled MED, a scheduled SURG, and a call-in patient who all want beds, in what *order* are they admitted to the beds? (For example, would they be admitted in the order they are listed above?)

These rules, or this system, define the flow of patients into the hospital as follows. As requests for admission from non-ER surgical patients arrive, they are scheduled for the day in the future which best coincides with the convenience of patient and physician, but subject to their not exceeding the surgical allowance for that date. Some urgent medical patients will also be scheduled, subject to the medical allowance: these medical patients may also choose to be on the waiting list. Other medical patients are put on a waiting list in the order that their request was received (or in some other order). Late each morning (or early afternoon) when the number of discharges is fairly well known, the admission office

1. calculates the number of empty OB beds and allocates as many as possible of the GYN patients who are scheduled for admission that day to the OB unit, keeping enough empty OB beds to maintain the OB allowance;

2. calculates the number of empty beds on the MED/SURG unit, and subtracts from this the number of patients scheduled for admission today (including the GYN who did not get allocated to OB) to get *net empty beds;*

3. compares number of net empty beds with the cancellation allowance; if it is less than the cancellation allowance, enough patients are cancelled to make the two numbers equal;

4. compares net empty beds with the census reduction allowance; if it is greater than the census reduction allowance, enough call-in patients are called in to make the two numbers equal, or to fill the call-in allowance, whichever is lower.

Throughout the day ICU/CCU, ER, and OB patients arrive and are admitted immediately unless facilities are full, in which case they are temporarily placed on an inappropriate unit or turned away, according to the appropriate policies. In addition, transfers are made throughout the day, although most take place in the morning.

We will call the set of rules the *system*, and call a specific set of numbers for the rules (like the example) a *schedule*. Thus there are many, many schedules possible for this system, and the schedules will be our decision variables. (Note that we have limited our decision variables to the schedules of *this* system; other systems with their schedules would also be candidates for decision variables and should be included if they are not already a subset of the chosen system. We will assume that the chosen system includes a sufficiently wide variety of schedules.)

The second step of the decision process is quantification. The $C_i$ and the $A_i$ must be established subjectively, while the functions must be quantified by simulation. As before, we will wait to determine the $C_i$ in the solution step. The $A_i$ are determined through consultation with the administration and the medical staff of the hospital. The $A_i$ should be treated at this point as initial approximations, allowing some adjustment once more information is known about how they interact with one another and with the objective function. An initial set for the 300-bed study hospital is shown in Figure 5.27.

Data for the simulation included the arrival distributions of

ER patients,
—ICU/CCU patients,

*Figure 5.27*

*Initial Quantification of Constraint Values*

$A_1 = .2$ ICU/CCU turnaways/week (TUI)
$A_2 = .5$ ER turnaways/week (TUE)
$A_3 = .2$ OB turnaways/week (TUO)
$A_4 = .5$ Cancellations/week (CAN)
$A_5 = 2$ Failed transfers/week (FAL)
$A_6 = 1.5$ Forced transfers/week (FOR)
$A_7 = 4$ (Ratio of surgical delay to medical delay) ⎱ (range for RAT)
$A_8 = 6$ (Ratio of surgical delay to medical delay) ⎰

—OB patients,
—requests for admission of surgical patients,
—requests for admission of medical patients,
—requests for admission of GYN patients,

and length of stay distributions of

—ER patients,
—ICU/CCU patients while in ICU/CCU,
—ICU/CCU patients after they are transferred to MED/SURG,
—OB patients,
—GYN patients,
—surgical patients, and
—medical patients.

These were gathered from hospital records from a one-year period. (A special computer program was later devised to generate most of the distributions directly from the widely used Professional Activity Study (PAS) data files.)

To evaluate the functions for each possible schedule $S$ would be unmanageable. Thus Steps 2 (quantification) and 3 (solution) were combined in a process that measures the effect of schedules only when they are believed to have some potential for improving the current schedule being evaluated. This is called a heuristic approach and proceeds as follows.

First, an *initial schedule* is determined (Figure 5.28). This may be done by taking the schedule currently used in the hospital (the schedule of our "system" which most closely approximates the current

*Figure 5.28*

*The Initial Schedule*

|  | Sun | Mon | Tue | Wed | Thurs | Fri | Sat |
|---|---|---|---|---|---|---|---|
| Surgical Allowance | 16 | 14 | 12 | 12 | 13 | 0 | 0 |
| Medical Allowance | 0 | 0 | 0 | 0 | 0 | 0 | 0 |
| Census Reduction Allowance | 23 | 12 | 11 | 11 | 11 | 14 | 31 |
| Cancellation Allowance | 7 | 7 | 7 | 7 | 7 | 7 | 7 |
| Call-in Allowance | 8 | 8 | 8 | 8 | 8 | 8 | 8 |
| OB Allowance | 8 | 8 | 8 | 8 | 8 | 8 | 8 |

| Priorities | A. Forced Transfers Allowed |
|---|---|
|  | B. Priorities for admission are ICU, ER, scheduled MED, scheduled SURG, then Call-in. |

*Figure 5.29*

## Baker Hospital Initial Solution

#### ···· MS UNIT SUMMARY STATISTICS ····

| TOT | SUN | MON | TUE | WED | THU | FRI | SAT | |
|---|---|---|---|---|---|---|---|---|
| 0.09 | 0.0 | 0.01 | 0.02 | 0.03 | 0.02 | 0.0 | 0.0 | AVG # OF CANCELLATIONS |
| 0.06 | 0.0 | 0.02 | 0.02 | 0.0 | 0.0 | 0.0 | 0.0 | AVG # OF EMG TURNAWAYS |
| 0.00 | 0.0 | 0.0 | 0.0 | 0.0 | 0.0 | 0.0 | 0.0 | AVG # OF ICU TURNAWAYS |
| 0.00 | 0.0 | 0.0 | 0.0 | 0.00 | 0.0 | 0.0 | 0.0 | AVG # OF GYN PTS. ADMITTED |
| 37.52 | 5.65 | 5.55 | 4.30 | 4.20 | 4.88 | 7.57 | 5.38 | AVG # OF CALLIN PTS. ADMITTED |
| 160.45 | 29.13 | 27.09 | 24.06 | 23.56 | 25.14 | 16.98 | 14.47 | AVG # OF ADMISSIONS |
| 160.45 | 20.79 | 16.45 | 21.58 | 23.81 | 25.63 | 25.37 | 26.81 | AVG # OF DISCHARGES & TRANSFERS TO ICU/CCU |
| 200.1 | 193.7 | 204.3 | 206.8 | 206.6 | 206.1 | 197.7 | 185.4 | AVG # OF BEDS OCCUPIED |
| 0.93 | 0.91 | 0.95 | 0.97 | 0.97 | 0.96 | 0.92 | 0.87 | AVG % OCCUPANCY |

#### ···· OB UNIT SUMMARY STATISTICS ····

| TOT | SUN | MON | TUE | WED | THU | FRI | SAT | |
|---|---|---|---|---|---|---|---|---|
| 0.01 | 0.0 | 0.0 | 0.0 | 0.00 | 0.0 | 0.0 | 0.0 | AVG # OF OB TURNAWAYS |
| 0.00 | 0.0 | 0.0 | 0.0 | 0.00 | 0.0 | 0.0 | 0.0 | AVG # OF GYNS TO MED/SURG |
| 42.04 | 6.38 | 6.15 | 6.42 | 6.65 | 6.45 | 5.08 | 4.90 | AVG # OF ADMISSIONS |
| 42.00 | 5.81 | 5.97 | 5.64 | 5.90 | 6.19 | 6.19 | 6.28 | AVG # OF DISCHARGES |
| 22.60 | 21.86 | 22.04 | 22.82 | 23.57 | 23.83 | 22.72 | 21.34 | AVG # OF BEDS OCCUPIED |
| 0.63 | 0.61 | 0.61 | 0.63 | 0.65 | 0.66 | 0.63 | 0.59 | AVG % OF OCCUPANCY |

#### ···· ICU UNIT SUMMARY STATISTICS ····

| TOT | SUN | MON | TUE | WED | THU | FRI | SAT | |
|---|---|---|---|---|---|---|---|---|
| 0.00 | 0.0 | 0.17 | 0.17 | 0.16 | 0.18 | 0.13 | 0.15 | AVG # OF ICU TURNAWAYS |
| 1.12 | 0.14 | 0.17 | 0.01 | 0.13 | 0.13 | 0.13 | 0.04 | AVG # OF FORCED TRANSFERS |
| 0.38 | 0.03 | 0.02 | 0.01 | 0.03 | 0.03 | 0.05 | 0.04 | AVG # OF DELAY TRANSFERS TO MED/SUR |
| 0.24 | 0.03 | 0.02 | 0.00 | 0.03 | 0.02 | 0.04 | 0.03 | AVG # OF DELAY ADMITTANCES |
| 0.20 | 0.03 | 0.02 | 0.00 | 0.01 | 0.01 | 0.01 | 0.01 | DELAYED IN EMERGENCY HOLDING AREA |
| 0.04 | 0.0 | 0.0 | 0.0 | 0.0 | 0.0 | 0.0 | 0.01 | DELAYED ON MED/SURG UNIT |
| 0.0 | | | | | | | | AVG # OF IN-HOUSE ADMISSIONS |
| 14.02 | 2.04 | 2.13 | 1.99 | 1.90 | 1.84 | 2.13 | 1.98 | AVG # OF DIRECT ADMISSIONS |
| 13.00 | 1.84 | 1.84 | 1.78 | 1.86 | 1.79 | 1.98 | 1.89 | AVG # OF TRANSFERS TO MED/SURG |
| 11.80 | 11.73 | 11.85 | 11.93 | 11.88 | 11.74 | 11.76 | 11.69 | AVG # OF BEDS OCCUPIED |
| 0.74 | 0.73 | 0.74 | 0.75 | 0.74 | 0.73 | 0.74 | 0.73 | AVG % OCCUPANCY |

#### ···· EHA UNIT SUMMARY STATISTICS ····

| TOT | SUN | MON | TUE | WED | THU | FRI | SAT | |
|---|---|---|---|---|---|---|---|---|
| 0.09 | 0.03 | 0.07 | 0.17 | 0.18 | 0.09 | 0.04 | 0.03 | AVG # OF BEDS OCCUPIED—TOTAL |
| 0.04 | 0.01 | 0.04 | 0.08 | 0.09 | 0.04 | 0.02 | 0.02 | AVG % OCCUPANCY—TOTAL |
| 0.06 | 0.0 | 0.05 | 0.15 | 0.15 | 0.03 | 0.0 | 0.0 | AVG # OF BEDS OCCUPIED BY EMERGENCY PTS. |
| 0.03 | 0.03 | 0.02 | 0.07 | 0.07 | 0.03 | 0.04 | 0.03 | AVG % OF BEDS OCCUPIED BY EMERGENCY PTS. |
| 0.03 | 0.03 | 0.02 | 0.08 | 0.08 | 0.02 | 0.04 | 0.03 | AVG # OF BEDS OCCUPIED BY ICU PTS. |
| 0.02 | 0.01 | 0.01 | 0.01 | 0.02 | 0.01 | 0.02 | 0.02 | AVG % OF BEDS OCCUPIED BY ICU PTS. |

DISTRIBUTION OF EHA CENSUS

| ZERO | ONE | >TWO |
|---|---|---|
| 0.94 | 0.02 | 0.03 |

#### ···· WAITING LINE STATISTICS ····

| | | SURG | MED | RATIO |
|---|---|---|---|---|
| LENGTH OF WAITING LINE | INITIAL | 250.00 | 25.00 | |
| | AVERAGE | 250.55 | 49.34 | 5.08 |
| | END | 253.00 | 9.00 | |
| DELAY (DAYS) | INITIAL | 26.52 | 8.33 | |
| | AVERAGE | 26.57 | 5.45 | 4.88 |
| | END | 26.80 | 3.00 | |

*Figure 5.30*

*Summary of Output Using Initial Schedule*

$$OCM = 93$$
$$OCI = 74$$
$$OCO = 63$$
$$SCM = 0$$

| | | | |
|---|---|---|---|
| TUI = | .00 | $A_1 =$ | .2 |
| TUE = | .06 | $A_2 =$ | .5 |
| TUO = | .01 | $A_3 =$ | .2 |
| CAN = | .09 | $A_4 =$ | .5 |
| FAL = | .38 | $A_5 =$ | 2 |
| FOR = | 1.12 | $A_6 =$ | 1.5 |

method), or by devising an initial schedule "theoretically" (for example, setting the ER allowance to the 95th percentile of the distribution of ER arrivals, etc.). A combination of these two was used for the 300-bed hospital of our example (again see Hancock et al. for details). It was decided to begin the search holding the medical scheduling allowance at zero, and then slowly to increase it as the search through schedules progressed.

The initial schedule was first evaluated by the simulation program (see Figure 5.29). All results of Figure 5.29 are weekly, based on a simulation run of 200 weeks. Figure 5.30 summarizes the relevant portions for our objective function and constraints. Our initial schedule achieves very good objective (occupancies) while easily keeping within our constraints. The search for better schedules continues heuristically. Small changes are made in the allowances which intuitively suggest better results, and the new schedule is evaluated by the simulation model. It was decided (heuristically) first to make changes and evaluate until the constraint terms seemed as low as possible, keeping

*Figure 5.31*

*The Intermediate Schedule*

| | Sun | Mon | Tue | Wed | Thurs | Fri | Sat |
|---|---|---|---|---|---|---|---|
| Surgical Allowance | 17 | 13 | 12 | 12 | 13 | 0 | 0 |
| Medical Allowance | 0 | 0 | 0 | 0 | 0 | 0 | 0 |
| Census Reduction Allowance | 20 | 11 | 11 | 11 | 11 | 13 | 26 |
| Cancellation Allowance | 4 | 4 | 4 | 4 | 4 | 4 | 4 |
| Call-in Allowance | 8 | 8 | 8 | 8 | 8 | 8 | 8 |
| OB Allowance | 8 | 8 | 8 | 8 | 8 | 8 | 8 |
| Priorities | (No change) | | | | | | |

## Figure 5.32

### Baker Hospital Intermediate Solution

```
            ···· MS UNIT SUMMARY STATISTICS ····
  TOT     SUN     MON     TUE     WED     THU     FRI     SAT
  0.02    0.0     0.02    0.0     0.00    0.0     0.0     0.0    AVG # OF CANCELLATIONS
  0.17    0.0     0.04    0.08    0.03    0.01    0.0     0.0    AVG # OF EMG TURNAWAYS
  0.00    0.0     0.0     0.0     0.0     0.00    0.0     0.0    AVG # OF ICU TURNAWAYS
  0.0     0.0     0.0     0.0     0.0     0.0     0.0     0.0    AVG # OF GYN PTS. ADMITTED
 38.37    5.52    5.38    4.04    4.26    4.67    7.64    6.86   AVG # OF CALLIN PTS. ADMITTED
160.77   30.11   26.18   23.55   23.51   25.36   16.43   15.61  AVG # OF ADMISSIONS
160.81   20.59   16.23   22.38   23.91   25.31   25.68   26.69  AVG # OF DISCHARGES & TRANSFERS TO ICU/CCU
200.7   195.8   205.7   206.9   206.5   206.6   197.3   186.2   AVG # OF BEDS OCCUPIED
  0.94    0.91    0.96    0.97    0.96    0.97    0.92    0.87   AVG % OCCUPANCY

            ···· OB UNIT SUMMARY STATISTICS ····
  TOT     SUN     MON     TUE     WED     THU     FRI     SAT
  0.08    0.0     0.02    0.01    0.0     0.03    0.00    0.01   AVG # OF OB TURNAWAYS
  0.0     0.0     0.0     0.0     0.0     0.0     0.0     0.0    AVG # OF GYNS TO MED/SURG
 42.36    6.34    6.32    6.42    6.48    6.38    5.38    5.03   AVG # OF ADMISSIONS
 42.32    5.92    6.10    6.19    5.94    5.79    6.22    6.15   AVG # OF DISCHARGES
 22.49   21.97   22.20   22.43   22.97   23.56   22.71   21.59  AVG # OF BEDS OCCUPIED
  0.62    0.61    0.62    0.62    0.64    0.65    0.63    0.60   AVG % OCCUPANCY

            ···· ICU UNIT SUMMARY STATISTICS ····
  TOT     SUN     MON     TUE     WED     THU     FRI     SAT
  0.00    0.0     0.0     0.0     0.0     0.00    0.0     0.0    AVG # OF ICU TURNAWAYS
  1.01    0.16    0.20    0.12    0.17    0.13    0.13    0.09   AVG # OF FORCED TRANSFERS
  0.12    0.0     0.02    0.03    0.04    0.02    0.0     0.0    AVG # OF DELAY TRANSFERS TO MED/SUR

  0.24    0.01    0.02    0.03    0.05    0.05    0.04    0.03   AVG # OF DELAY ADMITTANCES
  0.16    0.01    0.02    0.02    0.03    0.03    0.02    0.01   DELAYED IN EMERGENCY HOLDING AREA
  0.08    0.0     0.0     0.00    0.02    0.02    0.02    0.01   DELAYED ON MED/SURG UNIT

  0.0     0.0     0.0     0.0     0.0     0.0     0.0     0.0    AVG # OF IN-HOUSE ADMISSIONS
 13.70    2.06    2.01    1.95    1.92    1.71    2.06    1.99   AVG # OF DIRECT ADMISSIONS
 12.85    1.64    1.80    1.84    1.72    1.97    1.88    1.98   AVG # OF TRANSFERS TO MED/SURG
 11.82   11.86   11.89   11.96   12.02   11.65   11.70   11.63  AVG # OF BEDS OCCUPIED
  0.74    0.74    0.74    0.75    0.75    0.73    0.73    0.73   AVG % OCCUPANCY

            ···· EHA UNIT SUMMARY STATISTICS ····
  TOT     SUN     MON     TUE     WED     THU     FRI     SAT
  0.09    0.01    0.10    0.22    0.15    0.10    0.02    0.01   AVG # OF BEDS OCCUPIED   TOTAL
  0.05    0.01    0.05    0.11    0.08    0.05    0.01    0.01   AVG % OCCUPANCY—TOTAL
  0.07    0.0     0.08    0.19    0.12    0.07    0.0     0.0    AVG # OF BEDS OCCUPIED BY EMERGENCY PTS.
  0.03    0.0     0.04    0.10    0.06    0.04    0.0     0.0    AVG % BEDS OCCUPIED BY EMERGENCY PTS.
  0.02    0.01    0.02    0.02    0.03    0.03    0.02    0.01   AVG # OF BEDS OCCUPIED BY ICU PTS.
  0.01    0.01    0.01    0.01    0.02    0.01    0.01    0.01   AVG % OF BEDS OCCUPIED BY ICU PTS.

DISTRIBUTION OF EHA CENSUS
 ZERO    ONE    >TWO
 0.94    0.03    0.03
                        ···· WAITING LINE STATISTICS ····
                                             SURG     MED     RATIO
            LENGTH OF      INITIAL          250.00   25.00
            WAITING        AVERAGE          251.23   51.16    4.91
            LINE           END              255.00   11.00

            DELAY          INITIAL           26.52    8.33
            (DAYS)         AVERAGE           27.11    5.98    4.53
                           END               26.98    1.08
```

MED/SURG occupancy to 94 percent and keeping the scheduled medical allowance at zero.

Experience with the simulation showed that MED/SURG, OB, and ICU/CCU occupancy did not compete with one another in any significant way, allowing us to avoid the quantification of $C_1'$ and $C_2'$.

After evaluating approximately twelve schedules, the *intermediate* schedule of Figure 5.31 was determined, which seemed to come significantly close to minimizing the constraint factors while keeping OCM to 94 percent; its full evaluation is in Figure 5.32. Next, the initial medical allowance of Figure 5.33 was determined analytically (details in Hancock et al.). A second search through approximately twelve more schedules produced the final schedule of Figure 5.34 and its evaluation (Figure 5.35) which is summarized in Figure 5.36. It was found, incidentally, that SCM($S$) did not compete with OCM($S$)—they actually complemented one another—allowing the avoidance of the quantification of $C_3'$.

## Figure 5.33

### The Medical Allowance

|                  | Sun | Mon | Tue | Wed | Thurs | Fri | Sat |
|------------------|-----|-----|-----|-----|-------|-----|-----|
| Medical Allowance | 2   | 2   | 1   | 1   | 2     | 7   | 4   |

## Figure 5.34

### The Final Schedule

|                              | Sun | Mon | Tue | Wed | Thurs | Fri | Sat |
|------------------------------|-----|-----|-----|-----|-------|-----|-----|
| Surgical Allowance           | 17  | 12  | 12  | 12  | 13    | 0   | 0   |
| Medical Allowance            | 2   | 2   | 2   | 2   | 2     | 7   | 4   |
| Census Reduction Allowance   | 20  | 11  | 11  | 11  | 11    | 13  | 26  |
| Cancellation Allowance       | 3   | 3   | 3   | 3   | 3     | 3   | 3   |
| Call-in Allowance            | 10  | 10  | 10  | 10  | 10    | 10  | 10  |
| OB Allowance                 | 8   | 8   | 8   | 8   | 8     | 8   | 8   |
| Priorities                   | (No change) | | | | | | |

## Figure 5.35

### Baker Hospital Final Solution

```
                •••• MS UNIT SUMMARY STATISTICS ••••
TOT      SUN     MON     TUE     WED     THU     FRI     SAT
0.28     0.0     0.07    0.06    0.06    0.08    0.0     0.0     AVG # OF CANCELLATIONS
0.49     0.02    0.06    0.19    0.15    0.06    0.0     0.0     AVG # OF EMG TURNAWAYS
0.01     0.0     0.0     0.0     0.00    0.00    0.0     0.0     AVG # OF ICU TURNAWAYS
0.00     0.0     0.0     0.0     0.0     0.00    0.0     0.0     AVG # OF GYN PTS. ADMITTED
22.45    2.35    3.25    2.25    2.67    2.97    5.71    3.24    AVG # OF CALLIN PTS. ADMITTED
163.34   28.61   24.42   23.16   23.95   25.51   21.70   15.98   AVG # OF ADMISSIONS
163.31   21.02   16.77   22.35   24.11   25.51   26.69   26.84   AVG # OF DISCHARGES & TRANSFERS TO ICU/CCU
204.3    200.2   207.9   208.7   208.5   208.5   203.5   192.7   AVG # OF BEDS OCCUPIED
0.95     0.94    0.97    0.98    0.97    0.97    0.95    0.90    AVG % OCCUPANCY

                •••• OB UNIT SUMMARY STATISTICS ••••
TOT      SUN     MON     TUE     WED     THU     FRI     SAT
0.11     0.00    0.0     0.01    0.02    0.04    0.03    0.0     AVG # OF OB TURNAWAYS
0.00     0.0     0.0     0.0     0.0     0.00    0.0     0.0     AVG # OF GYNS TO MED/SURG
42.19    6.36    5.92    6.51    6.88    6.32    5.21    4.98    AVG # OF ADMISSIONS
42.16    5.97    6.02    6.13    5.85    5.73    6.16    6.29    AVG # OF DISCHARGES
22.61    22.04   21.93   22.32   23.84   23.94   22.99   21.68   AVG # OF BEDS OCCUPIED
0.63     0.61    0.61    0.62    0.65    0.66    0.64    0.60    AVG % OCCUPANCY

                •••• ICU UNIT SUMMARY STATISTICS ••••
TOT      SUN     MON     TUE     WED     THU     FRI     SAT
0.01     0.0     0.0     0.0     0.00    0.00    0.0     0.0     AVG # OF ICU TURNAWAYS
1.39     0.16    0.25    0.23    0.25    0.18    0.17    0.13    AVG # OF FORCED TRANSFERS
0.46     0.00    0.07    0.11    0.16    0.12    0.0     0.0     AVG # OF DELAY TRANSFERS TO MED/SUR

0.14     0.01    0.01    0.02    0.04    0.01    0.01    0.02    AVG # OF DELAY ADMITTANCES
0.14     0.01    0.01    0.02    0.04    0.01    0.01    0.02    DELAYED IN EMERGENCY HOLDING AREA
0.0      0.0     0.0     0.0     0.0     0.0     0.0     0.0     DELAYED ON MED/SURG UNIT

0.0      0.0     0.0     0.0     0.0     0.0     0.0     0.0     AVG # OF IN-HOUSE ADMISSIONS
13.83    2.05    2.10    1.98    1.89    1.75    2.09    1.96    AVG # OF DIRECT ADMISSIONS
13.09    1.84    1.75    1.73    1.65    2.06    2.08    1.97    AVG # OF TRANSFERS TO MED/SURG
11.92    11.71   11.93   12.11   12.25   11.97   11.81   11.67   AVG # OF BEDS OCCUPIED
0.75     0.73    0.75    0.76    0.77    0.75    0.74    0.73    AVG % OCCUPANCY

                •••• EHA UNIT SUMMARY STATISTICS ••••
TOT      SUN     MON     TUE     WED     THU     FRI     SAT
0.24     0.07    0.32    0.47    0.41    0.36    0.03    0.02    AVG # OF BEDS OCCUPIED—TOTAL
0.12     0.04    0.16    0.23    0.20    0.18    0.02    0.01    AVG % OCCUPANCY—TOTAL
0.22     0.06    0.30    0.44    0.36    0.34    0.02    0.0     AVG # OF BEDS OCCUPIED BY EMERGENCY PTS.
0.11     0.03    0.15    0.22    0.18    0.17    0.01    0.0     AVG % OF BEDS OCCUPIED BY EMERGENCY PTS.
0.02     0.01    0.01    0.02    0.04    0.01    0.01    0.02    AVG # OF BEDS OCCUPIED BY ICU PTS.
0.01     0.00    0.01    0.01    0.02    0.01    0.01    0.01    AVG % OF BEDS OCCUPIED BY ICU PTS.

DISTRIBUTION OF EHA CENSUS
ZERO     ONE     >TWO
0.86     0.04    0.10
                                •••• WAITING LINE STATISTICS ••••
                                              SURG     MED     RATIO
                        LENGTH OF   INITIAL   250.00   25.00
                        WAITING     AVERAGE   248.71   28.77   8.64
                        LINE        END       244.00   10.00

                        DELAY       INITIAL   26.52    8.33
                        (DAYS)      AVERAGE   25.51    4.36    5.85
                                    END       27.73    3.81
```

*Figure 5.36*

*Summary of Output Using Final Schedule*

OCM = 95
OCI = 75
OCO = 63
SCM = 21

| TUI = | .01 | $(A_1 = .2)$ |
|-------|------|------------------|
| TUE = | .49 | $(A_2 = .5)$ |
| TUO = | .11 | $(A_3 = .2)$ |
| CAN = | .28 | $(A_4 = .5)$ |
| FAL = | .46 | $(A_5 = 2 \; )$ |
| FOR = | 1.39 | $(A_6 = 1.5)$ |
| RAT = | 5.85 | $(4 \le RAT \le 6)$ |

Part of the sensitivity analysis had been made concurrently with the heuristic searches: each new run gave more information about possible trade-offs among the constraint elements, and between those elements and OCM($S$). For example, the trade-off between cancellations and ER turnaways was almost completely determined by the cancellation allowance, trade-offs between occupancy and cancellations almost completely determined by the reduction allowance, etc. Such trade-offs became a major element governing the heuristic search.

A second type of sensitivity is sensitivity to the length of the simulation run, i.e., sensitivity of results to the shape of certain of the arrival distributions, and to certain of the assumptions made in building the simulation program. These are detailed by Hancock et al., but Figure 5.37 summarizes the range of error due to "run variance" (measured by running the same schedule with different sets of random numbers).

The final schedule was implemented in the study hospital with very good results. In fact, the hospital was able to out-perform the simulation, being able to make last minute "fine tuning" adjustments on a day-by-day basis. The system has also been implemented in other hospitals.

The cost of the analysis for the initial hospital was considerable. Devising the system took more than two man-years. Writing the

*Figure 5.37*

*Sensitivity to Simulation Error*

OCM ± .5
CAN ± .2
TUE ± .2
TUI ± .01

FORTRAN computer program and debugging it took approximately ten more man-months. Gathering the data took another two man-months for the first hospital; however, data collection for subsequent hospitals took less than two weeks. The computer runs themselves were relatively inexpensive (about $5 per run), and related analysis time by the experienced team was less than two weeks. Thus while the cost of the first analysis was rather expensive, subsequent analyses were done with approximately one man-month of time and $200 in computer cost.

Now consider the benefits. Reduction of cancellations, turnaways, and failed transfers must be subjectively evaluated, but the value of the increased revenue to the hospital from higher occupancy is considerable. (Note that this must be taken as a proxy for the benefit to the community: the real benefit to the community is more efficient use of fixed resources which should in turn result in lower costs.)

## 5.6 A PLANNING EXAMPLE:
### ADMISSIONS SCHEDULING EXTENDED

The admissions scheduling example deals with a hospital whose beds are fixed in number and in configuration (that is, the number of beds assigned to medical, to surgical, to OB, etc.). A related problem is faced when a hospital

—must close beds because of a reduction of patient flow,

—must open beds because of an increase, or

—must shift beds from one service to another.

These decisions are major ones, because of both the amount of resources involved and the effect on physician behavior. A careful analysis is required to determine how many, if any, beds to close, open, or shift, and which ones are to be affected.

The Hospital Inpatient Census Control (HICC) model was developed as an extension to admission scheduling to address just these decisions. The model allows a hospital to define up to 30 types of patients (pediatric, orthopedic, neurosurgery, medical oncology, etc.), each divided into emergency, urgent, and elective arrival components. The hospital's nursing units are divided into as many as 30 units (not necessarily the same as the 30 patient types), up to 10 of which can be special care units (ICU, CCU, Burn Unit, etc.).

As in admission scheduling, arrival patterns for each type of patient by day of week, as well as length of stay, admission and transfer priorities, preference of unit by type of patient, etc., are gathered from hospital data sources (usually already on computer tape) and established for a base year. When the HICC model is run on this base year, activities of the base year are simulated, giving occupancy, turnaway, cancellation, and transfer implications.

The power of the model lies in its ability to facilitate development and evaluation of different scenarios involving closing, opening, or shifting of beds, and to evaluate the effects of predicted changes in patient flow. For example, once a base year's data are developed and the model is verified for that year, estimates of changes in patient arrival patterns are made. Let's say that for each patient type, a percentage change in arrival rates is determined from trend analysis and from talking with the clinical directors. These new arrival rates (say, for next year) are entered and a new data file called "next year" is created and stored. When run on the "next year" scenario, the HICC model predicts the effect on occupancy, turnaways, cancellations, transfers, etc., of changes in arrival patterns.

Using this information, the model can easily evaluate new scenarios involving bed shifting (say, take ten beds from pediatrics and move them to medical, close one of the surgical units, etc.). An "inventory" of scenarios, all saved on computer files, is developed over time; from this inventory new scenarios can be developed when new situations or questions arise.

The HICC model has been used to analyze such situations in several hospitals over the past few years, and has become a working part of the internal planning function for some of these installations.

## Exercises

5.1 Choose any flow process in a health care institution or organization (e.g., lab tests in lab, patients in neighborhood health clinic, patients in emergency room), and consider it as a queueing process.

a. Draw a detailed flow diagram showing
   —queues
   —servers
   —flow relationship between queues and servers.

b. Comment on the nature of
   —the arrival distribution to each service
   —the service time at each service
   —the service discipline
   —the maximum number of items or people that can be in the queueing system(s) at any one time.

c. How would you go about measuring the distributions in part b?

   d. Can this queue be "solved" analytically using queueing theory? Under what circumstances and making what simplifying assumptions? Comment on the usefulness of such a solution, if one is possible.

5.2 In planning a new hospital, a question arises concerning the number of emergency room (ER) physicians (and thus exam rooms, equipment, etc.) to make available around the clock to serve ER patients. A study indicates that the ER will serve about 8,750 patients a year for the next few years. Your quantitative specialist finds a study done at another hospital which had 17,500 arrivals last year. For the 200 hours over which the study was done at this hospital last year, the following distribution of the number of arrivals per hour was observed:

| Number arriving per hour | Number of hours observed |
|---|---|
| 0 | 30 |
| 1 | 50 |
| 2 | 58 |
| 3 | 34 |
| 4 | 17 |
| 5 | 10 |
| 6 | 1 |

Another study indicated that it took 30 minutes to examine and treat the average ER patient.

   a. What assumptions are necessary to use mathematically solvable queueing theory to analyze the decision?

   b. Make the necessary assumptions and provide as much data as possible upon which to base a decision.

5.3 Patient arrivals at your walk-in outpatient clinic follow a Poisson arrival process with $\lambda = 2$ per half hour. The Poisson distribution with $\lambda = 2$ is as follows:

| Number of arrivals per half hour | Probability |
|---|---|
| 0 | .13 |
| 1 | .27 |
| 2 | .27 |
| 3 | .18 |
| 4 | .09 |
| 5 | .04 |
| 6 | .02 |

The distribution of time required in an exam room is as follows:

| Hours | Probability |
|-------|-------------|
| .25   | .2          |
| .50   | .4          |
| .75   | .2          |
| 1.00  | .2          |

a. What criteria would you use to decide the number of exam rooms to provide? Which can be predicted from a simulation?

b. Use the random number table in the text to perform an 8 hour (16 half hour) simulation. How many exam rooms would you recommend? Why?

5.4 Patient arrivals at your hospital's two labor rooms occur according to the following distribution:

| Patients per hour | Probability of occurrence | Cumulative probability |
|-------------------|---------------------------|------------------------|
| 0                 | .755                      | .755                   |
| 1                 | .230                      | .985                   |
| 2                 | .015                      | 1.000                  |
| 3 or more         | .000                      | 1.000                  |

Patient stay in a labor room has the following distribution:

| Hours | Probability | Cumulative probability |
|-------|-------------|------------------------|
| 0     | .189        | .189                   |
| 1     | .133        | .322                   |
| 2     | .098        | .420                   |
| 3     | .131        | .551                   |
| 4     | .089        | .640                   |
| 5     | .047        | .687                   |
| 6     | .057        | .744                   |
| 7     | .041        | .785                   |
| 8     | .040        | .825                   |
| 9     | .003        | .828                   |
| 10    | .069        | .897                   |
| 11    | .017        | .914                   |
| 12    | .030        | .944                   |
| 13    | .016        | .960                   |
| 14    | .022        | .982                   |
| 15    | .008        | .990                   |
| 16    | .010        | 1.000                  |

Using a random number table, simulate the utilization of the two labor rooms for a start-up period of 24 hours, and then for another 72 hours of routine operation. Use the rooms in order (i.e., number them 1 and 2 and always place the arriving patient in the lowest numbered room which is vacant).

a. How many patients went through the system during start-up? During routine operation? What is the average occupancy (utilization) of each room during start-up? During the routine operation?

b. How many patients were forced to wait? What was the average waiting time for patients who had to wait? (Divide your analysis between start-up and routine time.)

c. What would have been the case if there were three rooms to meet the demand?

d. In what ways is the simulation unrealistic?

5.5 Use simulation to analyze Problem 5.2 by making two runs, each 24 hours long.

5.6 Suppose in Problem 5.2 that 50% of ER patients arrive between 4 P.M. and 12 midnight. Simulate a 24 hour day where there is one ER physician on duty between 12 midnight and 4 P.M., and two physicians between 4 P.M. and midnight.

5.7 You are the administrator of a 400-bed hospital in a metropolitan area of approximately 2 million people. Your hospital currently operates a small outpatient clinic where, at present, four physicians (aided by two RNs) see patients from 8:00 A.M. to 11:30 A.M. weekdays. The doctors are paid a flat fee per shift. Patients on their first visit to the clinic arrive on a "walk in" basis, but on subsequent visits they are usually given a future date on which they should come in. There is also a receiving clerk who takes demographic information from the patients, arranges schedules, and assigns patients to an appropriate physician. Four GPs cover the clinic so that two are on duty each day. The RNs are called on by the physicians as they are needed, and otherwise "stand by."

Having operated the clinic for three years, you are aware of the following:

—*Overall* demand for clinic services has been increasing on the order of 10% per year, and you expect it to continue increasing at this rate for the next five years.

—Some physicians complain that, at times, they are "wasting

their time" on clinic duties because they are idle; other times they are concerned because they are overloaded.

—Some physicians say that they are idle at times waiting for an RN; others say that the RNs are less productive here than on the wards, "where they are needed."

—Patients complain that they must wait for two or three hours to see a physician, and indeed sometimes have to return the following day after waiting past 11:30.

a. State appropriate overall objectives for the walk-in clinic. What are the costs associated with idle time? Are there "costs" associated with overflows, turnaways and patient delays? Can you measure these costs?

b. What are the decision variables (alternatives) of this problem?

c. How can simulation be used as an aid in the analysis of the problem?

d. What inputs must be supplied to the simulation analysis? What information would you expect to get as output from the simulation analysis?

e. If the clinic offers specialty physician care in the future, this will certainly complicate the scheduling problem. Would you wish to use simulation to analyze this situation? What new data would be required?

f. Do you think that the cost of a simulation analysis can be justified in the analysis of the clinic? (Why? Or why not?)

5.8 Your hospital's radiology department has six examining rooms, three of which have special equipment for non-routine examinations. The department does routine and non-routine exams on inpatients (emergency and non-emergency) and outpatients (emergency and non-emergency). Manpower to run the lab includes

      2 full time radiologists
      8 full time technologists (1 is chief technologist)
      4 medical secretaries
      2 clerks

The lab runs 8:00–4:30 daily, with stat coverage on evenings, nights and weekends (a technologist on duty, and a radiologist on call). Your opinion is that the present demand is beginning to tax the present capacity of the lab. Furthermore, a consulting firm gives you forecasts of a 20 percent growth in demand over the next ten years, most of it outpatient.

Other facts:

—The head of your management engineering group, who has just completed a study of the lab, points out the high efficiency of resource use, citing as evidence very low idle times for both equipment and personnel.

—Patients (especially outpatients) have been known to complain about quite long waits. ("This is the price you have to pay for efficiency: we want to minimize costs in this hospital," says the management engineer.)

—Some of your high-volume physicians complain of delay in getting reports back on inpatients. They sometimes must call down for results, which disturbs them and the radiologist as well.

—Your management engineering team suggests that since demand will increase by 20 percent over the next ten years, the hospital should plan on a 20 percent increase in facilities to keep up with demand but not to lose the current high efficiency in resource use.

a. Carefully formulate the objectives of the lab. Suggest measures of performance for each objective. Be specific.

b. What would you consider as decision variables in the *resource-size* portion (i.e., not scheduling) of the problem?

c. Construct a total cost equation of the resource-size problem. Be specific, showing the makeup of each component of the equation.

d. Discuss how you would go about measuring *each part* of each component of the TC equation (HINT: consider simulation).

e. Assume you are to use simulation. Discuss the *inputs* necessary to perform the simulation. Include how you would obtain the inputs.

f. What are the *outputs* you would expect from the simulation?

g. Can you justify simulation analysis in this problem? (How?)

h. How do you deal with the increasing demand question?

i. Discuss how you might use simulation to analyze different scheduling schemes. Include typical scheduling schemes you might consider.

5.9 Discuss the reasons why the queueing analysis of obstetrics (Tables 5.4 through 5.7) is different from the simulation analysis (Table 5.11). Why would you expect more agreement on some of the four phases (labor, delivery, recovery, postpartum) than on others? Discuss each phase separately.

## Additional Reading

*Technique*

Churchman, C. W., Ackoff, R. L. and Arnoff, E. L. *Introduction to Operations Research.* New York: John Wiley and Sons, 1957.

Warner, D. Michael. "Simulated Waiting Times for Certain Poisson Arrival, Gamma Service, Multiple Service Queueing Systems." Working Paper. Durham, N.C.: Department of Health Administration, Duke University, 1976.

Hillier, F. S. and Lieberman, G. J. *Introduction to Operations Research.* San Francisco: Holden-Day, 1974.

Naylor, T. H., Balintfy, J. L., Burdick, D. S. and Chu, K. *Computer Simulation Techniques.* New York: John Wiley and Sons, 1966.

Wagner, H. M. *Principles of Operations Research With Applications to Managerial Decisions.* Englewood Cliffs, N.J.: Prentice-Hall, 1969.

*Reviews of Applications*

Shuman, L. J., Speas, R. D. and Young, J. P. *Operations Research in Health Care.* Baltimore: Johns Hopkins Press, 1975.

Stimson, D. H. and Stimson, R. H. *Operations Research in Hospitals.* Chicago: Hospital Research and Educational Trust, 1972.

*Resource-Size Applications*

Goldman, J., Knappenberger, H. A. and Eller, J. C. "Evaluating Bed Allocation Policy with Computer Simulation." *Health Services Research,* Summer 1968, pp. 119–129.

Fetter, R. B. and Thompson, J. D. "Patient's Waiting Time and Doctor's Idle Time in the Outpatient Setting." *Health Services Research,* Summer 1966, pp. 66–90.

*Scheduling Applications*

Barnoon, S. and Wolfe, H. "Scheduling a Multiple Operating Room System: A Simulation Approach." *Health Services Research,* Winter 1968, pp. 272–285.

Briggs, G. *Inpatient Admissions Scheduling: Application to a Nursing Service.* Ph.D. dissertation, University of Michigan, 1971.

Hancock, W. M., Warner, D. M., Heda, S. and Fuhs, P. "Admissions Scheduling and Control Systems." In *Cost Control in Hospitals*, edited by John R. Griffith, Walton M. Hancock, and Fred C. Munson. Ann Arbor, Michigan: Health Administration Press, 1976.

Milsum, J. H., Turban, E. and Vertinsky, I. "Hospital Admission Systems: Their Evaluation and Management." *Management Science* 19 (February 1973): 646–666.

*Resource Size and Scheduling Combined*

Perry, P. "A Scheduling and Resource Allocation Model for a Radiology Department." In *Cost Control in Hospitals*, edited by John R. Griffith, Walton M. Hancock, and Fred C. Munson. Ann Arbor, Michigan: Health Administration Press, 1976.

Savas, E. S. "Simulation and Cost Effectiveness Analysis of New York's Emergency Ambulance Service." *Management Science* 15 (1969): B608–B627.

# 6

# Complex Deterministic Analysis

## 6.1 Introduction

There are two general types of complexity in the quantitative decision-making process. The first type of complexity occurs in the quantification step (Step 2), and we addressed it in the preceding chapter. The second is in the solution step, which is the focus of this chapter. This second complexity lies in the frequent existence of a very large number of alternatives from which the best is to be chosen. In most of the examples of Chapters 4 and 5 the solution step was straightforward because we had only one decision variable that took on only a small number of possible values. We were able to use the approximation or trial-and-error solution technique only because the number of alternatives was so limited. In the last chapter, we began to see the number of alternatives grow very rapidly. The OB merger problem, for example, had four decision variables: the number of labor beds (L), delivery beds (D), recovery beds (R), and postpartum beds (P). Each of these could take on several values —let's say they can take on values of 3, 4, 4, and 10, respectively. This means that there are $3 \times 4 \times 4 \times 10 = 480$ alternative configurations from which to choose the "best." Of course, we would normally try to reduce this number by ruling out certain values for each decision variable and/or by trying to analyze the four segments individually. Ideally, if a method that was not prohibitively time-consuming existed to evaluate all 480 (and even more) alternatives, we should employ it. For the OB problem no such method exists. (The same is true for the admissions scheduling problem, for which the number of theoretical alternative configurations is larger than $10^{30}$.) In these cases we must do what we did for the admissions scheduling problem: try to devise some heuristic scheme of intelligently searching through only a small set of alternatives to reach a "good" one, one with which we are satisfied.

There are some decisions, however, that lend themselves to a technique that allows the implicit evaluation of *all* alternatives and the identification of the "best" or optimal one, even though the number of alternatives is very large (even infinite). The technique is called, generally, *mathematical programming* (MP)—with linear programming, nonlinear programming, integer programming, transportation problems, and assignment problems as special cases. Although MP can be used to consider the stochastic nature of some decisions in a very limited sense (stochastic programming), we will not investigate this usage here; the interested reader is referred to any of the texts at the end of the chapter. Thus, the analysis in this chapter will be deterministic in nature. The reader should be alert to the important limiting assumptions necessary in many cases to make the analysis deterministic, and to what such assumptions "cost" in the way of limiting the usefulness of the results.

Much of MP involves mathematical sophistication that is beyond the scope of this text. We will focus heavily only on those parts of the analysis in which the administrator plays a dominant role: formulation (Step 1), evaluation of the results (including consideration of the limitations of MP and its assumptions), and, in general, the "management" of the analysis. We will examine the technical side only to gain an appreciation of the technique rather than attempt to equip the reader as a technical specialist. We begin with the type of MP easiest to formulate and solve: linear programming (LP). In Section 6.2 we will formulate problems and examine assumptions necessary to formulation, and in Sections 6.3 and 6.4 we will examine two approaches toward the solution of the formulation (i.e., identifying the optimal alternative). Then, in Section 6.5 we will look at other special cases of MP, focusing primarily on formulation. Finally, in the last section we look at several complete MP analyses which have been applied in the health field.

## 6.2 PROBLEM FORMULATION

It will be useful to view the processes for which decisions will be made in a "production" framework, as in Figure 6.1; resources, as inputs, are converted to outputs with "technology." For example, we can very generally view the hospital as a system in which resources (beds, personnel, equipment) are converted into a product, i.e., a change in health status for the discharged patient. On a smaller scale,

*Figure 6.1*

*The Production Process*

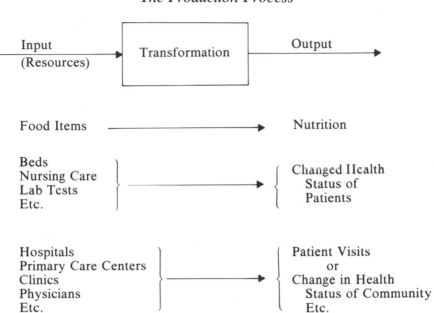

the dietary department might view its process as one in which different combinations and amounts of food items, as resources, are converted to nutrition—the product, or output. On a larger scale, the community health planner might regard community health production as the process in which physicians, nurses, other health personnel, clinics, hospitals, emergency facilities, etc., are converted to patient visits, discharges, etc., as the outputs. There are two ways to view decisions within this production framework:

—maximizing some expression of output, subject to using a fixed amount of resources, or

—minimizing the cost (of resources) of producing a fixed level of output.

(It is also possible to combine the two, as we will see below.)

## Maximizing Output Formulation

**Problem:** A hospital in a large metropolitan area is just about to open an additional 100 medical/surgical beds, making its total medical/surgical bed complement 400. It has not added additional operating rooms, laboratory, or X-ray facilities because none of these was being used to capacity with the present 300 beds, and it did not seem at the time that the 100-bed addition would overtax these services. The hospital and the medical staff have the ability to decide how the new beds will be used (what portion medical and what portion surgical), which depends on whom they add to the medical staff, the quotas per physician or service, etc. The problem is deciding how many of the additional 100 beds *should* be used for medical patients, and how many for surgical patients.

In the production framework we can regard the resources as (1) additional annual patient days available (the total is $100 \times 365$), (2) number of additional laboratory examinations that can be performed, (3) number of additional X-ray examinations that can be performed, and (4) number of additional surgical procedures that can be performed. (There are, of course, many other resources involved, but for the purpose of the example we will assume these are the relevant ones. Also, these four may not be completely fixed, although we will assume this to be the case for the present.)

What are the outputs? One might be the change in health status of discharged patients. A more easily measured output is the number of patients, medical and surgical, that can be treated by the additional 100 beds.

Let $M$ be the number of medical and $S$ be the number of surgical patients discharged annually from the 100 beds. (This formulation was developed by Dowling; see reference in Additional Reading.) Our objective function in this type of formulation is

$$\text{Maximize } Z\ (M,S),$$

where $Z$ is some appropriate function of $M$ and $S$. One function might be revenue. If the average medical patient generates \$2,000 revenue and the average surgical patient generates \$1,000, then we may want to

$$\text{Maximize } \$2,000M + \$1,000S.$$

Another possibility is simply to maximize the number of patients treated: $M + S$. There are many others. Let's adopt the revenue objective for our example.

The number of $M$ and $S$ that can be treated is limited by the available resources that they will consume. We know we have only 36,500 patient days available. If the average medical length of stay is 10 days and the average surgical length of stay is 6, then the following *constraint* must hold:

$$10M + 6S \le 36,500. \qquad \text{(B)}$$

If we use all the beds for medical patients, we can produce $36,500/10$ = 3,650 medical discharges generating $3,650 \times \$2,000 = \$7,300,000$ in revenue. If we use all beds for surgical patients, we can produce $36,500/6 = 6,083$ discharges generating $6,083 \times \$1,000 = \$6,083,000$. From the bed constraint alone, it looks as if we would be better off designating all beds as medical. (Would some combination of $M$ and $S$ give us higher revenue?)

There are other constraints, however. Suppose that a study of the laboratory sets the number of additional tests that could be handled there at 9,500 per year. Suppose further that the average $M$ uses 3 lab tests and the average $S$ only 1. Thus a second constraint on $M$ and $S$ is

$$3M + 1S \le 9,500. \qquad \text{(L)}$$

Now what combination of $M$ and $S$ generates the most revenue? There are two more constraints to add. Suppose the average $S$ uses 1.1 X-ray examinations per stay and the average $M$ uses 2.1, and that there is a maximum of 9,000 examinations per year available for the patients of the additional 100 beds. Finally, suppose there are only 3,500 additional surgical procedures that can be performed, and the average surgical patient uses 1 procedure (medical patients use none).

We can now state the complete problem:

*decision variables:* $M$ and $S$

*objective function:* Maximize $\$2,000M + \$1,000S$

$$\text{constraints} \begin{cases} \text{subject to:} & 10M + 6S \le 36,500 \quad \text{(B)} \\ & 3M + 1S \le 9,500 \quad \text{(L)} \\ & 2.1M + 1.1S \le 9,000 \quad \text{(R)} \\ & 0M + 1S \le 3,500. \quad \text{(U)} \end{cases}$$

Since we are considering only positive values for $S$ and $M$, we must add

$$constraints \begin{cases} \text{subject to:} & S \geq 0 \\ & M \geq 0. \end{cases}$$

Defining the problem in this way puts it in the mathematical programming formulation. To solve the formulation, we need to find values for $M$ and $S$ that simultaneously satisfy the six constraints *and* maximize $Z = 2,000M + 1,000S$. Before investigating how to solve this problem for optimal $M$ and $S$, we need to look at the second type of formulation.

## Minimizing Cost of Resources

**Problem:** The dietary department of a hospital feels that patients on a "regular" diet should obtain the following amount of nutrition daily:

—between 2,600 and 4,000 calories,
—at least 72 grams of protein,
—no more than 100 grams of fat, and
—at least 12 mg of iron.

(There would be other requirements, but these will suffice for our example.) The dietary department (let's suppose) has eight food items it can serve to meet these requirements. The cost per pound of each food item and its contribution to each of the four nutritional requirements are given in Figure 6.2 (the figures are not actual). What combination and amounts of the food items will provide the nutritional requirements *at lowest food cost*?

In this type of formulation, our decision variables are the resources—the eight food items. Let $X_i$ (where $i = 1$ to 8) be the amounts (in lbs.) of each food item to include in the diet. Let $C_i$ be the cost of item $i$ (per lb.). Then our objective function is

$$\text{Min} \sum_i C_i X_i.$$

To guarantee that the minimum amount of calories is provided, we require that

$860X_1 + 440X_2 + 500X_3 + 310X_4 + 280X_5 + 140X_6 + 402X_7 + 613X_8$

$\geq 2,600.$

## Figure 6.2

## Nutritional Requirements

| $i$ | $(X_i)$ Food Item | $(C_i)$ Cost/lb | $(a_{i1})$ Calories/lb | $(a_{i2})$ Protein/lb | $(a_{i3})$ Fat/lb | $(a_{i4})$ Iron/lb |
|---|---|---|---|---|---|---|
| 1 | Flour | .20 | 860 | 15 | 16 | 3 |
| 2 | Milk | .30 | 440 | 31 | 39 | 6 |
| 3 | Beef | 1.40 | 500 | 60 | 110 | 10 |
| 4 | Chicken | .50 | 310 | 63 | 84 | 14 |
| 5 | Kidney Beans | .10 | 280 | 51 | 12 | 8 |
| 6 | Spinach | .18 | 140 | 41 | 4 | 12 |
| 7 | Fish | .68 | 402 | 78 | 34 | 18 |
| 8 | Potatoes | .08 | 613 | 30 | 20 | 4 |

Let $j$ index the nutrients, and let $a_{ij}$ be the amount that each pound of food item $i$ contributes to nutrient $j$. For example, $j = 1$ refers to the calories, and $a_{11} = 860$, $a_{22} = 31$, etc. We can restate the constraint as

$$\sum_i a_{i1} X_i \geq 2{,}600.$$

We can state the maximum calories constraint as

$$\sum_i a_{i1} X_i \leq 4{,}000.$$

Also

$$\sum_i a_{i2} X_i \geq 72$$

$$\sum_i a_{i3} X_i \leq 100$$

$$\sum_i a_{i4} X_i \geq 12$$

$$X_i \geq 0$$

Mathematically, the problem is to find values for $X_i$ which meet all five constraints simultaneously, but do so at minimum cost (i.e., minimize the objective function).

The major differences between the two types should now be evident. In the *maximization* case, the decision variables are the outputs, and the constraints are given in terms of limited fixed resources. In the *minimization* case, the decision variables are the resources, and the constraints are stated in terms of output requirements. It is quite common for MP problems to reflect both types in the same formulation. Consider, for example, the added constraint on the first problem of maintaining a minimum of 3,000 surgical discharges from the 100 beds ($S \geq 3,000$)—an *output* constraint. Similarly, consider a constraint on the diet problem that the amount of meats must be less than or equal to 1.5 lbs a day ($X_3 + X_4 + X_7 \leq 1.5$)—a *resource* constraint. We will examine other examples of combining the two types later in the chapter.

What general assumptions have been made for these two formulations? First, we have formulated the problems around average figures, leaving out all stochastic considerations. Second, we have assumed that both the objective function and the constraints are linear. In the case of the objective function of the hospital problem, we assumed that $M$ and $S$ substitute for one another in a linear fashion—one $M$ is always "worth" two $S$. In the constraints of that problem, we assumed that $M$ and $S$ combined in a linear fashion to consume the resources; i.e., there were no economies of scale or of combination in the consumption process. A third assumption (which we imply by not stating otherwise) is that the decision variables are continuous, i.e., they can take on fractional values. Which of these might seriously restrict the usefulness of the results of the solution for each problem?

If we make these assumptions, we have formulated a linear programming (LP) problem. If we do not allow the decision variables to be continuous but require that they take on only integer values, we have an integer programming (IP) problem. If one or more of the equations (objective function or constraint) of the formulation is nonlinear, reflecting nonlinear relationships between the variables, we have a nonlinear programming (NP) problem. (There are, of course, nonlinear integer programming problems as well.)

Although most real-world decisions involve nonlinear relationships (quantity discounts, economies of scale, etc.) and are stochastic, we will begin our examination of mathematical programming (MP) with the linear programming (LP) formulation to demonstrate how MP formulations are solved. Very large LP problems (thousands of variables and hundreds of constraints) can be solved on a computer, but only relatively small NP and IP problems can be solved, and then only to a limited extent in most cases. Moreover, the solution techniques for NP and IP are much more complicated than those for LP. We will examine real-world NP and IP formulations later in the chapter.

Before we examine the solution of the LP, we should place MP in our original framework for decision making. The formulation stage of MP coincides with the model formulation stage of Step 1: the concepts of decision variables, objective functions, and constraints are the essence of the model formulation stage of Step 1. Step 2, quantification, is straightforward in this case, primarily because we avoid the problems of dealing directly with the stochastic nature of the decision. Thus the quantification step is one of determining the coefficients of the objective function (usually denoted as $c$) and the coefficients of the constraints (usually denoted as $a$). If nonlinear relationships are involved, the quantification step also includes establishing the nonlinear nature of such equations (which are sometimes approximated by linear equations). It is in Steps 3 and 4 that MP plays a new role as a solution technique (replacing trial and error, heuristic, and calculus), and as a technique of sensitivity analysis, as we shall see below.

## 6.3 SOLVING LINEAR FORMULATIONS—GRAPHICAL METHOD

Return to the maximization problem of the previous section. Figure 6.3 graphs different combinations of $M$ and $S$, i.e., each point on the graph corresponds to a value for $M$ and $S$. Considering only the constraints $M \geq 0$ and $S \geq 0$, possible solutions include all points in the upper right quadrant of Figure 6.3.

Now consider the patient-day constraint.

$$10M + 6S \leq 36,500. \quad (B)$$

If we produce only $M$ (and no $S$), we can produce a maximum of $36,500/10 = 3,650$ of them. If we produce only $S$ (and no $M$), we can produce a maximum of $36,500/6 = 6,083$. Line $B$ on Figure 6.4 shows the line between these two points. *Every* point on the line consumes all the 36,500 patient days, so that now feasible solutions are confined to the area *under* line $B$, including the line. By determining where they cross the $M$ and $S$ axes, each of the other constraints can be similarly represented—as in Figure 6.5. Now our feasible solution space is confined to all points within the shaded area of Figure 6.5.

Where is the optimal solution point, that point which maximizes $2,000M + 1,000S$? To find that point graphically, we use the concept of iso-objective lines. On an iso-objective line, we are indifferent between each point of the line, in terms of our objective. Consider

*Figure 6.3*

*Solution Space of* **M** ≥ *0 and* **S** ≥ *0*

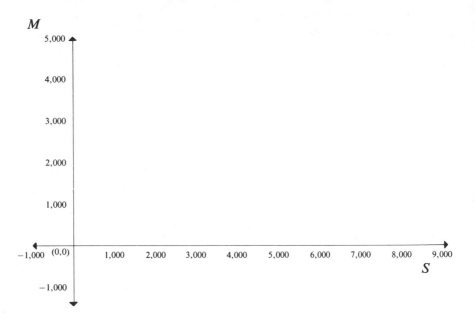

*Figure 6.4*

*Solution Space (Shaded) Including Bed Constraint*

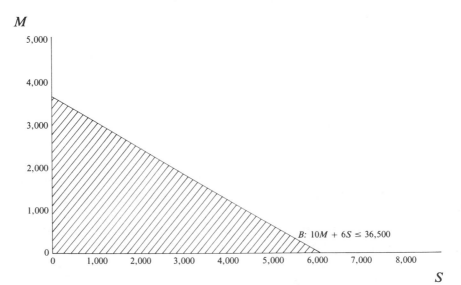

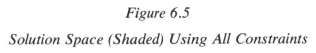

Figure 6.5

Solution Space (Shaded) Using All Constraints

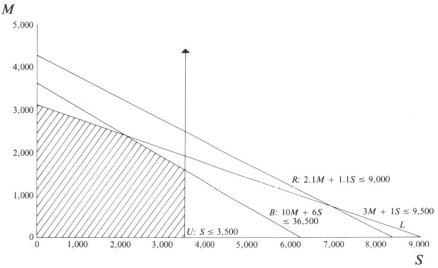

the line that goes through (0, 1,000) and (2,000, 0) in Figure 6.6. Any point on that line, when substituted into $2,000M + 1,000S$, gives 2,000,000. Consider the line parallel to it that goes through (0, 2,000) and (4,000, 0). It is also iso-objective, since each point on it produces 4,000,000 when substituted into $2,000M + 1,000S$. While we are indifferent between points on an iso-objective line, we are not indifferent to which iso-objective line we are on—we want to be on the iso-objective line as far as possible from (0, 0).

To maintain feasibility, however, we must also be in the feasible area. So the optimal iso-objective is that one which is as far out as possible but which still just touches the solution space, and the optimal point is the one where they touch: (2,000, 2,500) in Figure 6.6. If the iso-objective lines are parallel to an outside boundary of the solution space, then the optimal iso-objective will touch all along an edge, and any point (and all points) on the intersection are optimal.

The graphical solution technique is good for only two (or theoretically three) variables (why?), and its value does not lie in its ability to solve practical problems. Instead, it is useful to provide insight into how larger LP problems are solved (as well as IP and NP problems), and to give insight into some of the properties of the optimal solution.

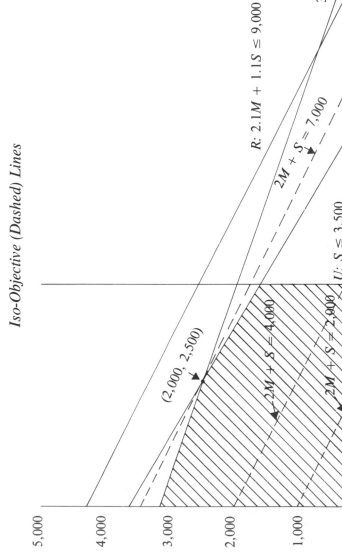

*Figure 6.6*

*Iso-Objective (Dashed) Lines*

First notice that the optimal solution must always be at a vertex of the solution space. This suggests that not all of the infinitely possible solutions of the solution space need be searched through—only those at the vertexes. Note also that if you were to "climb" the solution space from vertex to vertex, checking each vertex with the slope of the iso-objective lines, you would know when you had reached the optimal. (Try it.) This is because the solution space is *convex.* These two properties—the optimal solution is at a vertex and the solution space is convex—allow the LP to be easily solvable by a mathematical technique known as the simplex method.

Notice that only two of the constraints—*B* and *L*—"restrain" or "bind" the solution at the optimal point. The other constraints are said to be non-binding at that point. What is the effect of making available more surgical room capacity or more radiology examinations? (One of the constraints, *R*, does not even help define the solution space and is never binding. Such a constraint is called a redundant constraint.) One property of an optimal solution is that some of the constraints are binding, and thus if those constraints are relaxed (i.e., if more capacity were added), it would improve the optimal solution; others are non-binding and cannot improve the optimal solution by being relaxed. As you move up the solution space from vertex to vertex, note that some constraints become binding while others become non-binding; thus whether a constraint is binding or non-binding is a function of which vertex one is on.

Consider the value of relaxing a constraint. For binding constraints, relaxation allows an improvement in the objective function, while for non-binding ones, there is no improvement. We call the *change in the objective function associated with a unit change in the right side value of a constraint that constraint's "shadow price."* The shadow price is thus the opportunity cost of *not* increasing that resource by one unit. For example, if the shadow price on the bed-day constraint is equal to 125 (dollars, because the objective function is in terms of dollars), then the "value" of one more bed-day per year is $125, meaning that the hospital could discharge a small fraction more of a patient if it had one more bed-day available (i.e., 36,501 instead of 36,500). Fortunately, the value of each constraint's shadow price is an automatic by-product of the mathematical solution technique we will examine below—the simplex method.

Finally, notice that if you started at (0, 0) and moved to the right to the first vertex (3,500, 0), you include one of the variables (*S*) in the solution at a positive value, while the other variable (*M*) stays at 0. We will call variables which are in solution at a positive value *basic* variables, and those which are at value 0 *non-basic* variables. Thus at (0, 0) both $M$ and $S$ are non-basic, while at (3,500, 0) $S$ is basic and $M$ non-basic; at (0, 3,167) $M$ is basic and $S$ is not, while both are basic at the other vertexes.

## 6.4 SOLVING LINEAR FORMULATIONS—SIMPLEX METHOD*

We will now very briefly examine a mathematical technique for solving LP problems. Our development will be of the "cookbook" variety, and we refer the interested student to any of the texts at the end of the chapter for details. The intent of the development is to give some insight into the solution technique, not to prepare practitioners.

Recall our hospital problem:

Maximize $2,000M + 1,000S$

$$10M + \phantom{0}6S \le 36,500 \quad \text{(B)}$$

$$3M + \phantom{00}1S \le \phantom{0}9,500 \quad \text{(L)}$$

$$2.1M + \phantom{0}1.1S \le \phantom{0}9,000 \quad \text{(R)}$$

$$0M + \phantom{00}1S \le \phantom{0}3,500 \quad \text{(U)}$$

We found out that the $R$ constraint is redundant—it will never constrain our solution. We can thus ignore it and reduce the problem to

Maximize $2,000M + 1,000S$

$$10M + \phantom{0}6S \le 36,500 \quad \text{(B)}$$

$$3M + \phantom{00}1S \le \phantom{0}9,500 \quad \text{(L)}$$

$$0M + \phantom{00}1S \le \phantom{0}3,500 \quad \text{(U)}$$

We can convert the inequalities to equalities by adding a "slack" variable to each—to take up the slack between, for example, $10M + 6S$ and 36,500. Again for example, if $M = S = 0$, then the slack variable inserted into that constraint to take up the slack would equal 36,500. These slack variables have no "value," so they show up in the objective function with coefficient 0:

---

*This section may be omitted without seriously disturbing the continuity of the chapter; the reader should, however, read the last part of this section, "Simplex Computer Programs."

Maximize $2,000M + 1,000S + 0B + 0L + 0U$

$$10M + \quad 6S + 1B \qquad\qquad\qquad = 36,500 \;\; \text{(B)}$$

$$3M + \quad 1S \qquad + 1L \qquad\qquad = 9,500 \;\; \text{(L)}$$

$$0M \qquad\qquad\qquad\qquad\qquad + 1U = 3,500 \;\; \text{(U)}$$

Now, let $Z$ be the value of the objective function, so that

$$Z = 2,000M + 1,000S + 0B + 0L + 0U$$

or

$$Z - 2,000M - 1,000S - 0B - 0L - 0U = 0.$$

Add this version of the objective function to the constraints to get

$$Z - 2,000M - 1,000S - 0B - 0L - 0U = \qquad 0$$

$$10M + \quad 6S + 1B \qquad\qquad\qquad = 36,500 \qquad \text{(B)}$$

$$3M + \quad 1S \qquad + 1L \qquad\qquad = 9,500 \qquad \text{(L)}$$

$$0M + \quad 1S \qquad\qquad\qquad + 1U = 3,500 \qquad \text{(U)}$$

Not counting the $Z$, we now have five variables (two real ones and three slack).

We begin our search through the vertexes by starting at the origin. At the origin $M$ and $S$ are both zero. If $M$ and $S$ are zero, then mathematically $B$ must $= 36,500$, $L = 9,500$, and $U = 3,500$. (Why?) Our basic variables at this point (those not $= 0$) are thus the slack ones, and the $M$ and $S$ are non-basic. The value of the objective function $Z$ at this point ($M = 0$ and $S = 0$) is 0. We will be able to tell which variables are basic in our current solution from the tableau of numbers by noticing which variables have a 1 as a coefficient in one constraint and a 0 as a coefficient in all other constraints—variables $B$, $L$, and $U$ in our initial tableau. The *value* of the basic variables can always be read as the current right-side value: $B = 36,500$, $L = 9,500$ and $U = 3,500$.

How can we improve the solution? We must bring one of the non-basic variables into the group of basic variables (called the *basis*). Which one: $S$ or $M$? The $M$ is more profitable because of the $2,000 instead of the $1,000 in the first equation of the tableau. So Rule 1 is to try to bring in the non-basic variable which has the *lowest* number above it in the top equation (lowest because they are negative: −2,000 is lower than −1,000). If there is no variable with a coefficient less than 0, then *no* variable should be brought in (in which case we have the optimal solution).

How much $M$ can we bring into the solution? In the B constraint, if we set $S$ and $B$ equal to 0, we could bring in as much as $36,500/10 = 3,650\ M$. Similarly, if we look at the L constraint and set $S$ and $L$ equal to 0, we could bring in $9,500/3 = 3,167\ M$. Finally, according to the U constraint, we can bring in as many $M$ as we like, since each $M$ uses none of it. (How are these points—3,650, 3,167, and ∞—interpreted on the graph of the preceding section?) Since we must satisfy all constraints at once, we can only bring in the *smallest* amount of $M$ allowable by any one constraint: 3,167 in the L constraint. So Rule 2 is to bring the variable of Rule 1 into the most binding constraint, found by dividing the right side by the coefficient of the variable in that constraint (36,500/10; 9,500/3; etc.).

Remember that the basic variables are noted by having a coefficient of 1 in one constraint and a 0 in all others. We now "force" the tableau to conform to this notation by

1. dividing row $L$ by 3 (converts the coefficient of $M$ to 1), and

2. adding or subtracting multiples of row $L$ to the other rows so that there are zeros in the column for $M$, except in row $L$.*

Dividing row $L$ by 3 gives

$$1M + 1/3S + 1/3L = 3,167. \qquad \text{(L)}$$

We can make the "10$M$" of row B into a "0$M$" by subtracting 10 times row $L$ from row $B$:

$$(10 - 10)M + (6 - 10/3)S + (1 - 0)B + (0 - 10/3)L = (36,500$$

$$- 31,670) \qquad \text{(B)}$$

or

---

*How can we do this without upsetting the basic equality relationship of our equations? Look at it this way. Suppose A = B. Divide both sides by C: A/C = B/C. The equality still holds, so Step 1 does not disturb the equality. Now suppose A = B and C = D. First multiply C = D by E: CE = DE. Equality still holds. Now add A = B to CE = DE: A + CE = B + DE. Since A = B, C = D and E = E, the equality still holds.

$$0M + 8/3S + 1B - 10/3L = 4{,}830. \qquad \text{(B)}$$

Finally, adding 2,000 times row $L$ to the first row gives

$$0M - 333S + 0B + 667L + 0U = 6{,}334{,}000$$

$$0M + 8/3S + 1B - 10/3L + 0U = \quad 4{,}830 \qquad \text{(B)}$$

$$1M + 1/3S + 0B + 1/3L + 0U = \quad 3{,}167 \qquad \text{(L)}$$

$$0M + \quad 1S + 0B + \quad 0L + 1U = \quad 3{,}500 \qquad \text{(U)}$$

Now our basic variables are $M$, $B$, and $U$ ($L$ has left the basis, being replaced by $M$). Moreover, the current solution is

$$M = 3{,}167,$$

$$B = 4{,}830,$$

$$U = 3{,}500,$$

$$S \text{ and } L = \quad 0,$$

giving us an objective value of $6,334,000. (Where are we on the graph?)

Now we are ready for a second iteration. Rule 1 says that our most profitable variable is now $S$ (with a top-line coefficient of $-333$). So $S$ is our candidate to enter the basis. At which constraint should it come in? (Which is most binding?)

$$\text{Row } B: \quad 4{,}830 \div 8/3 = 1{,}811.25.$$

$$\text{Row } L: \quad 3{,}167 \div 1/3 = 9{,}501.$$

$$\text{Row } U: \quad 3{,}500 \div \quad 1 = 3{,}500.$$

Thus $B$ is the most binding. Dividing row $B$ by $8/3$ gives

$$0M + 1S + 3/8B - 10/8L + 0U = 1{,}811.25. \qquad \text{(B)}$$

Adding 333 times row $B$ to the first row gives the new top row:

$$Z = 0M - 0S + 125B + 250L + 0U = 6{,}937{,}146.25.$$

Subtracting $1/3$ times row $B$ from row $L$ gives the new row $L$ as

$$1M + 0S - 1/8B - 2/24L = 2{,}563.25. \qquad \text{(L)}$$

Finally, subtracting row $B$ from row $U$ gives

$$0M + 0S - 3/8B + 10/8L + 1U = 1,688.75, \quad \text{(U)}$$

thus giving our new tableau as

$$Z + 0M + 0S + 125B + 250L + 0U = 6,937,146.25$$

$$0M + 1S + 3/8B - 10/8L + 0U = \quad 1,811.25 \quad \text{(B)}$$

$$1M + 0S - 1/8B - 2/24L + 0U = \quad 2,563.25 \quad \text{(L)}$$

$$0M + 0S - 3/8B + 10/8L + 1U = \quad 1,688.75 \quad \text{(U)}$$

Our new solution is now

$$S = 1,811.25,$$

$$M = 2,563.25,$$

$$U = 1,688.75,$$

$$\text{and } B \text{ and } L = \quad 0,$$

giving us an objective value of 6,937,146.25. (Where is this point on the graph?)

For the next iteration, Rule 1 says to pick the smallest of the negative coefficients in the top row as the new variable to come in. No coefficient is negative, so we're through! We have identified the optimal solution.

What does $U = 1,688.75$ mean? Recall that $U$ is the slack variable for the operating room. Thus, at the optimal solution, there will be 1,688.75 operating procedures not used. (Where is this on the graph?) The $B = 0$ and $L = 0$ mean that all of the patient days and laboratory tests will be used—these are binding constraints, and they have 0 slack.

Now for the magic part—consider the top row of the final tableau. Recall that throughout the solution, the top row coefficients gave the opportunity cost of keeping each of the variables out, with the minus sign ignored—we used it only for convention. That is, we brought in the one which had the largest absolute value because it was "worth" the most. Now if at the last tableau we were to *force in* one unit of $B$ (i.e., require one bed-day a year to be idle or slack), it would *cost* us $125. On the other hand, if we could have obtained one more bed-day a year—36,501 instead of 36,500—we could *generate* $125 more revenue. This is the definition of the shadow price. So the top line of the final tableau automatically gives the shadow prices as follows:

coefficient of $B$ = shadow price of constraint $B$,

coefficient of $L$ = shadow price of constraint $L$,

etc.

(Why is the shadow price of $U$ equal to 0?) While an additional bed-day may not be warranted at only \$125 increase in revenue, what about the value of some additional laboratory tests? The shadow prices thus give us an opportunity for a cost-benefit decision on adding more resources.

## Using Linear Programming Techniques for PERT/CPM Networks

PERT networks, as discussed in Chapter 3, are easily amenable to analysis and solution using linear programming modeling. However, large projects which require considerable modifications in time and task specifications could be dealt with more efficiently by using a computer package for PERT rather than for LP. The reasoning behind this recommendation should become evident.

PERT networks and crashing techniques can be analyzed as linear programming problems. If $T_{exp(i)}$ is the time expected to reach a task end node $i$, then the objective function is to find the critical path which minimizes the time from node $o$ to the end node of the project:

$$\text{Minimize } Z = T_{exp(n)} - T_{exp(o)},$$

where

$T_{exp(n)}$ = expected time to the end of the project, and

$T_{exp(o)}$ = expected time at the beginning of the project.

The constraints are set by virtue of the fact that the time for any activity, $A$, starting at node $i$ and ending at node $j$, is made up of the time to complete the activity plus any available slack time for the activity. The constraints are:

$$T(j) - T(i) \geq T(A),$$
$$T(j) - T(i) = T(A) + T_{slack}(A).$$

To illustrate the use of linear programming for PERT networks, we will use the crashing example presented in Section 3.5. The following notation will be used:

$D$        = specified deadline for project,

$T(A)$   = time for activity $A$ (under normal conditions),

$T'(A)$  = time for activity $A$ (under crashing conditions),

$T(i)$    = time to reach node $i$,

$R(A)$   = amount of crash time used for activity $A$,

$C(A)$   = crashing cost per time unit.

As in the example presented earlier, the project manager would like the project done in the least costly manner while completing it within 26 weeks. The objective function is thus to minimize $\sum_A R(A)C(A)$, or to minimize crashing costs. The constraints are as follows:

1. Meet the deadline of 26 weeks:

$$T_{(n)} - T_{(o)} \le 26 \text{ weeks.}$$

2. Abide by the constraint on amount of time available for any activity:

$$T_{(j)} - T_{(i)} \ge T(A) - R(A).$$

3. The limits on crash time are defined by the project manager and can't exceed those specifications:

$$R(A) \le T(A) - T'(A).$$

$T(A)$, $T'(A)$, $C(A)$, and $D$ are all set by the project manager; all equations for the program are thus described in terms of $R(A)$ and $T(i)$. Formulating the crashing example used in Section 3.5, the objective function becomes:

Minimize $Z = \$50,000 + (\$100/\text{wk} \times R(\text{space})) + (\$200/\text{wk} \times R(\text{Radiologists})) + (\$200/\text{wk} \times R(\text{Equipment})) + (\$300/\text{wk} \times R(\text{Remodel})) + (\$100/\text{wk} \times R(\text{Install})) + (\$200/\text{wk} \times R(\text{Nurses})) + (\$200/\text{wk} \times R(\text{Train})) + (\$300/\text{wk} \times R(\text{Publicity})) + (\$200/\text{wk} \times R(\text{Final}))$

Subject to:

1. $T_n - T_o \le 26$.
2. Predecessor tasks determine the structural constraints on the amount of time available for any activity:

$(A_i)$ refers to event node preceding activity $A$,

$(A_j)$ refers to event node following activity $A$.

$T(\text{Remodel}_i) - T(\text{Begin}_j) \geq 14 - R(\text{Space})$

$T(\text{Equipment}_i) - T(\text{Begin}_j) \geq 16 - R(\text{Radiologist})$

$T(\text{Install}_i) - T(\text{Radiologist}_j) \geq 12 - R(\text{Equipment})$

$T(\text{Install}_i) - T(\text{Radiologist}_j) \geq 6 - R(\text{Remodel})$

$T(\text{Final}_i) - T(\text{Equipment}_j) \geq 2 - R(\text{Install})$

$T(\text{Train}_i) - T(\text{Begin}_j) \geq 5 - R(\text{Nurse})$

$T(\text{Final}_i) - T(\text{Nurse}_j) \geq 4 - R(\text{Train})$

$T(\text{Final}_i) - T(\text{Begin}_j) \geq 11 - R(\text{Publicity})$

$T(\text{End}_i) - T(\text{Install}_j) \geq 3 - R(\text{Final})$

3. Limits on the crashing:

$R(\text{Space}) \leq 6$

$R(\text{Radiologist}) \leq 4$

$R(\text{Equipment}) \leq 6$

$R(\text{Remodel}) \leq 1$

$R(\text{Install}) \leq 1$

$R(\text{Nurse}) \leq 2$

$R(\text{Train}) \leq 2$

$R(\text{Publicity}) \leq 1$

$R(\text{Final}) \leq 1$

$T(i) \geq 0$

The computer-based solution coincides with the manual PERT crashing solution presented in Section 3.5, with total cost of the project equal to $51,300. To identify the critical path, the constraints that result in no slack variables ($T_{slack} = 0$), and therefore are an equality in the solution $T(j) - T_{(i)} = T(A)$, have corresponding surplus (negative) variables equal to zero.

**Simplex Computer Programs**

Solving any but the smallest problems by the simplex method is tedious by hand but not by computer. In fact, very large problems can be solved in short running times by computer, and simplex programs are available on all but the smallest computers. Not only are the shadow prices automatically available for sensitivity analysis (Step 4 of our decision-making framework), but most programs also give information concerning sensitivity of the solution to the coefficients of the objective function, and to the right-side values of the constraints.

Consider the right-side value of the constraints and examine the graph of the previous section. Will the shadow price of the *B* constraint remain equal to $125 no matter how many bed days we add above 36,500? No—there comes a point when another constraint would bind the solution from moving further out. Thus each right-side constraint value has a *range* over which its shadow price remains constant. This range is also an automatic by-product of most simplex computer programs. Figure 6.7 shows the output of a typical simplex computer program, and Figure 6.8 interprets the output of Figure 6.7.

## 6.5 OTHER FORMS OF MATHEMATICAL PROGRAMMING

Reconsidering the maximization problem of the previous sections, suppose that there are fewer laboratory tests available, and also suppose that because of "reverse" economies of scale, the laboratory can perform *fewer* tests if all tests are either only on *M* patients, or only *S* patients, and *more* tests if there is a mixture of *M* and *S* type tests. Something similar to the nonlinear constraint of Figure 6.9 results, showing a convex "production possibility" curve for laboratory tests. Now consider the resulting solution space. Although it is still convex, the optimal solution is no longer at a vertex; and searching through all vertexes (which the simplex method does) would not turn up the optimal solution. What would happen with a nonlinear objective function—especially if it were "bumpy," having both convex and concave sections?

Nonlinear programming formulations are much more difficult to solve than LP formulations primarily because of the shape of the solution space and/or the objective function. (Although it is impossible to imagine the 4 + space graph of a formulation, an analogous difficulty results for all size formulations.) A limited number of NP problems of limited size, however, can be solved to a limited degree, with useful solutions resulting in many cases; we will examine one in Section 6.6. (There are also "tricks" that can be used in some cases to approximate curved lines with segmented linear ones; or it may not be too serious to assume a relationship is linear over some limited range.)

Now reconsider the diet problem of Section 6.2. A more practical formulation for an ongoing dietary department is the menu problem—selecting from a set of menu items (instead of food items) the least

## Figure 6.7

### Output of Computer Program for Linear Programming

LINEAR PROGRAMMING CODE WITH SENSITIVITY ANAYLSIS AND UPPER BOUNDING OPTION

INPUT MATRIX WITH SLACKS

| ROW | B-VEC | 1 | 2 | 3 | 4 | 5 | |
|---|---|---|---|---|---|---|---|
| | *** | *** | *** | *** | *** | *** | |
| 0 | 0.0 | 2000.0 | 1000.0 | 0.0 | 0.0 | 0.0 | (1) |
| 1 | 36500.0 | 10.0 | 6.0 | 1.0 | 0.0 | 0.0 | |
| 2 | 9500.0 | 3.0 | 1.0 | 0.0 | 1.0 | 0.0 | |
| 3 | 3500.0 | 0.0 | 1.0 | 0.0 | 0.0 | 1.0 | |

BEGIN PHASE I (2)

BEGIN PHASE II

| # | 1 | VAR IN 1 | VAR OUT 4 | |
|---|---|---|---|---|
| # | 2 | VAR IN 2 | VAR OUT 3 | (3) |
| | | 2 ITERATIONS | | |

OPTIMUM SOLUTION AND SHADOW PRICES

OPTIMAL OBJECTIVE = 6937498.000

| VAR | X | ROW | SP | (4) |
|---|---|---|---|---|
| 2 | 1812.502 | 1 | 125.000 | |
| 1 | 2562.501 | 2 | 250.000 | |
| 5 | 1687.498 | 3 | 0.000 | |

FEASIBILITY RANGES FOR B-VECTOR

| B-VECT POS | ORIGINAL VALUE | VAR MADE NEGATIVE | LOWER LIM LEVEL | UPPER LIM LEVEL | VAR MADE NEGATIVE | |
|---|---|---|---|---|---|---|
| 1 | 36500.00 | 2 | 31666.66 | 40999.99 | 5 | (5) |
| 2 | 9500.00 | 5 | 8150.00 | 10950.00 | 2 | |
| 3 | 3500.00 | 5 | 1812.50 | 999999900.00 | 0 | |

INDIFFERENCE RANGES FOR OBJECTIVE FUNCTION COEFFICIENTS

| VAR NAME | ORIGINAL COEF | LOWER COEF LIMIT | LOWER LIM VECT TIE | UPPER COEF LIMIT | UPPER LIM VECT TIE | |
|---|---|---|---|---|---|---|
| 2 | 1000.00 | 666.67 | 3 | 1200.00 | 4 | (6) |
| 1 | 2000.00 | 1666.67 | 4 | 3000.00 | 3 | |
| 5 | −0.00 | −200.00 | 4 | 333.33 | 3 | |

## Figure 6.8

### Interpretation of Linear Programming Output

(1) Shows initial tableau, with right hand side as first row (the top row has been multiplied by −1 leaving all coefficients positive, as they were read in).

(2) If needed, program puts in artificial variables and solves Phase I (result is a feasible solution or the message "no feasible solution").

(3) Phase II begins. Activity at each interation is shown.

(4) Optimal solution. Thus $X_1 = 2{,}562.501$, $X_2 = 1{,}812.502$, and $X_5$ (the slack in constraint #3) = 1,687.498. Row refers to constraints, SP to shadow price.

(5) Feasibility range for right hand side (B) values, by constraint. Thus for the first constraint, the shadow price of 125 is relevant for decreases in the right hand side down to 31,666.67 (from 36,500) and up to 40,500. At the lower limit, Variable 2 would become negative if the right hand side were forced lower than 31,666.67,

and Variable 5 would go negative if the right hand side were forced higher than 40,500.

(6)  Interpretation: If the coefficient of Variable 2 (which was 1,000 as inputted) were reduced to lower than 666.67, Variable 3 would become more attractive and would replace 2 in the basis. If the coefficient were forced higher than 1,200, Variable 4 would come into the basis.

cost solution which maintains nutritional requirements.* Suppose the dietary department can serve only the eight menu items of Figure 6.10, which includes the cost of each item and its contribution to the four nutritional requirements (the figures are not actual, but made up for the example). Since each of the items is a "serving," it no longer makes sense to allow fractional values in our solution (.376 of a serving of Chicken à la King?). Thus we add an additional requirement that *only integer values* of the variables be allowed. Our complete formulation is now:

$$\text{Minimize} \quad \sum_i C_i X_i$$

$$\text{Subject to} \quad \sum_i a_{i_1} X_i \geq 2{,}600$$

$$\sum_i a_{i_1} X_i \leq 4{,}000$$

$$\sum_i a_{i2} X_i \geq \quad 72$$

$$\sum_i a_{i3} X_i \leq \quad 100$$

$$\sum_i a_{i4} X_i \geq \quad 12$$

$$X_i \text{ is an integer.}$$

We cannot graph eight menu items, so to demonstrate the difficulties of solving integer programming problems of this sort, suppose we had only two menu items to choose from: Roast Pork and Apple Pie. Figure 6.11 shows the solution space for this problem. But now our solution must be one of the "lattice points" (dots) indicating integer solutions. While it would seem that this *reduces*

---

*This formulation is a much simplified version of a successful application by Balintfy— see reference in Additional Reading.

## Figure 6.9

### A Nonlinear Constraint

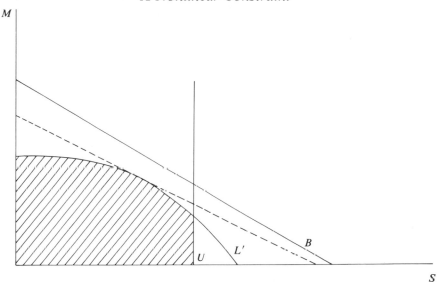

the number of possible solutions that would have to be searched through for the optimal, observe that the optimal solution is not a vertex of the solution space, so that an orderly search through the vertexes no longer finds the optimum. If the values that the decision variables take on are large—for example, like those of the hospital problem where $M$ and $S$ are $> 1,000$—then rounding the LP result is not a serious problem. But when the values of the decision variables are, for example, 0, 1, 2, or 3, rounding can be very serious (examine the nurse-staffing or scheduling problem of the next section). Like nonlinear programming (NP) formulations, only small integer programming (IP) formulations can be easily solved, and then only to a limited degree in most cases. However, like NP formulations, useful results are often available. We will look at two applications of IP in Section 6.6.

There are two special types of IP formulations that can be easily solved even for very large problems, and, furthermore, there are many real-world decisions that can be formulated in these two special ways: the assignment formulation and the transportation formulation.

### The Assignment Formulation

**Problem:** The nursing supervisor responsible for the night shift of the OB, MED, SURG, and Nursery (NUR) units

## Figure 6.10
### Cost and Nutritional Content of Menu Items

| $(X_i)$ Menu Item | $(C_i)$ Cost/Serving | $(a_{i1})$ Calories/Serving | $(a_{i2})$ Protein/Serving | $(a_{i3})$ Fat/Serving | $(a_{i4})$ Iron/Serving |
|---|---|---|---|---|---|
| Chicken à la King | .74 | 397 | 13.0 | 8.0 | 1.8 |
| Roast Pork | .90 | 591 | 18.5 | 12.6 | 2.3 |
| Baked Ham | .81 | 416 | 16.0 | 9.0 | 1.4 |
| Roast Beef | 1.40 | 340 | 14.0 | 7.8 | 1.7 |
| Brabant Potatoes | .24 | 180 | 4.2 | 3.1 | .6 |
| Creole Rice | .16 | 210 | 5.0 | 3.8 | 1.4 |
| Fruit Cup | .36 | 100 | 6.0 | .4 | .2 |
| Apple Pie | .30 | 433 | 10.0 | 11.3 | 3.0 |

## Figure 6.11

### Feasible Solution Points for Menu Problem

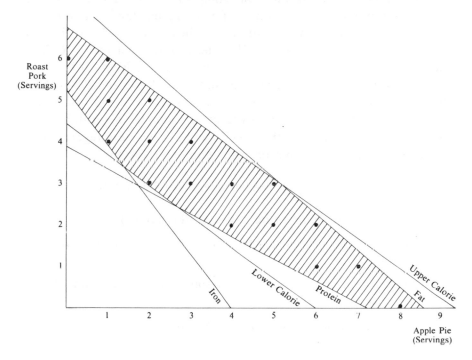

must appoint head nurses for the night shift on each unit. These are new positions for which four nurses were hired: RNA, RNB, RNC, and RND. The problem is to assign each nurse to a unit so that the overall resulting assignment is optimal. Having a healthy respect for quantification, the supervisor has interviewed each nurse, considered the background of each, and developed a "cost scale" of 0 to 100 to be used in the assignment. A 0 for nurse RNA being assigned to the OB unit means that she is completely suited to that unit because of background, personality, preference, etc. On the other hand, a 90 for nurse RNA being assigned to the MED unit means she is not suited for that unit for the same type of reasons. Table 6.1 gives the complete set of cost figures that the supervisor felt represented the possible assignments. How shall she assign the four nurses to the four units?

How many ways can four nurses be assigned to four units? (Or thirty nurses to thirty units!) The solution to the problem is to find the best one without evaluating all $4 \times 3 \times 2 = 24$ ways to assign four nurses to four units. Try assigning the best nurse to OB, then of the other three nurses the best one to MED, then of the two nurses left the best to SUR, leaving the last to NUR. You should get a total cost of 190. Now try assigning RNA to her best unit, assigning RNB to a remaining unit, then RNC and RND. You should get 180. (The optimal assignment has a cost of 170.) Although assignment problems can be solved by the simplex algorithm when formulated as below (and the results will always be integer), there are faster methods available on many computer systems.

Mathematical Formulation of Assignment Problem (Optional)

Let $i$ index the items to be assigned (the nurses).

Let $j$ index the spaces to which the items are to be assigned (the units).

Let $X_{ij} = 1$ if item $i$ is to be assigned to space $j$, and 0 otherwise.

Let $C_{ij}$ be the cost of assigning item $i$ to space $j$.

The objective function is

$$\text{Minimize} \sum_i \sum_j C_{ij} X_{ij}.$$

The constraints are

$$\sum_i X_{ij} = 1 \text{ for each } j,$$

$$\sum_j X_{ij} = 1 \text{ for each } i,$$

and

$$X_{ij} = 0 \text{ or } 1 \text{ (the } integer \text{ constraints) for all } i \text{ and } j.$$

## Transportation Formulation

**Problem:** The four blood banks in a large metropolitan area are coordinated through a central office which coordinates

## Table 6.1

### Cost of Assigning Nurses (Rows) to Units (Columns)

|      | OB  | MED | SUR | NUR |
|------|-----|-----|-----|-----|
| RNA  | 50  | 20  | 10  | 50  |
| RNB  | 30  | 10  | 40  | 60  |
| RNC  | 60  | 80  | 40  | 80  |
| RND  | 100 | 50  | 50  | 100 |

blood delivery to the ten hospitals in the area. Figure 6.12 shows the location of the four banks (A, B, C, and D) and the ten hospitals (1, 2, ..., 10). The cost to ship a "shipment" of blood from bank $i$ ($i = 1, 2, 3, 4$) to hospital $j$ ($j = 1, 2, ..., 10$) is designated $C_{ij}$ and is given in Table 6.2. Also given are the biweekly number of shipments of blood needed at each hospital, and the biweekly number of shipments available at each bank. How many shipments should be made from bank $i$ to hospital $j$ each biweekly period so that total shipment costs are minimized?

Let $X_{ij}$ be the (integer) number of shipments from bank $i$ to hospital $j$. Our objective is to

$$\text{Minimize} \sum_i \sum_j C_{ij} X_{ij}.$$

We have only $B_i$ shipments available at bank $i$, however, so that

$$\sum_j X_{ij} \leq B_i \quad \text{for each } i.$$

Also, we need a minimum of $H_j$ shipments to hospital $j$, so that

$$\sum_i X_{ij} \geq H_j \quad \text{for each } j.$$

Without adding the constraints that $X_{ij}$ be integer, we have an LP problem with $4 \times 10 = 40$ variables and $10 + 4 = 14$ constraints. It turns out that because of special properties of the transportation (and assignment) formulation, the integer constraints are not required— we could use the simplex technique to solve the transportation problem and the solution would automatically be integer. There is, how-

*Table 6.2*

### Cost to Ship a "Shipment" of Blood from Banks (Rows) to Hospitals (Columns)

| | | | | | Hospital | | | | | | $(B_i)$ |
| Bank | 1 | 2 | 3 | 4 | 5 | 6 | 7 | 8 | 9 | 10 | Total Available |
|---|---|---|---|---|---|---|---|---|---|---|---|
| A | 40 | 36 | 34 | 20 | 20 | 13 | 10 | 14 | 10 | 18 | 4,000 |
| B | 54 | 46 | 30 | 8 | 8 | 12 | 11 | 6 | 19 | 29 | 6,000 |
| C | 18 | 9 | 4 | 8 | 7 | 6 | 10 | 21 | 21 | 13 | 5,000 |
| D | 3 | 4 | 4 | 13 | 13 | 7 | 6 | 26 | 21 | 3 | 8,000 |
| Total Needed | | | | | | | | | | | |
| $(H_j)$ | 86 | 140 | 190 | 230 | 600 | 100 | 250 | 300 | 200 | 160 | |

*Figure 6.12*

### Location of Blood Banks (Letters) and Hospitals (Numbers)

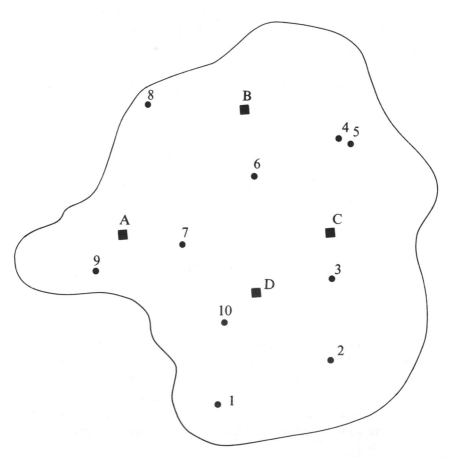

ever, a special algorithm that has been developed for solving transportation problems, also available on most large computers, that is very fast and efficient. Most programs also offer the ability to require that no more than a fixed amount be shipped from $i$ to $j$ (the capacitated transportation problem), or that some of the $j$ destinations can become transhipment points (the transhipment problem), where, of the items that are shipped to $j$, some are left at $j$ and the rest shipped on to another destination $\neq j$. The algorithm is detailed in the texts at the end of the chapter and is easy to use to solve small problems by hand.

## Goal Programming

In addition to linear and nonlinear programming, there is another form of mathematical programming that deserves attention because of the likelihood of its growing use. Goal programming (GP) addresses problems with multiple goals that cannot be reduced to one dimension. Goals are ranked by the decision maker and sequentially satisfied by the algorithm. Instead of trying to directly minimize or maximize one objective function which is an aggregate of multiple goals and objectives, as in LP or NP, the differences between the goals and what can be achieved given certain constraints are minimized.

## Model Formulation

Often, a decision maker must make trade-offs in the goals related to a particular project. But she does not have to eliminate any goals if she can order those goals, in which case this "satisficing" model can be formulated as a goal-programming problem. The objective function is expressed in terms of deviations from the maximum achievement of the goal. The slack variables of the constraints, as we know them in the LP formulation, take on new significance in goal programming in that they are minimized. Mathematically, the model is expressed as:

$$\text{Minimize } Z = \sum_{i=1}^{m} w_i (d_i^+ + d_i^-)$$

Subject to

$$\sum_{j=1}^{n} a_{ij} x_j + d_i^- - d_i^+ = b_i \text{ for all } i,$$

and

$$x_j, d_i^-, d_i^+ \geq 0 \text{ for all } i, j;$$

where

$$d_i^- \times d_i^+ = 0 \left.\right\} \text{(over- and underachievement}$$
$$d_i^-, \ d_i^+ \geq 0 \left.\right\} \text{cannot occur simultaneously),}$$

$x_j$ represents the decision variable, the goal,

$d$  represents the overachievement ($+$) or underachievement ($-$) of the goal, and

$w$  represents the ordinal and/or cardinal weights of each goal.

The goal-programming algorithm moves $d^-$ and $d^+$ as close to zero as possible within the constraints of the model. Once formulated, goal programming is almost identical computationally to the simplex method of LP.

### Example: Single Goal

Let us modify and extend the maximization problem from the earlier section into a single satisfying goal-programming model.

**Problem:** The administrator is adding 100 beds but cannot decide how to distribute medical ($M$) and surgical ($S$) beds among the 100-bed addition. She decided that her goal, given the constraints, was to maximize revenue; thus, the objective function became

$$\text{Maximize } Z = \$2,000M + \$1,000S$$
$$\text{under } 10M + 6S \leq 36,500$$
$$3M + 1S \leq 9,500$$
$$1S \leq 3,500.$$

The optimal solution was

$$S = \quad 1,811.25$$
$$M = \quad 2,563.25$$

$$\text{Revenue} = \$6,937,146.25,$$

which called for

1,811 discharges/year $\times$ 6 days/discharge $\div$ 365 days/year
       = 30 surgical beds

and

2,563 discharges/year $\times$ 10 days/discharge $\div$ 365 days/year
       = 70 medical beds.

Now, however, the corporation is considering a major reorganization and feels that maximizing revenue is not a realistic objective, although it does wish to achieve some satisfactory level of revenue. Management feels that an annual revenue of $6 million is satisfactory and wants to determine, given the same constraints, what the mix of medical and surgical beds should be. This now changes from an LP problem to a GP problem.

To incorporate the $6 million satisficing revenue goal into the model, deviational variables must be defined:

$d_1^- = $ the $ amount of underachievement of the revenue goal,
  and

$d_1^+ = $ the $ amount of overachievement of the revenue goal.

The revenue goal constraint is specified, but as a *target*, not an absolute requirement:

$$2,000M + 1,000S + d_1^- - d_1^+ = 6,000,000.$$

The model now becomes:

$$\text{Minimize } Z = d_1^- + d_1^+$$

subject to

$$10M + 6S \le 36,500,$$
$$3M + 1S \le 9,500,$$
$$0M + 1S \le 3,500,$$
$$2,000M + 1,000S + d_1^- - d_1^+ = 6,000,000,$$

and

$$M, S, d_1^-, d_1^+ \ge 0.$$

In this model the weights assigned to $d^+$ and $d^-$ are equal, which means that the manager wants over- and underachievement equally. If she felt that overachievement was three times more important than underachievement, the objective function would be $Z = 3d^- + d^+$, with the same constraints. Also, since both $d^+$ and $d^-$ appear in the model, it is clear that management wants to achieve the objectives exactly.

To solve graphically, plot the resource constraints as before in the LP problem (see Figure 6.13). Now, plotting the goal constraint and realizing that revenue can be equal to, greater than, or less than 6,000,000, it becomes clear that the feasible solution can be on either

side of the goal constraint line within the shaded feasible space defined by the resource constraints. The objective function tells us our
goal is to minimize $d^+$ and $d^-$ to zero. To achieve this, our optimal
feasible solution must lie at any point between and including points
A and B. This means we will be able to satisfy the manager's $6 million
goal with only convex combinations of medical and surgical discharges
between M = 1,250, S = 3,500; and M = 3,000, S = 0.

This example graphically illustrates a one-goal model. As noted
earlier, using the simplex method on this type of problem is computationally similar to and less time-consuming than a graphical solution.
But the power of goal programming is derived from its ability to deal
with the multiple goals and subgoals of a decision maker.

*Figure 6.13*

*GP Single Goal*

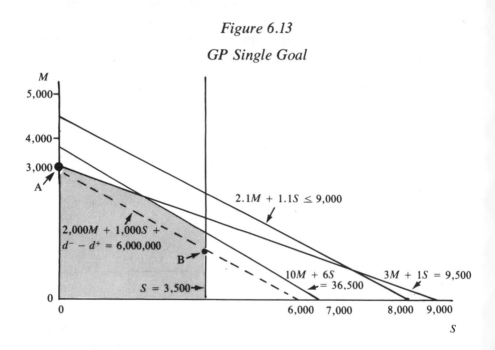

### Example: Multiple Goals and Subgoals

Let us assume now that the corporate reorganization effort is
complete and the manager would like to see an annual revenue of $8
million. It is clear that some of the constraints set earlier must be
violated. In examining the constraints, it appears that there have been
scheduling problems in the surgery and laboratory departments but
that if personnel are instructed properly, over- and underscheduling

can be eliminated. It is also observed that the costs of overscheduling in surgery are two times greater than in the laboratory.

The manager has been instructed to define and prioritize her goals related to these issues:

$P_1$: achieve an annual revenue of \$8,000,000;

$P_2$: minimize overscheduling in the laboratory and surgery departments;

$P_3$: minimize costs of overscheduling in the surgery department;

$P_4$: reduce unnecessarily long lengths of stay.

The objective function which illustrates these prioritized goals includes the following factors:

$P_1\ (d_1^- + d_1^+)$ indicates that our manager wants to achieve the first-priority goal exactly, as in our first example.

$P_2\ (d_2^+ + d_3^+)$ indicates that minimizing the total overscheduling that occurs in the lab and in surgery has second priority.

$2P_3\ d_3^+ + P_3\ d_2^+$ indicates the double cost of overscheduling in the surgery department.

$P_4\ d_4^+$ indicates the desire to minimize lengths of stay that are longer than optimal.

The goal-programming formulation appears as such:

Minimize $Z = P_1(d_1^- + d_1^+) + P_2(d_2^+ + d_3^+) + 2P_3d_3^+ + P_3\ d_2^+ + P_4d_4^+,$

subject to these goals (rather than constraints):

$$2{,}000M + 1{,}000S + d_1^- - d_1^+ = 8{,}000{,}000,$$

$$3M + 1S + d_2^- - d_2^+ = 9{,}500,$$

$$0M + 1S + d_3^- - d_3^+ = 3{,}500,$$

$$10M + 6S + d_4^- - d_4^+ = 36{,}500;$$

where

$d_1^-, d_1^+$ = underachievement and overachievement of target revenue goal (respectively),

$d_2^-, d_2^+$ = underscheduling and overscheduling in the laboratory (respectively),

$d_3^-, d_3^+$ = underscheduling and overscheduling in the surgery department (respectively),

$d_4^-, d_4^+$ = lengths of stays under and over the optimum for patient care quality (respectively),

$S$ = surgical discharges/year,

$M$ = medical discharges/year.

In the model, the priorities of the goals have been specified: $P_1 > P_2 > P_3 > P_4$. There is no value by which a lower priority can be weighted which would change its overall priority. For example, in the above model, $P_1 > P_2 > P_3 > P_4$ holds, even though $P_3$ is weighted three times greater by virtue of the multiplicand. Different weights and priorities have been assigned within goals and between goals.

Solving graphically, see Figure 6.14. Any point on the revenue line meets our first goal. Next we search for a point which satisfies both our second goal *and* our first goal. In this case we are after the point which minimizes the sum of the overscheduling in both departments. There are two likely options—points K and N. At point K, the total deviation is 2,100; at point N, it is 250. At no other point but N are all the priorities on our list met. The optimal solution is thus $S = 3,500$, $M = 2,250$. We have achieved the $8,000,000 exactly and come close to meeting the other goals as well.

Goal programming is being applied in many fields, including health care. Common examples include portfolio analysis, advertising planning, capital budgeting, manpower planning, and production scheduling. The reader is referred to the references for illustrations of its usefulness.

## 6.6 APPLICATIONS OF MATHEMATICAL PROGRAMMING

Mathematical programming is important for our purposes in two ways. First, the formulation of decisions as mathematical programming problems is the essence of the model formulation stage of Step 1 of the decision-making framework developed in Chapter 2; formulation entails determining alternatives (decision variables), relating the al-

### Figure 6.14

### GP Multiple Goals

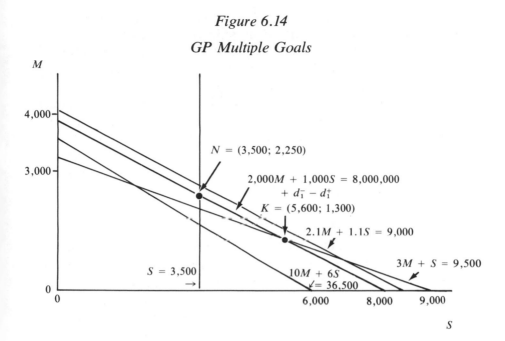

M

4,000 —

3,000 —

$N = (3,500; 2,250)$

$2,000M + 1,000S = 8,000,000$
$+ d_1^- - d_1^+$

$K = (5,600; 1,300)$

$2.1M + 1.1S = 9,000$

$3M + S = 9,500$

$S = 3,500$

$10M + 6S$
$= 36,500$

0

6,000    8,000    9,000

S

ternatives to our objectives (the objective function), and specifying which constraints must be respected. In this way MP, like our decision-making framework, is useful as a way to structure decisions for orderly analysis. Of course, many times this is as far as MP can be useful. Most problems in the health care delivery area involve stochastic elements that cannot be ignored and cannot be solved mathematically, unlike the type of MP formulation we have examined in this chapter.

When the decision *can* be analyzed as deterministic, MP is important in the second way—as a solution technique. It is a powerful solution technique when the relationships of the decision variables are linear and the variables continuous, and less powerful but still useful if they are not.

Although a significant amount of research applying MP to planning and operations decisions in the health field has been undertaken, and many MP models have been formulated addressing decisions in many areas in health care delivery, MP has not reached its full potential in the health field. There are relatively few applications that have been fully implemented and are operational, and these are mainly of the scheduling type. The major influence of MP to date has been in the area of structuring decisions. Some of the obstacles in achieving full implementation of MP in the health field are discussed in Shuman, Speas, and Young (see reference at end of chapter). Many researchers feel that MP is still in the experimental stage, as is evidenced by the fact that most of the literature describes experiments by researchers rather than by practitioners: most researchers to date do not attempt to implement results fully.

In this final section we will examine representative examples of MP formulations in three important areas: area-wide health facilities planning, resource allocation within hospitals, and personnel staffing and scheduling. The reader should keep in mind which assumptions are being made, how much they limit the usefulness of the analyses, and what would be necessary to relax them in the formulations.

### Area-Wide Planning*

Consider the problem of location and necessary size of primary-care centers within an area, shown in Figure 6.15. The area is divided into $N$ population divisions. Assume that the need for primary care for the $N$ populations has been assessed (a large measurement problem!). Let $B_i$, $i = 1, 2, ..., N$ be the number of annual primary-care visits needed by the population in area $i$. After carefully considering possible sites for primary-care centers (including existing ones), the $M$ sites shown as *s on Figure 6.15 are selected as feasible sites.

Now a decision is made as to whether site $j$ ($j = 1, 2, ..., M$) offers "adequate access" to population $i$. "Access" is used in the context of distance and time, not in terms of sufficient size of the facility. Adequacy is decided subjectively. (We will use different degrees of adequacy below to "price out" adequacy.) Let $a_{ij} = 1$ if site $j$ offers adequate access to population $i$, and let $a_{ij} = 0$ if it does not. Let $X_{ij}$ be the number of visits at site $j$ to be provided to population $i$. Finally, let $Y_j$ be the "size" of the facility to be provided at site $j$, in terms of the total number of annual visits it can accommodate.

To guarantee that population $i$ is offered adequate access to $B_i$ visits, we require

$$\sum_j a_{ij} X_{ij} \geq B_i \quad \text{for each } i;$$

and to guarantee adequate facilities at $j$, we require

$$\sum X_{ij} \leq Y_j.$$

---

*This example is a somewhat simplified combination of several studies: see references at end of chapter.

*Figure 6.15*

*Population Divisions (Letters) and*
*Location of Hospitals (Asterisks)*

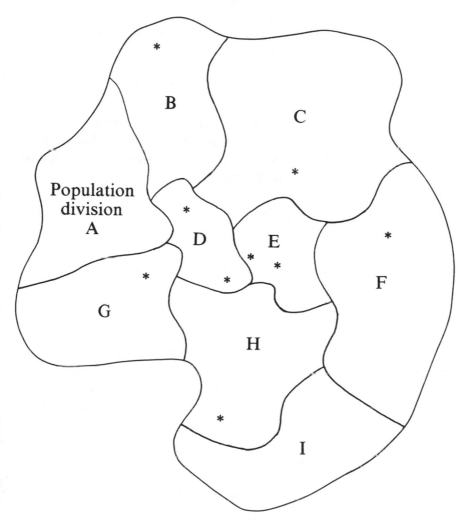

Now let $f_j (Y_j)$ be the cost of providing $Y_j$ visits at site $j$. This function is certainly nonlinear, reflecting economies of scale. Also, for those sites *already* offering a certain amount of facilities, the costs of $Y_j$ up to the present level is very low relative to a new site. A major quantification task is to derive the $f_j (Y_j)$ functions, because few types of nonlinear functions are amenable to existing nonlinear programming solution techniques.

The complete problem is as follows:

$$\text{Minimize } Z = \sum_j f_j(Y_j)$$

$$\text{Subject to } \quad \sum_j a_{ij} X_{ij} \geq B_i \text{ for each } i, \text{ and}$$

$$\sum_i X_{ij} \leq Y_j \quad \text{for each } j.$$

Solving this problem gives the minimum cost solution relative to our "adequate access" assessment of the $a_{ij}$. Now let $a'_{ij}$ reflect a more liberal (or a more conservative) assessment of adequacy of access as we solve the problem again:

$$\text{Minimize } Z' = \sum_j f_j(Y_j)$$

$$\text{Subject to } \quad \sum_j a'_{ij} X_{ij} \geq B_i \quad \text{for each } i, \text{ and}$$

$$\sum_i X_{ij} \leq Y_j \quad \text{for each } j.$$

Now note the difference between $Z$ and $Z'$: this difference is the "cost" of supplying a different level of adequacy. By solving several problems reflecting several levels of adequacy of access, planners gradually acquire a sense of the optimal placement and size of facilities, and also an ability to "price out" adequacy of access. (The literature listed at the end of this chapter discusses some of the quantification problems of this example.)

### Resource Allocation within Hospitals*

Consider a classification scheme that classifies potential patients of a hospital into one of $M$ mutually exclusive classes:

1. All patients within a class are approximately equally desirable in terms of the utility of treating them in the hospital. (The measure of utility can be based on whatever criteria the hospital

---

*This extension of the "hospital" problem in previous sections is from Baligh and Laughhunn: see Additional Reading.

board, administration, and medical staff wish to establish—another measurement problem.)

2. All patients within a class *also* require approximately the same amount of each of the hospital's $K$ types of resources (laboratory tests, X-ray tests, bed days, nursing hours, etc.).

Let $i$ index the $M$ patient classes, so that $i = 1, 2, ..., M$. Let $w_i$ be the relative value of treating a patient of class $i$. Let $X_i$ be the number of *paying* patients from class $i$ who will be admitted to the hospital, and $Y_i$ be the number of *indigent* patients from that class. Assuming that equal emphasis is placed on paying and indigent (an assumption that can be easily modified), our objective function is

$$\text{Maximize} \sum_i w_i (X_i + Y_i).$$

There are several types of constraints that we can consider, and we will examine four types. The first are constraints imposed by fixed resources. Divide the $K$ types of resources into fixed resources and variable resources. Examples of fixed resources are bed-days, operating rooms, etc., while manpower, supplies, etc., are variable. Let $j$ index the types of resources as follows: $j = 1, 2, ..., L$ are fixed resource types while $j = L - 1, L + 2, ..., K$ are variable resource types. Now let $T_j$, for $j = 1, 2, ..., L$ be the amount of fixed resource type $j$ available for the time period of interest (e.g. one year), and let $a_{ij}$ be the amount of resource $j$ that a class $i$ patient consumes. Thus we must require that

$$\sum_i a_{ij} (X_i + Y_i) \le T_j \quad \text{for } j = 1, 2, ..., L.$$

There are no resource constraints for the variable resources since they are not fixed.

The second type of constraint is budgetary. Let $r_i$ be the amount of revenue generated by a class $i$ patient. Let $c_i$ be the cost of the *variable* resources consumed by a class $i$ patient. Let $F$ be the cost of the fixed resources. Let $S$ be any subsidy the hospital receives and $G$ be its profit goal. (In some cases, either or both $G$ and $S$ will be zero.) Total income is thus

$$S + \sum_i r_i X_i$$

and total expenses are

$$F + \sum_i c_i (X_i + Y_i).$$

We require as our budgetary constraint that

$$S + \sum_i r_i X_i \geq G + F + \sum_i c_i (X_i + Y_i).$$

The third type of constraint is patient availability. Let $B_i$ be the total number of patients of class $i$ available for the planning period:

$$X_i + Y_i \leq B_i \quad \text{for each } i.$$

The final type of constraint is a policy one. Let $D_i$ be the minimum number of patients of type $i$ that the hospital, by policy, wants to admit:

$$X_i + Y_i \geq D_i \quad \text{for each } i.$$

Furthermore, let $V$ be the minimum number of indigent patients that should be treated:

$$\sum_i Y_i \geq V.$$

Now the complete formulation can be stated as:

$$\text{Maximize} \quad \sum_i w_i (X_i + Y_i)$$

$$\text{Subject to} \quad \sum_i a_{ij} (X_i + Y_i) \leq T_j \quad \text{for } j = 1, 2, \ldots, L,$$

$$S + \sum_i r_i X_i \geq G + F + \sum_i c_i (X_i + Y_i),$$

$$X_i + Y_i \leq B_i \quad \text{for each } i,$$

$$X_i + Y_i \leq D_i \quad \text{for each } i, \text{ and}$$

$$\sum_i Y_i \geq V.$$

The above is an LP problem, which of course includes assumptions of linearity, especially in the objective function and the resource constraints. (There is, however, a complicated way to restate the resource constraint that reduces the seriousness of the assumption somewhat.) Moreover, there are significant measurement problems, plus the problem of devising the $M$ patient equivalence classes. These problems are discussed to a greater extent in the Baligh and Laughhunn reference.

## Personnel Staffing and Scheduling

The greatest amount of effort in this area has been concerned with nursing personnel in the hospital—their salary cost is approximately one-third of the total budget. We will look at examples from two of the three following stages of decision.

1. *The staffing decision:* an annual decision, specifying the number of full-time equivalent *positions* of each skill level to be funded for each unit. The skill levels are registered nurse (RN), practical nurse (LPN), and nurse's aide (AIDE).

2. *The scheduling decision:* a four-week decision, specifying when each nurse on unit $i$ will be on duty and off duty for the next four weeks, taking into account weekend policy, requests for days off, and the minimum number of nurses of each skill class that must be on duty during each day and shift.

3. *The reallocation decision:* a shift-by-shift decision (three times a day) specifying how a float pool of nurses is to be allocated among various units to compensate for unforecastable changes in the need for nursing care, and for absenteeism. (A float nurse is a nurse who does not report directly to a unit when she arrives for work, but reports to the nursing office which allocates her to where the need is greatest on that shift.)

The Staffing Decision

In this application of the staffing decision (taken from Wolfe and Young; see Additional Reading), we divide the patient care tasks that nurses perform into $J$ categories and let $j = 1, 2, \ldots, J$ index them. For example, Figure 6.16 gives a classification of $J = 16$ categories. Let $i$ index the skill classes of nurses (e.g., $i = 1 = \text{RN}$, $i = 2 = \text{LPN}$, etc.). Now let $X_{ij}$ be the *fraction* of a nurse shift (8 hours) of a skill class $i$ nurse performing task $j$.

## Figure 6.16

### Classification of Nursing Tasks

| Task Type | Description |
|-----------|-------------|
| 1 | Highly technical tasks made on high care patients |
| 2 | Highly technical tasks made on intermediate care patients |
| 3 | Highly technical tasks made on self care patients |
| 4 | Less highly technical tasks made on high care patients |
| 5 | Less highly technical tasks made on intermediate care patients |
| 6 | Less highly technical tasks made on self care patients |
| 7 | Evaluation of patient need and assignment |
| 8 | Supervising and teaching |
| 9 | Tasks preparatory to highly technical tasks |
| 10 | Tasks preparatory to less highly technical tasks |
| 11 | Clerical tasks directly related to patient |
| 12 | Clerical tasks less directly related to patient |
| 13 | Medical record notation |
| 14 | Housekeeping |
| 15 | Escorting and emergency errands |
| 16 | Maintenance, checking, ordering |

Finally, let $B_j$ be the total number of nurse shifts needed for task $j$ over an eight-hour period. Then the constraints

$$\sum_i X_{ij} \geq B_j \quad j = 1, 2, \ldots, J$$

provide that task $j$ will be covered. We must also require that $\sum_j X_{ij}$ be an integer.

However, some nurse skill classes cannot perform certain tasks and can perform other tasks only at some "cost" of loss in patient care quality. For example, it may be that AIDEs cannot perform *any* of the first six tasks, and can perform the seventh task at a level of quality below what an RN would do. To account for this, let $c_{ij}$ be the loss of quality cost of a nurse of skill class $i$ performing task $j$. Thus $c_{11}$ (an RN performing task 1) will be zero, while $c_{31}$ (an AIDE performing task 1) will be very large, etc. The $c_{ij}$ are the cost of skill $i$ nurse performing task $j$ for 8 full hours.

Let $s_i$ be the salary cost of a skill $i$ nurse for an 8-hour shift. Our decision is then to

$$\text{Minimize} \sum_i \sum_j (s_i + c_{ij}) X_{ij}.$$

The $c_{ij}$ must be measured subjectively by nursing administration, the medical staff, and hospital administration. What are the units of measurement of $c_{ij}$? To answer this question, first observe how all such costs due to loss of quality can be avoided—by providing all RNs, i.e., by spending money. So the unit of measure of the $c_{ij}$ must also be in dollars. Like the facilities location decision above, we can first solve the problem for "conservative" $c_{ij}$, then more "liberal" $c_{ij}$, and then observe the resulting changes in the objective function to "cost out" our $c_{ij}$.

The problem is an IP problem because of the last constraint. Since the formulation is relatively small—in our case $4 \times 16$ variables, (minus those variables with extremely high $c_{ij}$) and 16 constraints (not counting the integer ones)—good solutions can be obtained by using available techniques of solution for IP formulations. Using LP and rounding the results, however, may leave us far from the optimal staff.

## Nurse Scheduling

In this discussion of scheduling taken from Warner (see Additional Reading) we consider a two-week scheduling horizon and the problem of scheduling only the *day* shift (i.e., assume that nurses work on only one shift and ignore the evening and night shift for now). Now suppose that there are $R$ RNs, $L$ LPNs, and $A$ AIDEs on the unit to be scheduled for the two-week horizon on the day shift. Let

$i = 1, 2, \ldots, R$ be RNs,

$i = R + 1, R + 2, \ldots, R + L$ be LPNs, and

$i = R + L + 1, R + L + 2, \ldots R + L + A$ be AIDEs.

Now consider nurse $i$. There are a finite number of schedules that nurse $i$ can work in a two-week period. Suppose she must work the "end" weekend, must be off the "middle" weekend, and that she is *already* scheduled to work Friday and Saturday *before* the two weeks begin, and the Sunday *after* (see top of Figure 6.17). Now also suppose that nurse $i$ works exactly 5 days each week. There are exactly 25 ways nurse $i$ can be scheduled for the two-week period, shown in Figure 6.17.

Now nurse $i$ is not indifferent about the 25 schedules—she likes short work stretches and 3-day weekends. Suppose each nurse is asked to divide 50 "aversion weights" among the following conditions which might show up in her schedule (the numbers in parentheses are nurse $i$'s weights):

—a single day on                                                                (10)

—a single day off                                                               (4)

—a stretch of 6 days                                                            (3)

—a stretch of 7 days                                                            (6)

—a stretch of 8 days                                                            (13)

—a stretch of 6 days that includes a 3-day weekend          (0)

—a stretch of 7 days that includes a 3-day weekend          (6)

—a stretch of 8 days that includes a 3-day weekend          (8)

(The number 50 is arbitrary.) By nurse $i$'s giving the above division of weights, it means she was twice as averse (6) to a stretch of 7 days with a 3-day weekend as to a stretch of 6 days (3), etc. Using this scheme, we can weight nurse $i$'s 25 schedules as in Figure 6.17.

Now suppose we generate schedules for *all* $R + L + A$ nurses (they won't be the same for each nurse, but will reflect restrictions on each nurse's schedule such as weekends, a request to be off, class, etc.). Let $N_i$ be the number of such schedules for nurse $i$. Also suppose each nurse has given her "aversion weight spread," so that we can weight her schedules according to her aversions. Let $j$ index the potential schedules for each nurse; that is, nurse $i$'s schedules are $j = 1, 2, \ldots, N_i$. Let $c_{ij}$ be the aversion that nurse $i$ has to working her $j$th schedule. Finally, let $X_{ij} = 1$ if nurse $i$ is to work her $j$th schedule, and 0 if she is not. Our objective could be stated as

$$\text{Minimize} \sum_i \sum_{j=1}^{Ni} c_{ij} X_{ij}.$$

To build the constraint that a minimum number of nurses should be on duty each day, let $k$ index the 14 days of the scheduling period. Let $BR_k$ be the minimum number of RNs needed on day $k$, $BRL_k$ be the minimum number of RNs *plus* LPNs needed on day $k$, and let $BRLA_k$ be the minimum number of RNs plus LPNs plus AIDEs needed.

Now let $a_{ijk} = 1$ if nurse $i$'s $j$th schedule has her on duty on

Figure 6.17

## Alternative Two-Week Schedules

| Restrictions Schedule | Weight | Previous Week | | SU | MO | TU | WE | TH | FR | SA | SU | MO | TU | WE | TH | FR | SA | Next Week |
|---|---|---|---|---|---|---|---|---|---|---|---|---|---|---|---|---|---|---|
| Restrictions | | D | D | D | | | | | X | X | X | | | | | | D | D |
| 1 | 4 | D | D | D | D | X | D | D | D | D | X | X | X | D | D | D | D | D |
| 2 | 4 | D | D | D | D | D | X | D | D | D | X | X | X | D | D | D | D | D |
| 3 | 4 | D | D | D | D | D | D | X | D | D | X | X | X | D | D | D | D | D |
| 4 | 3 + 10 + 4 | D | D | D | D | D | D | D | X | X | X | X | D | D | D | D | D | D |
| 5 | 6 | D | D | D | D | D | D | D | X | D | X | X | D | D | D | D | D | D |
| 6 | 10 + 4 + 4 | D | D | D | D | X | D | D | D | D | X | X | X | X | D | D | D | D |
| 7 | 10 + 4 + 4 | D | D | D | D | D | X | D | D | D | X | X | X | X | D | D | D | D |
| 8 | 10 + 4 + 4 | D | D | D | D | D | D | X | D | D | X | X | X | X | D | D | D | D |
| 9 | 4 + 4 + 3 + 10 + 10 | D | D | D | D | D | D | D | X | X | X | X | D | D | D | D | D | D |
| 10 | 6 + 10 + 4 | D | D | D | D | D | D | D | D | D | X | X | X | D | D | D | D | D |
| 11 | 4 + 4 | D | D | D | D | X | D | D | D | D | X | X | D | D | D | D | D | D |
| 12 | 4 + 4 | D | D | D | D | D | X | D | D | D | X | X | D | D | D | D | D | D |
| 13 | 4 + 4 | D | D | D | D | D | D | X | D | D | X | X | D | D | D | D | D | D |
| 14 | 3 + 10 + 4 + 4 | D | D | D | D | D | D | D | X | X | X | X | D | D | D | D | D | D |
| 15 | 6 + 4 | D | D | D | D | D | D | D | X | D | X | X | D | D | D | D | D | D |
| 16 | 4 + 4 | D | D | D | D | X | D | D | D | D | X | X | D | D | D | D | D | D |
| 17 | 4 + 4 | D | D | D | D | D | X | D | D | D | X | X | D | D | D | D | D | D |
| 18 | 4 + 4 | D | D | D | D | D | D | X | D | D | X | X | D | D | D | D | D | D |
| 19 | 3 + 10 + 4 + 4 | D | D | D | D | D | D | D | D | D | X | X | D | D | X | X | X | D |
| 20 | 6 + 4 | D | D | D | D | D | D | D | D | D | X | X | D | D | D | X | X | D |
| 21 | 4 + 4 | D | D | D | D | X | D | D | D | D | X | X | D | D | D | D | X | D |
| 22 | 4 + 4 | D | D | D | D | D | X | D | D | D | X | X | D | D | D | D | X | D |
| 23 | 4 + 4 | D | D | D | D | D | D | X | D | D | X | X | D | D | X | D | X | D |
| 24 | 3 + 10 + 4 + 4 | D | D | D | D | D | D | D | D | D | X | X | D | D | D | X | X | D |
| 25 | 6 + 4 | D | D | D | D | D | D | D | D | D | X | X | D | D | D | D | X | D |

day $k$, and $= 0$ if she is off. For example, suppose nurse $i$'s $j$th schedule is

$$(k =)\ 1\ 2\ 3\ 4\ 5\ 6\ 7\ 8\ 9\ 10\ 11\ 12\ 13\ 14$$

$$(\text{day})\ \ S\ M\ T\ U\ T\ F\ S\ S\ M\ T\ W\ T\ F\ S$$

$$X\ D\ D\ D\ D\ X\ D\ D\ X\ D\ D\ D\ D\ X.$$

Then $a_{ij1} = 0$, $a_{ij2} = 1$, $a_{ij3} = 1$, etc. Consider the constraints

$$\sum_{i=1}^{R} \sum_{j=1}^{Ni} a_{ijk} x_{ij} \geq BR_k \quad k = 1, 2, \ldots, 14.$$

Consider just the $a_{ijk}\ X_{ij}$ part. If nurse $i$ is working her $j$th schedule, then $X_{ij} = 1$. If nurse $i$'s $j$th schedule has her working on day $k$, then $a_{ijk} = 1$, and if both of these are true the product then adds one RN toward meeting the required $BR_k$ for day $k$. If nurse $i$ is *not* working her $j$th schedule ($X_{ij} = 0$) or if her $j$th schedule does not have her on duty on day $k$ ($a_{ijk} = 0$) then the product $= 0$. Now the constraint is to sum over all RNs (over $i = 1$ to $R$) and over all possible schedules for each nurse (over $j = 1$ to $N_i$), and make sure the minimum $BR_k$ is upheld for $k = 1, 2, \ldots, 14$.

Finally, to guarantee that nurse $i$ works exactly one of her $N_i$ schedules,

$$\sum_{j=1}^{Ni} X_{ij} = 1 \text{ for each } i, \text{ and}$$

$$X_{ij} = 0 \text{ or } 1 \text{ for each } i \text{ and } j.$$

Our complete integer programming problem is

Minimize $$\sum_{i} \sum_{j=1}^{Ni} c_{ij}\, X_{ij}$$

Subject to $$\sum_{i=1}^{R} \sum_{j=1}^{Ni} a_{ijk}\, X_{ij} \geq BR_k \qquad \text{for each } k,$$

$$\sum_{i=1}^{R+L} \sum_{j=1}^{Ni} a_{ijk}\, X_{ij} \geq BRL_k \qquad \text{for each } k,$$

$$\sum_{i=1}^{R+L+A} \sum_{j=1}^{Ni} a_{ijk}\, X_{ij} \geq BRLA_k \text{ for each } k,$$

$$\sum_{j=1}^{Ni} X_{ij} = 1 \qquad \text{for each } i, \text{ and}$$

$$X_{ij} = 0 \text{ or } 1 \qquad \text{for each } i \text{ and } j.$$

This is a much simplified version of the system Warner developed and has implemented in several hospitals over the last several years. The actual problem has the following extensions:

1. Nurses often *rotate* among shifts, so that the problem for all three shifts (day, evening and night) has to be solved together and $k = 1, 2, \ldots, 42$ ($14 \times 3$). Moreover, a rotating nurse has many more possible schedules than non-rotating ones, as do part-time nurses. The implemented system generates up to 600 possible schedules per nurse, weights them according to nursing preference, and keeps up to the 50 best schedules per nurse as input for the MP model. Thus if there are 30 nurses on a unit and they average 25 possible schedules each, the number of $X_{ij}$ is $25 \times 30 = 750$. Also, there are 42 constraints of the $BR_k$ type, 42 of the $BRL_k$ type, and 42 of the $BRLA_k$ type—a total of 128.

2. Nurses asked for schedule preferences have more things to be averse to if they work an uneven amount of times each week (e.g., six and four rather than five and five), if nurses on the unit do not have every other weekend off, or if the nurses rotate. The implemented system measures nurses' aversions to the additional items in Figure 6.18.

3. There are some times when it is not possible to find a solution that guarantees all minimum personnel requirements by day and by shift (e.g., Christmas, times of heavy vacation, periods when a unit is temporarily under its budgeted level, instances when the minimums are too high, and many other occasions). Moreover, a shortage of two nurses is much more than twice as serious as a shortage of one nurse. The implemented system uses a nonlinear *seriousness of shortage* objective function that it then minimizes, until all constraints are met as closely as possible. Only then does the minimization of the aversion objective function begin. Moreover, in order to place such shortages where they will do the least amount of harm, nursing administration is asked to "rank" days for shortage (see Figure 6.19) so that the nonlinear seriousness of shortage objective function can place shortages where they will do the least harm.

## Figure 6.18

### Scheduling Pattern Aversions

---

**INDIVIDUAL AVERSION TO WORK STRETCH AND DAYS OFF PATTERNS**

NAME  _Hake_  UNIT  _Sue_  DATE  4/8/78

Please arrange a total of 50 "aversion weights" among the work stretch and days off patterns below to indicate the relative aversion you have to working them. The more weight you place on a particular pattern, the higher your aversion to working it.

Single day on  _12_  (off-on-off)

Single day off  _6_  (on-off-on)

| | Without a 3- or 4-Day Weekend | If the Stretch Allows a 3- or 4-Day Weekend |
|---|---|---|
| Stretch of 6 days | 4 | 0 |
| Stretch of 7 days | 8 | 2 |
| Stretch of 8 days | 15 | 3 |

---

**UNIT-WIDE AVERSION TO CERTAIN ROTATING SITUATIONS**

UNIT  _Surgical_  DATE  4/8/78

After reviewing the aversion weights on work stretch indicated by all nurses on the unit, the following situations that might occur for *rotating* nurses should be assigned penalties for the "typical" rotating nurse on the unit. The weights assigned should be relative to both one another and the average or typical aversions on work stretch. For example, if EWWD is typically "twice as bad" as six day stretch, and the average weight placed on six day stretches is 10, then EWWD should be assigned 20. If then EV is "110% as bad" as EWWD, it should have a 22, etc. Use as much weight as appropriate keeping in mind the balance of the weights below with the work stretch weights.

EWWD (to E before weekend off)  _14_

DWWN (to N after weekend off)  _8_

ER (to E before a requested day off)  _15_

RN (to N after a requested day off)  _18_

EV (to E before a vacation day off)  _20_

VN (to N after a vacation day off)  _24_

DE (to E without a day off in between)  _1_

ND (back to D without a day off in between)  _1_

4. Often there are enough nurses that extra nurse shifts (above minimum) need to be scheduled. To ensure that such extra nurse shifts are distributed evenly over the schedule and that they are scheduled on days where they will be put to best use, an *overage* element is included in the objective function as measured in Figure 6.19.

5. Since nurses do not like to rotate, there is also an element in the objective function that equalizes rotation—not only total rotation, but also rotation to the night shift.

The system was programmed for real-time interaction on the computer. The schedulers (payroll clerks at one of the hospitals where the system was implemented, nursing personnel at others) first put all restrictions for a specific four-week period on a planning sheet (Figure 6.20). The nurses' names, which shifts they work, how often they work (full-time, part-time, etc.), their aversions, and how much they have rotated in the past is kept on a permanent computer file and updated when necessary. The minimum coverage data of Figure 6.19 is also kept on permanent file. At a computer terminal, the scheduler types in the restrictions from the planning sheet; and this information plus the "permanent" data allow the computer to generate up to 600 potential schedules for each nurse and to rank them with the aversion weights. As much or as little restriction as desired can be placed on the planning sheet—the computer generates schedules around the restrictions for each nurse. Then the computer program builds the MP problem (a non-linear integer one) and solves it with a special algorithm which obtains good results very quickly. The scheduler and the head nurse can then make minor improvements to the resulting schedule. A typical schedule generated by the system is given in Figure 6.21.

At one hospital where the system has been scheduling nurses on sixteen units for several years, the amount of time spent on the scheduling decision was reduced an average of 75 percent. Nurses were able to observe that rotation was being fairly distributed, as were weekends off—both of considerable importance to nurses. Moreover, the coverage was more "even" with the computer system and the patterns of rotation improved. Head nurses especially liked the new system, because they had previously spent a large, unpleasant part of each month doing the scheduling "by hand," only to find that many nurses on the staff believed that favoritism was reflected in the schedules produced, no matter how hard the head nurse tried to avoid favoritism.

## Figure 6.19

## Coverage Policy Data for a 46-Bed Surgical Unit

UNIT: Surgical     COVERAGE POLICY    DATE: 4/8/78

|  |  | S | M | T | W | T | F | S |
|---|---|---|---|---|---|---|---|---|
| MINIMUM | D | 3 | 4 | 4 | 4 | 4 | 4 | 3 |
| RN | E | 2 | 3 | 3 | 3 | 3 | 3 | 2 |
| COVERAGE | N | 2 | 2 | 2 | 2 | 2 | 2 | 2 |
| MAXIMUM | D | 2 | 2 | 2 | 2 | 2 | 2 | 2 |
| *ADDITIONAL* RN | E | 2 | 2 | 2 | 2 | 2 | 2 | 2 |
| COVERAGE | N | 1 | 1 | 1 | 1 | 1 | 1 | 1 |
| MINIMUM | D | 5 | 7 | 7 | 7 | 7 | 7 | 5 |
| RN + LPN | E | 4 | 5 | 5 | 5 | 5 | 5 | 4 |
| COVERAGE | N | 2 | 3 | 3 | 3 | 3 | 3 | 2 |
| MAXIMUM | D | 2 | 2 | 2 | 2 | 2 | 2 | 2 |
| *ADDITIONAL* RN + LPN | E | 2 | 2 | 2 | 2 | 2 | 2 | 2 |
| COVERAGE | N | 1 | 1 | 1 | 1 | 1 | 1 | 1 |
| MINIMUM | D | 6 | 9 | 9 | 9 | 9 | 9 | 6 |
| TOTAL | E | 4 | 6 | 6 | 6 | 6 | 6 | 4 |
| COVERAGE | N | 4 | 5 | 5 | 5 | 5 | 5 | 4 |
| MAXIMUM | D | 1 | 2 | 2 | 2 | 2 | 2 | 1 |
| *ADDITIONAL* TOTAL | E | 1 | 2 | 2 | 2 | 2 | 2 | 1 |
| COVERAGE | N | 0 | 0 | 0 | 0 | 0 | 0 | 0 |
| DAYS/SHIFTS WHICH CAN MOST | D |  |  | 4 | 4 |  |  |  |
| EASILY SUSTAIN A SHORTAGE | E | 3 |  |  |  |  |  |  |
| OF ONE NURSE (0–5)* | N |  |  |  |  |  |  |  |
| DAYS/SHIFTS WHERE EXTRA | D |  | 1 |  |  |  | 1 | 1 |
| (ABOVE MINIMUM) PERSONNEL | E |  |  |  |  |  |  |  |
| ARE DESIRED (0–5) | N |  |  |  |  |  |  |  |

*Rate on a scale of 0 to 5, where 0 is least and 5 is most.

N = night shift, the first shift of the day in this hospital (midnight to 8 A.M.), D = day shift (8 A.M. to 4 P.M.), and E = evening shift (4 P.M. to midnight)

The complete computer system consists of over 6,000 FORTRAN program statements which took several man-years to develop fully. The system, however, is now adaptable to a wide variety of hospitals and situations, is easily implemented in a hospital (one or two days' effort), and it costs only $5 to $10 per unit per month to run.

**Exercises**

6.1 Using only Spinach and Potatoes, solve the diet problem of Section 6.2 graphically. What is the interpretation of the shadow prices for the constraints of this problem?

6.2 Formulate a management problem in the hospital as an assignment problem. What limiting assumptions need to be made to use the assignment formulation? What measurement problems would occur if you actually tried to apply the formulation?

6.3 Do the same as in 6.2 but use the transportation formulation. Answer the two questions of 6.2.

6.4 Contrast the differences in formulating a linear programming and a goal programming problem.

6.5 You are interested in updating your lab by automating some of the testing. You have singled out 4 types of tests which lend themselves to automation. Looking at data from the past year, the average (weekday) daily demand for these 4 types of tests is:

| | |
|---|---|
| Test 1: | 450/day |
| Test 2: | 900/day |
| Test 3: | 360/day |
| Test 4: | 300/day |

(Weekend demand is considerably lower, never reaching these averages.)

Because your hospital's laboratory does all the lab work for several nearby hospitals, the daily variance is not too large. In fact, rarely (less than 1% of the time) did daily demand exceed 120% of these averages.

There are several automated lab machines on the market, but you have narrowed your choice down to two machines which

# Figure 6.20

## Input to Computer Scheduling Program
## Nurse Scheduling Planning Sheet

| UNIT | Name | Shift | W1 | W2 | W3 | W4 | Date of Request | PRE | 10 S | 11 M | 12 T | 13 W | 14 T | 15 F | 16 S | 17 S | 18 M | 19 T | 20 W | 21 T | 22 F | 23 S | 24 S | 25 M | 26 T | 27 W | 28 T | 29 F | 30 S | 1 S | 2 M | 3 T | 4 W | 5 T | 6 F | 7 S | NEXT | P1 SHT | P1 MIN | P1 MAX | P2 SHT | P2 MIN | P2 MAX | PER 1 | PER 2 |
|---|---|---|---|---|---|---|---|---|---|---|---|---|---|---|---|---|---|---|---|---|---|---|---|---|---|---|---|---|---|---|---|---|---|---|---|---|---|---|---|---|---|---|---|---|---|
| 1 | Hake | D | 5 | 5 | 5 | 5 | | 2 | D | | | | | X | X | | | | | | | D | D | | | | | | X | X | | | | | | | D 1 | | | | | | | | |
| | ∶ | | | | | | | | | | | | | | | | | | | | | | | | | | | | | | | | | | | | | | | | | | | | |
| 9 | Cheslik | DN | 1 | 5 | 5 | 5 | | 1 | R | | V | V | V | V | R | D | D | X | | | | X | X | C | C | C | | X | X | | | | | | | X | | | | | | | | |
| 10 | Menifee | DR | 5 | 5 | 2 | 5 | | 1 | • | N | | | | X | X | • | • | X | | | | • | • | C | C | X | X | X | | | | | | | • 1 | | | | | | | | |
| | ∶ | | | | | | | | | | | | | | | | | | | | | | | | | | | | | | | | | | | | | | | | | | | | | |
| 45 | Green | DE | 5 | 3 | 2 | 5 | | 3 | • | | | | R | R | B | V | | | | | • | • | | C | C | C | X | | | | | | | | • 1 | | | | | | | | |
| 46 | Greisbeck | DR | 5 | 5 | 5 | 5 | | X N | | | | | • | • | | V | | | | X | X | | | C | C | C | X | X | | | | | | | X | | | | E | 2 | 3 | 20 | |
| | ∶ | | | | | | | | | | | | | | | | | | | | | | | | | | | | | | | | | | | | | | | | | | | | |
| 60 | McMillon | DE | 5 | 5 | 5 | 5 | | 1 E | | | | | X | R | | | | | | • | • | | | | X | X | | | | | | | • 1 | | | | | | | | |
| 61 | Schmidt | DE | 5 | 5 | 5 | 5 | | X | | | | | X | X | | | | | X | X | | | | X | X | 4 | | | | | | | • 1 / • 1 | | | | | | | | |
| | ∶ | | | | | | | | | | | | | | | | | | | | | | | | | | | | | | | | | | | | | | | | | | | | |
| 82 | Steward | N | 5 | 5 | 5 | 5 | | N | N | | N | N | N | | N | N | N | N | N | N | N | | N | N | N | N | N | N | N | N | N | N | N | | | | | | | | | |
| | ∶ | | | | | | | | | | | | | | | | | | | | | | | | | | | | | | | | | | | | | | | | | | | | |

Legend:

- UNIT
- DATE
- X—off
- •—on
- N—night
- D—day
- E—evening
- N—not N ©
- D—not D $
- E—not E #
- R—request
- G—granted request
- V—vac.
- C—class
- B—birthday
- H—hol. off
- O—orien.

Input to Computer Scheduling Program, including weekend coverage as specified by the weekend policy decision, granted days off (R or X), hospital business, class or conference (C), vacation (V), and other restrictions imposed on feasible schedules. Requests, when "weighted" (see text), are done so either on the day for a single day off (see Nurse Schmidt for July 2), or in the final column for multiple days off (see Nurse Green). Explanation of column titles: WORKLOAD— number of days of shifts to be worked each of the four weeks; PREvious—number of consecutive shifts worked immediately prior to this schedule; NEXT—number of consecutive shifts to be worked at the beginning of the next schedule; ROTATION—PERiod I is the first two weeks, etc.; SHIFT—shift to be rotated to; MINimum and MAXimum—range of days to rotate (if left blank, default is an "equalizing" number).

# *Figure 6.21*

## *Four-Week Schedule for a 46-Bed Surgical Unit*

SUR SCHEDULE FOR PERIOD BEGINNING JUN 10 1978

| Nurse | Shift | 10 SU | 11 MO | 12 TU | 13 WE | 14 TH | 15 FR | 16 SA | 17 SU | 18 MO | 19 TU | 20 WE | 21 TH | 22 FR | 23 SA |
|---|---|---|---|---|---|---|---|---|---|---|---|---|---|---|---|
| 1 HAKE | D | D | D | | D | D | D | | | D | D | D | | D | D |
| 2 FRANK | D | | D | D | D | D | | D | D | D | | D | D | D | |
| 4 BRAUN | N | — | — | — | | N | N | | N | N | N | N | N | | |
| 5 BOYD | N | N | | | N | N | N | N | B | | | — | — | — | — |
| 6 HAMMER | N | N | N | | | | | | | N | N | | | | N |
| 7 COLLINS | DE | D | | E | E | E | E | | | E | E | | D | D | D |
| 8 REID | DN | | N | N | | D | D | D | • | — | — | C | | N | N |
| 9 CHESLIK | DN | • | — | — | — | — | • | D | D | D | | N | N | N | |
| 10 MENIFEE | DR | D | | N | N | D | D | | | D | D | D | D | | D |
| 12 TURNEY | DR | | D | D | D | D | | N | N | D | D | | D | D | |
| 14 SCHMITZ | DR | | D | D | D | | D | E | E | E | | D | D | D | |
| 20 GREGARIO | E | E | E | | E | E | E | • | • | — | E | E | | E | E |
| 21 LAYOS | E | E | E | E | | E | E | • | • | — | E | E | E | | E |
| 22 POLIDO | E | | E | E | E | E | | E | E | E | | E | E | E | |
| 23 DALY | D | | D | D | D | | D | D | D | | D | D | D | D | |
| 24 THORBECK | DE | | D | D | D | D | D | | | D | D | | E | E | E |
| 40 JOHNSON | N | | N | N | N | N | N | | | N | — | — | — | — | • |
| 45 GREEN | DE | D | E | E | | D | D | • | • | B | — | | D | D | D |
| 46 GRIESBECK | DR | | D | D | D | | D | D | D | | N | N | N | N | |
| 47 SALITZ | DE | D | D | D | | E | E | | D | D | D | D | • | • | • |
| 60 MCMILLON | DE | E | | D | D | D | D | | • | D | D | D | | D | D |
| 61 SCHMIDT | DE | | D | D | D | D | D | | | E | E | E | E | | D |
| 62 VOKOVICH | E | | E | E | E | E | • | E | E | E | • | E | E | E | |
| 63 DAVIS | E | E | E | E | | | E | | | | E | | E | E | E |
| 70 CUTLER | E | | | | E | | | E | E | E | | | | | |
| 80 DOOD | N | N | N | | | | N | N | N | N | | | | N | N |
| 82 STEWARD | N | N | N | N | N | N | | | N | N | N | N | N | | |
| 88 STAPLES | N | | | N | N | N | N | N | | | N | N | N | N | N |
| 89 HURD | D | | | D | D | D | D | D | | | D | D | D | D | D |
| 90 CSICSAY | D | D | D | D | D | D | | | D | D | D | D | D | | |
| 91 GLOVER | E | | E | | E | | E | | | E | | E | | E | |
| 92 WILLIAMS | E | | | E | E | E | E | E | | | E | E | E | E | E |
| RNS | NITE | 2 | 2 | 2 | 2 | 2 | 2 | 2 | 2 | 2 | 2 | 2 | 2 | 2 | 2 |
| | DAY | [illegible] | 6 | 5 | 6 | 6 | 6 | 4 | 3 | 6 | 5 | 5 | 6 | 6 | 3 |
| | EVEN | [illegible] | 3 | 3 | 3 | 4 | 3 | 2 | 2 | 3 | 3 | 3 | 3 | 3 | 3 |
| RN + LPN | NITE | [illegible] | 3 | 3 | 3 | 3 | 3 | 2 | 2 | 3 | 3 | 3 | 3 | 3 | 2 |
| | DAY | [illegible] | 9 | 9 | 9 | 9 | 10+ | 5 | 5 | 8 | 7 | 7 | 7 | 8 | 6 |
| | EVEN | 4 | 6 | 6 | 5 | 6 | 5 | 4 | 4 | 6 | 5 | 5 | 6 | 5 | 4 |
| TOTAL | NITE | 4 | 5 | 5 | 5 | 5 | 5 | 4 | 4 | 5 | 5 | 5 | 5 | 5 | 4 |
| | DAY | [illegible] | 10 | 11 | 11 | 11 | 11 | 6 | 6 | 9 | 9 | 9 | 9 | 9 | 7 |
| | EVEN | [illegible] | 7 | 7 | 7 | 7 | 7 | 5 | 4 | 7 | 6 | 7 | 7 | 7 | 5 |

| Nurse | 24 SU | 25 MO | 26 TU | 27 WE | 28 TH | 29 FR | 30 SA | 1 SU | 2 MO | 3 TU | 4 WE | 5 TH | 6 FR | 7 SA | RO/%N | WE | RG | RM | #W |
|---|---|---|---|---|---|---|---|---|---|---|---|---|---|---|---|---|---|---|---|
| 1 HAKE | D | D | | D | D | D | | | D | D | D | | D | D | | 50 | 0 | 0 | 28 |
| 2 FRANK | | D | D | D | D | | D | D | D | D | D | D | | | | 50 | 0 | 0 | 12 |
| 4 BRAUN | | N | N | N | | N | N | N | N | N | | N | N | | | 51 | 0 | 0 | 28 |
| 5 BOYD | — | | | N | N | N | N | N | | | N | N | N | N | | | 0 | 0 | 28 |
| 6 HAMMER | N | N | N | | • | • | • | • | • | N | N | | | | | 51 | 40 | 40 | 28 |
| 7 COLLINS | D | | D | D | | D | D | D | D | | D | D | D | • | 26 | 48 | 5 | 5 | 28 |
| 8 REID | N | N | | | N | D | D | D | D | | D | D | D | | 27 | 48 | 5 | 5 | 28 |
| 9 CHESLIK | | D | D | D | D | | D | D | D | D | | D | D | | 23 | 50 | 12 | 12 | 28 |
| 10 MENIFEE | D | | E | C | C | C | | | E | E | E | E | | D | 27/10 | 50 | 0 | 0 | 28 |
| 12 TURNEY | | D | D | E | E | | E | E | E | E | | D | D | | 28/ 9 | 50 | 0 | 0 | 28 |
| 14 SCHMITZ | | D | D | C | C | C | | | N | D | D | D | | N | 25/10 | 51 | 0 | 0 | 28 |
| 20 GREGARIO | E | E | | E | E | E | | | E | E | E | | E | E | | 50 | 10 | 10 | 28 |
| 21 LAYOS | E | E | E | | E | E | • | • | H | — | — | — | — | • | | 51 | 35 | 35 | 28 |
| 22 POLIDO | | E | E | E | | E | E | E | | E | E | E | E | | | 50 | 0 | 0 | 28 |
| 23 DALY | | D | D | D | D | D | | | D | D | D | | D | D | | 53 | 0 | 0 | 8 |
| 24 THORBECK | E | | D | D | D | D | | | D | D | | E | E | E | 27 | 51 | 0 | 5 | 28 |
| 40 JOHNSON | • | — | N | N | N | N | | | N | N | N | N | N | | | | 6 | 6 | 28 |
| 45 GREEN | D | D | | C | C | C | | | E | E | | D | D | D | 25 | 50 | 13 | 13 | 28 |
| 46 GRIESBECK | | D | E | E | | D | D | D | D | | D | D | D | | 26/10 | 50 | 0 | 0 | 28 |
| 47 SALITZ | • | • | D | D | D | D | | | | D | E | E | | D | 24 | 51 | 11 | 11 | 28 |
| 60 MCMILLON | E | E | | D | D | D | | | D | D | D | | D | D | 23 | 50 | 5 | 6 | 28 |
| 61 SCHMIDT | D | D | D | | D | D | | | • | D | D | D | D | E | 25 | 51 | 5 | 5 | 28 |
| 62 VOKOVICH | | E | E | E | E | • | E | E | E | • | E | E | E | | | 50 | 5 | 5 | 28 |
| 63 DAVIS | E | E | | | E | E | | | | E | | E | E | E | | 50 | 0 | 0 | 28 |
| 70 CUTLER | | | | | | E | E | E | E | | | | | | | 50 | 0 | 0 | 28 |
| 80 DOOD | N | N | | | | N | N | N | N | | | | N | N | | | 0 | 0 | 28 |
| 82 STEWARD | N | N | N | N | N | | | N | N | N | N | N | | | | | 0 | 0 | 28 |
| 88 STAPLES | | | N | N | N | N | N | | | N | N | N | N | N | | | 0 | 0 | 28 |
| 89 HURD | | | D | D | D | D | D | | | D | D | D | D | D | | | 0 | 0 | 28 |
| 90 CSICSAY | D | D | D | D | D | | | D | D | D | D | D | | | | | 0 | 0 | 28 |
| 91 GLOVER | | E | | E | | E | | | E | | E | | E | | | | 0 | 0 | 28 |
| 92 WILLIAMS | | | E | E | E | E | E | | | E | E | E | E | E | | | 0 | 0 | 28 |
| RNS NITE | 2 | 3 | 2 | 2 | 2 | 2 | 2 | 2 | 2 | 2 | 2 | 2 | 2 | 2 | | | | | |
| RNS DAY | 3 | 6 | 7+ | 6 | 5 | 5 | 4 | 4 | 7+ | 6 | 6 | 6 | 6 | 3 | | | | | |
| RNS EVEN | 3 | 3 | 3 | 3 | 3 | 3 | 2 | 2 | 3 | 4 | 3 | 3 | 3 | 2 | | | | | |
| RN + LPN NITE | 2 | 3 | 3 | 3 | 3 | 3 | 2 | 2 | 3 | 3 | 3 | 3 | 3 | 2 | | | | | |
| RN + LPN DAY | 5 | 9 | 9 | 8 | 8 | 9 | 5 | 5 | 9 | 9 | 9 | 9 | 10+ | 6 | | | | | |
| RN + LPN EVEN | 5 | 6 | 5 | 5 | 5 | 5 | 4 | 4 | 6 | 6 | 5 | 6 | 5 | 4 | | | | | |
| TOTAL NITE | 4 | 5 | 5 | 5 | 5 | 5 | 4 | 4 | 5 | 5 | 5 | 5 | 5 | 4 | | | | | |
| TOTAL DAY | 6 | 10 | 11 | 10 | 10 | 10 | 6 | [illegible] | 10 | 11 | 11 | 11 | 11 | 7 | | | | | |
| TOTAL EVEN | 5 | 7 | 6 | 7 | 6 | 7 | 5 | 4 | 7 | 7 | 7 | 7 | 7 | 5 | | | | | |

• REQUEST:—VACATION: C HOSPITAL BUSINESS: B BIRTHDAY: H HOLIDAY OFF

Nurses 1 through 24 are RNs, 40 through 70 LPNs, and 80 through 92 AIDs (AIDs work a fixed cyclical pattern in this hospital.) The columns of letters directly after the names indicate the shift(s) each nurse works according to the rotation policy decision. (N = night shift, the first shift of the day in this hospital—midnight to 8 AM; D = day shift—8 AM to 4 PM; and E = evening shift—4 PM to midnight). The numbers at the bottom indicate the number of nurses scheduled on duty each day and shift by skill class. A plus after a number indicates more than the minimum plus additional coverage, and a minus indicates less than minimum coverage. The columns of numbers to the right are interpreted as follows (all are based on accumulated data for the last #W weeks the last column): RO is the percentage of time the nurse has spent on other than her home shift. %N is the percentage of time on the night shift. WE is the percentage of weekend days the nurse was off duty. RG is the number of requests granted, divided by the total number of times the nurse has worked. RM is a similar ratio for the number of requests made.

have the same quality, and perform tests of similar quality. These are "multi-channel" machines, multi-channel in that they can perform tests simultaneously and independently. (They are actually like 4 separate machines, except that they come as a unit, sharing a common power supply, electronic interface with your computer, etc.)

The specifications on the two machines are below.

*Machine A:*                     $3,400 each

   *Daily* capacities of each type of test *per machine:*

|         |        |
|---------|--------|
| Test 1: | 42/day |
| Test 2: | 72/day |
| Test 3: | 39/day |
| Test 4: | 27/day |

*Machine B:*                     $2,700 each

   Daily capacity of each type of test per machine:

|         |        |
|---------|--------|
| Test 1: | 45/day |
| Test 2: | 39/day |
| Test 3: | 18/day |
| Test 4: | 36/day |

You are interested in converting to automation as cheaply as possible, and your automated lab must meet daily demand for these four types of tests (at least 99% of the time).

a. Formulate a linear programming model to solve the above problem.
   1. Identify the variables.
   2. Construct the objective function.
   3. Construct and identify the constraints.

b. What is the "linearity" assumption in this case? Are you comfortable in making it?

c. Solve the problem graphically.

d. What would the shadow prices tell you in this case, and how could you use them? (Give an example.)

e. What problems do you foresee with the linear programming formulation? (i.e., what problems would you have in using the LP solution to the above formulation?)

6.6 For medium-range planning purposes, you would like to establish a policy on the number of major and minor surgery procedures to which your hospital will commit itself for the next few years.

You have established, from historical data, that major procedures take an average of 2 hours to perform (including all clean-up time, etc.) while minor procedures take 1 hour. Moreover, your operating suite, with 2 major surgery rooms and 1 minor, plus 2 others which could be used for either major or minor, operates 8 hours a day, six days a week. (Minor procedures can be performed in any of the 5 rooms.)

You have committed 126 beds to surgical patients, and over the last two years major surgical patients averaged 8.9 days' stay in the hospital, while minor surgical patients averaged 3.5 days.

Major procedures require one anesthetist and two nurses constantly attending during the procedure, while minor procedures require no anesthetist and an average of 1.2 nurses per procedure. (Again, because of cleaning and setup, the nurses and anesthetists are needed for 2 hours per major and one hour per minor procedure.) You are willing to commit to the operating suite 9 full-time equivalent nurses (40 working hours per week) and 4 full-time anesthetists. (Assume all personnel figures represent 100% utilization; coverage for lunch, sick leave, vacation, etc., is included in the "full-time" concept.)

After consultations with your medical staff and board of trustees, they agree that major procedures contribute three times as much as do minor ones to the goals of the hospital.

a. Formulate an objective function for determining the mix of major vs. minor procedures; identify the production coefficients; and state the constraints as inequalities (label the constraints clearly).

b. Solve the problem graphically, indicating the solution space by shading. Which constraints are binding at the optimal solution? (To solve graphically, you will need to do a neat job on the graph; use *all* of an 8-1/2" × 11" sheet).

c. 1. Do you agree with the conceptual idea of determining the number of surgical procedures in this manner? If not, suggest another formulation of the problem.
   2. Are there other constraints that should be included?
   3. What are the major weaknesses of this model?
   4. Would you do this in a real situation? Why (or why not)?

6.7 a. Using a simplex computer program, solve for the optimal mix of major and minor procedures in Problem 6.6.

   b. What is the worth (and what does "worth" mean) of:

   1. One more *hour* of nursing time per year; one more *nurse* per year?

   2. One more *hour* of anesthetist time per year; one more *anesthetist* per year?

   3. One more *patient day* capacity annually; one more surgical *bed?*

   4. Purchasing the necessary equipment to change the minor OR room into a major-or-minor one?

   c. Later consultation with the medical staff and board of trustees establishes the relative contribution of major and minor procedures at 4 and 1, respectively. Can you still use the above solution?

6.8 Consider exercise 6.6. Suppose that two more goals have been expressed by the management. Management has learned that (1) surgical patients will now be reimbursed on a per case basis rather than per diem and (2) the nurses are expecting overtime hours because of the upcoming holidays. Management has expressed to you its additional goals of minimizing overtime hours in the surgery department. Reconstruct this exercise as a goal programming problem.

   a. Formulate the objective function.
   b. Solve graphically.

6.9 In planning the construction of a new 100-bed addition to the hospital, administration has indicated the following goals, with no indication of order of importance:

—Provide additional space for admissions
—Create jobs in the community
—Expand the type of services offered
—Generate revenue for the corporation
—Attract new physicians
—Meet community needs

In order to determine the ranking of the goals, you meet with the chairman of the board and compare all goals on a two-by-two basis.

   a. How many comparisons will there be?
      (Answer: 15)

b. Are the following noted comparisons sufficient to prioritize goals?

| | | |
|---|---|---|
| 1 > 2 | 2 < 4 | 3 > 6 |
| 1 < 3 | 2 < 5 | 2 < 3 |
| 1 < 4 | 2 < 6 | 3 < 5 |
| 3 < 4 | 4 > 6 | 1 < 5 |
| 4 > 5 | 1 > 6 | 5 > 6 |

c. If yes, rank-order the manager's preferences.

d. If no, what additional comparisons are needed?

## Additional Reading

*Technique*

Churchman, C. W., Ackoff, R. L. and Arnoff, E. L. *Introduction to Operations Research*. New York: John Wiley and Sons, 1957.

Dantzig, G. *Linear Programming and Extensions*. Princeton, N.J.: Princeton University Press, 1963.

Hillier, F. S. and Lieberman, G. J. *Introduction to Operations Research*. San Francisco: Holden-Day, 1974.

Ignizio, J. P. *Goal Programming and Extensions*. Lexington, Mass.: D.C. Heath, 1976.

Lee, A. M. and Nicely, R. "Goal Programming for Marketing Decisions: A Case Study." *Journal of Marketing* 38, no. 1 (1974): 24-32.

Lee, S. M. *Goal Programming for Decision Analysis*. Philadelphia: Auerback, 1972.

Wagner, H. M. *Principles of Operations Research With Applications to Managerial Decisions*. Englewood Cliffs, N.J.: Prentice-Hall, 1969.

*Reviews of Applications*

Shuman, L. J., Speas, R. D. and Young, J. P. *Operations Research in Health Care*. Baltimore: Johns Hopkins Press, 1975.

Stimson, D. H. and Stimson, R. H. *Operations Research in Hospitals*. Chicago: Hospital Research and Educational Trust, 1972.

*Resource Allocation within the Hospital*

Baligh, H. H. and Laughhunn, D. J. "An Economic and Linear Model of the Hospital." *Health Services Research* 4 (Winter 1969): 293 – 303.

Dowling, W. "The Application of Linear Programming to Decision Making in Hospitals." *Hospital Administration* (Summer 1971), pp. 66–75.

## Area Wide Planning

Abernathy, W. J. and Hershey, J. C. "A Spatial Allocation Model for Regional Health Services Planning." *Operations Research* 20 (1972): 629–642.

Gross, P. F. "Urban Health Disorders, Spatial Analysis, and the Economics of Health Facility Location." *International Journal of Health Services* 2 (1972): 63–84.

Morrill, R. L. and Earickson, R. "Locational Efficiency of Chicago Hospitals: An Experimental Model." *Health Services Research* 4 (1969): 128–141.

Toregas, C., Swain, R., ReVelle, C. and Bergman, L. "The Location of Emergency Service Facilities." *Operations Research* 19 (1971): 1363–1373.

Warner, D. Michael. *The Optimal Location and Size of Primary Care Centers*. Department of Health Administration, Durham, N.C.: Duke University, 1975.

## Personnel Staffing

Wolfe, H. and Young, J. P. "Staffing the Nursing Unit: Part I." *Nursing Research* 14, no. 3 (1965): 236–243, "Staffing the Nursing Unit: Part II." *Nursing Research* 14, no. 4 (1965): 299–303.

## Personnel Scheduling

Warner, D. Michael. "Scheduling Nursing Personnel According to Nursing Preference: A Mathematical Programming Approach." *Operations Research* 24 (1976): 842–856.

## Reallocation of Nursing Personnel

Trivedi, Vandan. *Optimal Allocation of Float Nurses Using Head Nurse Perceptions*. Doctoral dissertation, University of Michigan, 1974.

Warner, D. Michael and Prawda, Juan. "A Mathematical Programming Model for Scheduling Nursing Personnel in a Hospital." *Management Science* 19 (1972): 411–422.

*Menu Planning*

Balintfy, J. L. "Linear Programming Models for Menu Planning." In *Hospital Industrial Engineering*, edited by Smalley and Freeman. New York: Reinhold, 1966.

# Part III

# Forecasting and Measurement

*In Part I the concept of modeling a process was introduced, and in Part II models of many types were developed. In all the examples in Part II we assumed that a great deal of data had already been gathered: that many phenomena had been* measured *(turned into numbers) and that many* forecasts *of what may happen to these phenomena had been made. However, the concepts and techniques of forecasting and measurement were not directly addressed. In this part we investigate these concepts in some detail and discuss an extremely important related area,* information systems *(and the computers and organizations that support them). While decision making (Part II) and control (Part IV) are the main emphases of this text, neither can be undertaken effectively without some skill in forecasting and measurement, and an understanding of information systems.*

# 7

# Forecasting Demand

## 7.1 INTRODUCTION

Forecasting the demand for health services plays an essential role in decision making and control since the objectives of decision and control processes are almost always closely linked with meeting that demand. The decision to build new facilities, hire additional people, or begin new programs rests significantly on meeting the demand for facilities, personnel services, or program services. Meeting demand in an adequate manner is a central theme of control in the health field. Demand, for our purposes, consists of the amount of services (inpatient days, X-ray exams, outpatient visits, nursing hours of care, etc.) which will be sought directly by patients or indirectly by their physicians. There clearly is an important difference between *demand* for services and *need* for services. The diagram of Figure 7.1 separates the total amount of services into

Area A = services both needed and sought,

Area B = services needed but not sought, and

Area C = services sought but not needed.

It would be desirable to determine what part of Area B was attributable to an inappropriate amount and/or arrangement of services offered, so that we could include that portion with Area A in decision making and control. This, however, is beyond the scope of this text. Reducing Area C is a control problem. In this chapter we will deal with forecasting demand as defined by Areas A plus C: services sought.

*Figure 7.1*

*Services Needed Compared to Services Sought*

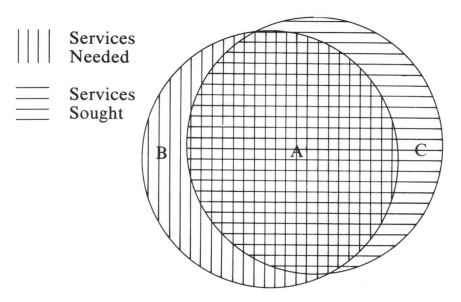

Forecasting future demand is essentially a two-stage process. First, the appropriate *measure* of demand must be identified. For example, demand may be expressed in terms of inpatient admissions to the hospital (by year, by month, etc.), total inpatient days, hours of nursing care, hours of LPN care, etc. The appropriate measure of demand depends upon how demand will be used in the decision or control process, in which the amount and arrangement of resources are planned to meet that demand. If we are analyzing the nurse-staffing decision, demand must be in terms of hours of RN, LPN, and AIDE time. If we are analyzing the decision of how many beds to build, the appropriate measure of demand is the number of inpatient days. The measure of demand must be carefully established in view of its role in the decision or control process. Note that in the list of measures above, each of the latter measures are derivatives of the preceding measures. We may consider forecasting such derivative measures either directly or by forecasting a "parent" measure and the derivative *relationship*. For example, we may forecast inpatient days directly, or we may forecast both admissions and the derivative relationship "average length of stay" (which when multiplied together give inpatient days). Such forecasting is discussed at the end of Section 7.2, Concluding Remarks.

The second stage of forecasting demand, to which the remainder of this chapter is devoted, is projecting the selected appropriate measure of demand into the future. There are essentially three ways to make such forecasts:

1. basing the forecast of future behavior of demand on observed past behavior,

2. basing the forecast of future behavior of demand on subjective (expert) opinion, or

3. basing the forecast on a combination of 1 and 2.

If the case of interest (for example, emergency arrivals) is one that has a past history, we may want to base our forecast of future behavior on past behavior. For example, if emergency arrivals have increased exactly 10 percent for the past eight years, a preliminary forecast for next year would be another 10 percent increase. If, however, there are no precedents that can govern the prediction, for example, forecasting the number of visits to a proposed facility designed to treat a newly treatable disease, the opinion of experts (such as physicians who will treat the disease) may be the only available predictor. A case that would fall somewhere between the above two types would be a process which is new to the institution (for example, a new burn center), but which has a prior history in similar institutions. In this case, it may be possible to combine projected behavior from the similar institution with a comparison of the institutions and their environment—along with expert opinion.

In basing a forecast of future behavior on past behavior (the first method, above), there are two important hypotheses:

—demand has exhibited some measurable trend in the past, and

—the trend will continue into the future.

We will see that we can test the first hypothesis statistically and obtain measurable confidence (in the statistical sense) regarding whether or not it is true. *There is no way, however, to test the second hypothesis.* Thus we will be uncomfortable in using the first method alone and will always temper our forecast based on method 1 with the best available subjective opinion.

A final distinction among forecasts is the length of time into the future for which forecasts will be made. The distinction is important because separate techniques exist for different horizons. We will thus consider three *types* of forecasts:

1. Long-term forecast: (arbitrarily) over one year.

2. Intermediate-term forecast: several months to a year.

3. Short-term forecast: a few hours to a few months.

The type of forecast appropriate for use will depend primarily upon the ability to manipulate the resources to be allocated and/or arranged to meet projected demand. Since building new beds (or new hospitals or additions to hospitals) is usually a process requiring several years, and the consequences of building or not building are significant for many more years, long-term forecasting of demand for new beds is necessary. On the other hand, nurses may be allocated among units on a shift-by-shift basis, requiring very short-term forecasts of the demand for nursing care services by skill class by nursing unit. Hiring additional nurses requires more time, so that intermediate-term forecasting of overall demand for nursing care services is appropriate. For all three types of forecasting, however, our basic procedure is the three-step process outlined above: (1) establish a past pattern, (2) project that pattern into the future, and (3) reconcile that projection with other available knowledge or opinion.

## 7.2 LONG-TERM FORECASTING

**Problem:** A 400-bed hospital established a Cardiac Care Unit (CCU) with 8 beds eight years ago. Until recently, the unit had easily handled demand for CCU beds; but during the last year there were several instances where the CCU was full and cardiac patients had to be put in Intensive Care beds, which are themselves approaching maximum utilization. The hospital would like to consider expanding the CCU unit if necessary, but is not sure whether last year was only an unusually heavy year, or if last year was an indication of a need for more CCU beds. In either case it wants to determine how many new beds will be required over the next 5 years.

Table 7.1 gives the annual number of patient CCU days consumed in the hospital over the past eight years. It is clear that demand has increased over the period, but the question is, Is there a *pattern*

*Table 7.1*

*The Annual Number of CCU Patient Days
for Past Eight Years*

| Year ($t$) | CCU PD | Average Census |
|:---:|:---:|:---:|
| 1 | 360 | 1.0 |
| 2 | 648 | 1.8 |
| 3 | 720 | 2.0 |
| 4 | 756 | 2.1 |
| 5 | 1,080 | 3.0 |
| 6 | 1,008 | 2.8 |
| 7 | 980 | 2.7 |
| 8 | 1,296 | 3.6 |

in the increase that we might project into the future? By displaying
the data graphically, Figure 7.2 indicates that a possible pattern is
a *linear* trend. Specifically, we might hypothesize from Figure 7.2
that there is an underlying linear increase in CCU patient days, with
some random fluctuation around that linear increase.

*Figure 7.2*

*Hypothesized Linear Trend in CCU Patient Days
from Year to Year*

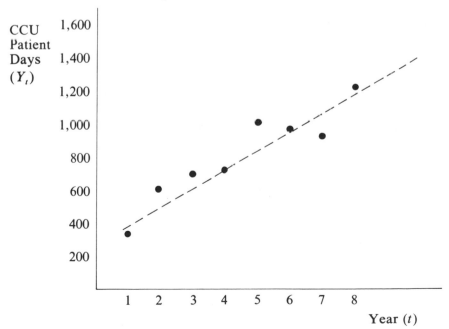

Note that there are many possible linear trends (or lines) that could be said to "fit" the data (see Figure 7.3). We will develop below the criteria to establish a "best" fit, but first we must introduce mathematical notation. Let

$Y_t$ be the *actual* number of CCUPD (CCU patient days) demanded in year $t$, and let

$\hat{Y}_t$ be the *estimated* or hypothesized or "trend" value of $Y$ for year $t$ (the $\hat{}$ will be used to refer to "estimated").

We can define any straight line by specifying its slope ($b$) and the point where it crosses the vertical axis ($a$). We can thus define our hypothetical trend line to explain past behavior as

$$\hat{Y}_t = a + bt,$$

*Figure 7.3*

*Alternative Hypothesized Linear Trends
in CCU Patient Days from Year to Year*

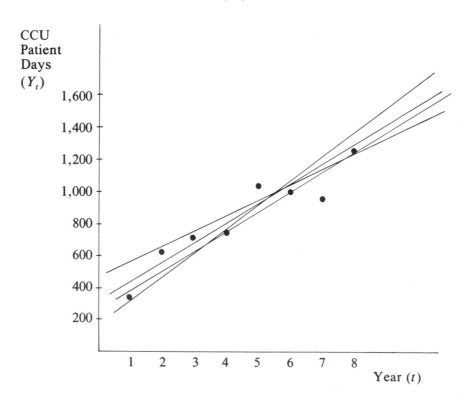

where $t$ refers to the year. Now we need to find the specific equation (i.e., specific values for $a$ and $b$) for the line that best fits the actual data $Y_t$ and $t$ of Table 7.1. We here arbitrarily define "best" as that line which minimizes the sum of squared deviations (or distances) of the actual data points $(Y_t)$ from their corresponding hypothesized value $(\hat{Y}_t)$. These deviations are shown as the vertical lines of Figure 7.4.

We can define the sum of squared deviations for $n$ points as follows:

$$S = \sum_{t=1}^{n} (Y_t - \hat{Y}_t)^2.$$

Or, since $\hat{Y}_t = a + bt$,

$$S = \sum_{t=1}^{n} (Y_t - a - bt)^2.$$

*Figure 7.4*

*Linear Trend that Minimizes the Sum of the Squared Deviations (Vertical Lines)*

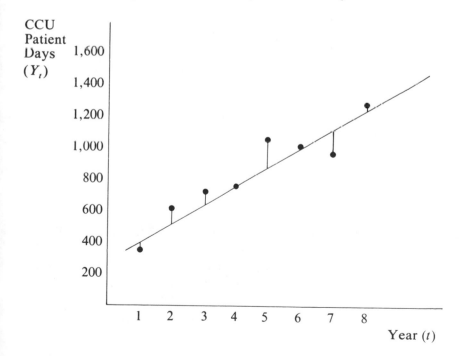

Skipping the calculus derivation of the minimum of $S$,* $S$ is minimized when (to simplify, let $\Sigma$ imply $\Sigma_{t=1}^{n}$),

$$b = \frac{n \Sigma t Y_t - (\Sigma t)(\Sigma Y_t)}{n \Sigma t^2 - (\Sigma t)^2}, \text{ and}$$

$$a = \bar{Y} - b(\bar{t}),$$

where $\bar{Y}$ is the average of the $Y$ (i.e., $\Sigma Y_t / n$) and $\bar{t}$ is the average of the $t$ (i.e., $\Sigma t / n$).

Table 7.2 calculates the necessary terms for the right side of the equations for $a$ and $b$ of our example (ignore the last column for the moment). Substitute into the equations for $a$ and $b$:

$$b = \frac{(8)(35,516) - (36)(6,848)}{8(204) - (36)^2} = \frac{37,600}{336} = 111.9,$$

$$a = 856 - (111.9)(4.5) = 352.4,$$

and our hypothesized regression line is

$$\hat{Y}_t = a + bt = 352.4 + 111.9t.$$

By our criteria of minimum least squares, this is the linear trend

### Table 7.2

*Calculations Required to Obtain Regression Coefficients a and b with Linear Trend*

| Year $t$ | $Y_t$ | $(Y_t)(t)$ | $t^2$ | $Y_t^2$ |
|---|---|---|---|---|
| 1 | 360 | 360 | 1 | 129,600 |
| 2 | 648 | 1,296 | 4 | 419,904 |
| 3 | 720 | 2,160 | 9 | 518,400 |
| 4 | 756 | 3,024 | 16 | 571,536 |
| 5 | 1,080 | 5,400 | 25 | 1,166,400 |
| 6 | 1,008 | 6,048 | 36 | 1,016,064 |
| 7 | 980 | 6,860 | 49 | 960,400 |
| 8 | 1,296 | 10,368 | 64 | 1,679,616 |
| 36 | 6,848 | 35,516 | 204 | 6,461,920 |
| $\Sigma t$ | $\Sigma Y_t$ | $\Sigma Y_t t$ | $\Sigma t^2$ | $\Sigma Y_t^2$ |

$$\bar{Y} = \Sigma Y_t / n = 6,848/8 = 856$$
$$\bar{t} = \Sigma t / n = 36/8 = 4.5$$

---

*The minimum $S$ is found by taking the partial derivatives of $S$ in terms of $a$ and $b$ and setting them equal to 0. The above equations for $a$ and $b$ are in a form convenient for computation.

that best fits the data. But how good is *best?* What is needed is an absolute measure of how likely it is that the equation $\hat{Y}_t = 352.4 + 111.9t$ actually reflects a past trend, against the possibility that in fact there has been *no trend* in the past.

## Testing the Linear Fit

What we have done so far is to try to explain how, in the past, annual CCU patient days $(Y_t)$ have changed with time $(t)$. To do this, we have implied that the past behavior of $Y$ *can* to some extent be explained by time. This we can test statistically, and to do so we set up the null hypothesis—

$$H_0: b = 0 \text{ (there is no temporal trend in } Y_t)$$

and the alternate hypothesis

$$H_a: b \neq 0 \text{ (there is a linear trend)}—$$

and try to reject $H_0$. The evidence against $H_0$ is the past data.

As we are aware, there are many factors influencing the past behavior of $Y_t$; for example, there are new physicians, changes in the population, the economy, the weather, etc. We divide all the factors which could (theoretically) be used to explain the past behavior of $Y_t$ into two groups:

1. those that we are going to put into our regression equation, called the independent variables (in our example we have only one; $t$), and

2. all others, which we refer to as *chance.*

To be more specific, let us examine the difference between $Y_t$ and $\bar{Y}$. These differences are depicted by vertical lines in Figure 7.5. We can divide this total deviation into two parts: deviation explained by time (i.e., by our regression line), and deviation unexplained by time (or due to chance). Consider Figure 7.6. The total deviation, for any $t$, is

$$(Y_t - \bar{Y}) = (\hat{Y}_t - \bar{Y}) + (Y_t - \hat{Y}_t);$$

total deviation = explained deviation + unexplained deviation.

The dashed vertical lines in Figure 7.6 show $(Y_t - \hat{Y}_t)$, the unexplained deviation. A part of the total deviation $(Y_t - \bar{Y}_t)$ is explained by $Y_t$, our predicted CCU patient days, and is shown by $(\hat{Y}_t - \bar{Y})$.

*Figure 7.5*

*Total Deviation of* $Y_t$ *from* $\overline{Y}$

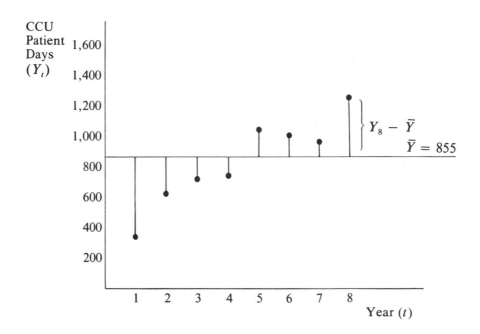

Note that in the right side of the above equation, $\hat{Y}_t$ has simply been added and subtracted, making it equal to the left side.

Without going through the steps, by squaring the deviations above and summing over $t$, it can also be shown that

$$\Sigma\,(Y_t - \overline{Y})^2 = \Sigma\,(\hat{Y}_t - \overline{Y})^2 + \Sigma\,(Y_t - \hat{Y}_t)^2,$$

or that total variation = explained variation + unexplained variation where variation is defined as the sum of the squared deviations.

Now if $H_0$: $b = 0$ is true, the following ratio will follow the $F$ distribution:

$$F = \frac{\text{variance explained by regression}}{\text{unexplained variance}}$$

with 1 and $n - 2$ degrees of freedom where $n$ is the number of observations. To get these *variances* from the *variations* above, each variation must be divided by its corresponding degrees of freedom (the usual formula for variance). However, an easier formula for hand calculations is

*Figure 7.6*

*Total Deviation Separated into*
*Unexplained Deviation and Explained Deviation*

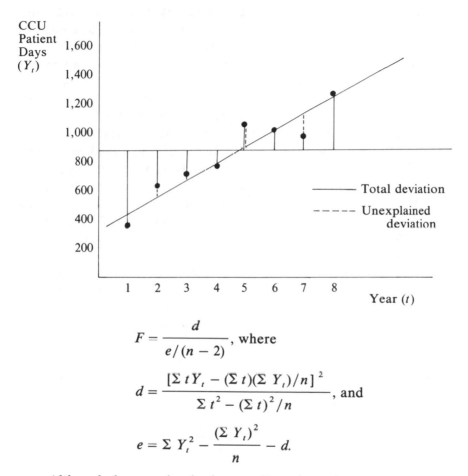

$$F = \frac{d}{e/(n-2)}, \text{ where}$$

$$d = \frac{[\Sigma\, tY_t - (\Sigma\, t)(\Sigma\, Y_t)/n]^2}{\Sigma\, t^2 - (\Sigma\, t)^2/n}, \text{ and}$$

$$e = \Sigma\, Y_t^2 - \frac{(\Sigma\, Y_t)^2}{n} - d.$$

Although the equation looks complicated, we have all the necessary terms for our example in Table 7.2, so that

$$d = \frac{[35{,}516 - (36)(6{,}848)/8]^2}{204 - (36)^2/8} = \frac{(4{,}700)^2}{42} = 525{,}952.4,$$

$$e = 6{,}461{,}920 - \frac{(6{,}848)^2}{8} - 525{,}952.4 = 74{,}079.6, \text{ and thus}$$

$$F = \frac{525{,}952.4}{74{,}079.6/6} = 42.6.$$

Since the 99th percentile of the $F$ distribution for 1 and $n - 2 = 6$ degrees of freedom (see Table II at end of text) is 13.74, it is clear that we may reject $H_0$. Our linear trend as derived above is presently our only alternative (we'll consider others below), and so we accept it as our $H_A$. Other (nonlinear) trends may give better evidence (a larger $F$) against $H_0$, and we use the $F$ test as a measure of the "quality" of the trend we offer as evidence against $H_0$. We can thus in this way use the $F$ test to choose among alternative candidates (linear and nonlinear) for explaining the past trend.

A common way to display the two types of variation (explained and unexplained) is in an Analysis of Variance (ANOVA) Table such as Table 7.3. The first column refers to the source of variation. The explained portion is called the Regression, and the unexplained, the About Regression or Error. The second column gives the equations for calculating the sum of squares associated with each type of variation. We have labeled the Regression sum of squares $d$, and the About Regression (or Error) sum of squares $e$. Note that $e$ is calculated by subtracting $d$ from the equation for Total sum of squares. The third column gives degrees of freedom, and the fourth column the Mean Square, or the sum of squares divided by the degrees of freedom. The $F$ ratio or statistic is then defined as the Regression Mean Square divided by the About Regression (Error) Mean Square. The lower part of Table 7.3 gives the calculated values from our example.

If we cannot reject $H_0$ at a "comfortable" level of confidence (the degree of comfort depends on the situation—95 percent and

### Table 7.3

### Analysis of Variance

| Source | Sum of Squares | Degrees of Freedom | Mean Square |
|---|---|---|---|
| Regression (explained) | $d = \dfrac{[\Sigma\, t Y_t - (\Sigma\, t)(\Sigma\, Y_t)/n]^2}{\Sigma\, t^2 - (\Sigma\, t)^2/n}$ | 1 | $d$ |
| About Regression or Error (unexplained, or residual) | $e = \Sigma\, Y_t^2 - \dfrac{(\Sigma\, Y_t)^2}{n} - d$ | $n - 2$ | $e/n - 2$ |
| TOTAL | $\Sigma\, Y_t^2 - \dfrac{(\Sigma\, Y_t)^2}{n}$ | $n - 1$ | $F \text{ ratio} = \dfrac{d}{e/(n - 2)}$ |
| Regression | 525,952.4 | 1 | 525,952.4 |
| About Regression | 74,079.6 | 6 | 12,346.6 |
| TOTAL | 600,032.0 | 7 | $F \text{ ratio} = 42.6$ |

99 percent being commonly used), then we must look for other (nonlinear) trends. If we find no good evidence against $H_0$ (linear or nonlinear), we must fail to reject $H_0$ and use $\hat{Y}_t = \bar{Y}$ as the trend line that best explains past data (this is called "no trend").

## The Coefficient of Determination and the Coefficient of Correlation

The *proportion* of the total variation that is *explained* is

$$R^2 = \frac{\Sigma(\hat{Y}_t - \bar{Y})^2}{\Sigma(Y_t - \bar{Y})^2}.$$

We call the proportion of variation explained by regression *the coefficient of determination* and denote it $R^2$. It gives us a measure of the strength of the regression line.

The square root of $R^2$ is called the *coefficient of correlation* and is another measure of how well $Y_t$ can be explained by $t$. $R$ has the same sign as $b$; if $R$ is positive, we say there is positive correlation between $Y_t$ and $t$, and if $R$ is negative, we say that there is negative correlation.

The above equation for $R^2$ is cumbersome for calculations. A much easier equation for calculating $R$ is

$$R = \frac{n(\Sigma\, tY_t) - (\Sigma\, t)(\Sigma\, Y_t)}{\sqrt{[n(\Sigma\, t^2) - (\Sigma\, t)^2]\,[n(\Sigma\, Y_t^2) - (\Sigma\, Y_t)^2]}}.$$

For our example,

$$R = \frac{8(35,516) - (36)(6,848)}{\sqrt{[(8)(204) - (36)^2]\,[(8)(6,446,304) - (6,848)^2]}}$$

$$= \frac{284,128 - 246,528}{\sqrt{(336)(4,800,256)}} = \frac{37,600}{40,160.75} = .936$$

and $R^2 = (.936)^2 = .877$.

Thus 87.7 percent of the total variation of $Y_t$ can be explained by $t$ (a rather high proportion). This, together with the high $F$ statistic would give us a fair amount of confidence in a linear trend in which time is able to explain the past behavior of CCU patient days.

To sum up so far, we first determined the linear trend $\hat{Y}_t = a + bt$ which best explains the past behavior of $Y_t$ (specifically for our example $\hat{Y}_t = 352.4 + 111.9t$). We then tried to reject the hypothesis that there is no significant trend ($b = 0$) by using as evidence the $F$ statistic. If we could not have rejected $H_0$, we would have had either to look for other (nonlinear) trends to explain $Y_t$ or use $\hat{Y}_t = \bar{Y}$ as our factor that explains past behavior. Given a satisfactory $F$ test outcome, we then calculated $R^2$ as a measure of the "strength" of our explanatory equation.

One final consideration is the examination of the unexplained deviations $(Y_t - \hat{Y}_t)$, sometimes called residuals and sometimes called errors—assuming of course that the regression line is "correct." In performing the regression analysis, we have assumed the errors have zero mean, are independent, have a constant variance, and (for the $F$ test) are normally distributed. We should examine the

## Figure 7.7

### Residuals Plotted against Time

| $t$ | $Y_t$ | $\hat{Y}_t$ | $Y_t - \hat{Y}_t$ |
|-----|-------|-------------|-------------------|
| 1 | 360 | 464 | −104 |
| 2 | 648 | 570 | 72 |
| 3 | 720 | 688 | 32 |
| 4 | 756 | 800 | −44 |
| 5 | 1,080 | 911 | 169 |
| 6 | 1,008 | 1,023 | −15 |
| 7 | 980 | 1,135 | −155 |
| 8 | 1,296 | 1,247 | 49 |

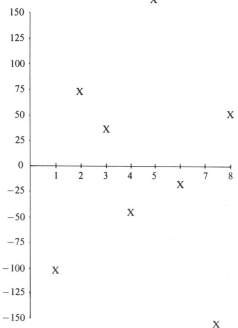

residuals to see if our assumptions hold. This can be done graphically. It is easy to do and usually reveals instances when our assumptions do not hold. A more complete discussion is found in Draper and Smith.

The residuals should at least be plotted against time, the independent variable, as shown in Figure 7.7. We should get an impression of a horizontal band of residuals equally placed above and below zero. The band should not be gradually increasing or decreasing, nor should it have a rainbow shape. Plotting often reveals calculation errors quickly when done by hand and might best be done before calculating $F$ and $R^2$. The residuals represent the sum of all the factors we have not explained by our regression, and therefore are important to examine.

Several warnings are appropriate before we continue. First, we have considered only linear trends to explain past behavior. Second, we have only tried to explain *past* behavior: we still have to deal with projecting past behavior into the future. Finally, we cannot infer that changes in $Y_t$ are *caused* by changes in $t$, no matter how high the $R^2$ and $F$. We can only say that they are related, or that, in the past, the behavior of $Y_t$ can be *explained* by $t$. To establish a cause and effect relationship, logical, not statistical, arguments must be used.

### Nonlinear Trends

It may be possible to obtain a better fit to past data (i.e., higher $F$ and $R^2$) by trying curved (nonlinear) trends to explain past behavior (see Figure 7.8). Although many types of nonlinear trends can be considered, we will examine only one type: exponential growth trends of the form

$$\ln \hat{Y}_t = a + bt,$$

where ln denotes the *natural log*. An exponential trend is likely to give a better fit in those cases where $Y_t$ appears to be increasing at an increasing rate over time.

The calculation of $a$, $b$, $F$, and $R^2$ is the same as above, except we use $\ln Y_t$ instead of $Y_t$. Table 7.4 gives the necessary components to calculate $a$, $b$, $F$, and $R^2$ for the nonlinear trend, along with

$$\overline{\ln Y} = 53.514/8 = 6.689 \text{ and}$$

$$\bar{t} = 4.5,$$

so that

*Figure 7.8*

**Hypothesized Curved (Nonlinear) Trend
in CCU Patient Days from Year to Year**

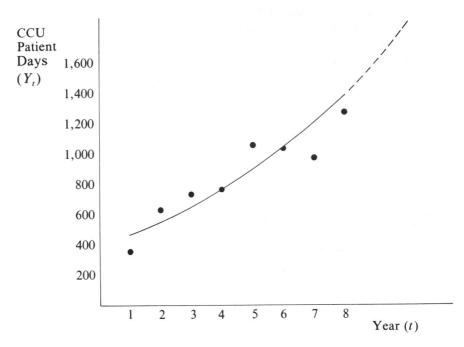

*Table 7.4*

**Calculations Required to Obtain Regression
Coefficients a and b with Exponential Trend**

| Year $t$ | $\ln Y$ | $(\ln Y)(t)$ | $t^2$ | $(\ln Y)^2$ |
|---|---|---|---|---|
| 1 | 5.886 | 5.886 | 1 | 34.646 |
| 2 | 6.474 | 12.948 | 4 | 41.911 |
| 3 | 6.579 | 19.738 | 9 | 43.287 |
| 4 | 6.628 | 26.512 | 16 | 43.931 |
| 5 | 6.985 | 34.924 | 25 | 48.786 |
| 6 | 6.916 | 41.494 | 36 | 47.827 |
| 7 | 6.879 | 48.155 | 49 | 47.326 |
| 8 | 7.176 | 57.336 | 64 | 51.366 |
| 36 | 53.514 | 246.994 | 204 | 359.080 |
| $\Sigma t$ | $\Sigma \ln Y$ | $\Sigma (\ln Y)(t)$ | $\Sigma t^2$ | $\Sigma (\ln Y)^2$ |

$$b = \frac{(8)(246.994) - (36)(53.514)}{(8)(204) - (36)^2} = \frac{49.448}{336} = .147 \text{ and}$$

$$a = 6.689 - (.147)(4.5) = 6.028.$$

Our explanatory trend line is thus

$$\ln \hat{Y}_t = a + bt = 6.028 + .147t.$$

To convert $\ln \hat{Y}_t$ to $\hat{Y}_t$ we must take the anti-ln—that is, raise $e$ to the power of $\hat{Y}_t$: $e^{\hat{Y}_t}$. For example, our estimate $\hat{Y}_3$ for year 3 is

$$\text{anti-ln } [6.028 + (.147)(3)] = \text{anti-ln } [6.469] = e^{6.469} = 644.8.$$

(This line is plotted in Figure 7.8.)
    As before

$$F = \frac{d}{e/(n-2)} \text{ where}$$

$$d = \frac{[246.994 - (36)(53.514)/8]^2}{204 - (36)^2/8} = \frac{38.205}{42} = .9096, \text{ and}$$

$$e = 359.080 - \frac{(53.514)^2}{8} - .9096 = .202, \text{ so that}$$

$$F = \frac{.9096}{.202/6} = 27.$$

Also,

$$R = \frac{(8)(246.994) - (36)(53.514)}{\sqrt{[(8)(204) - (36)^2][(8)(359.080) - (53.514)^2]}}$$

$$= \frac{49.448}{\sqrt{(336)(8.892)}} = \frac{49.448}{54.659} = .905$$

and $R^2 = .8184.$

Note that the linear fit is slightly superior to the exponential fit in terms of both $F$ and $R^2$.

**Making the Forecast**

Having established a past trend for the behavior of CCU patient days, the next step is to project that trend into the appropriate future, and finally to reconcile that projection with subjective data or opinion about the process $Y_t$. To project a linear trend to year 10 for our example, we simply calculate

$$\hat{Y}_{10} = a + b(10) = 352.4 + 111.9(10) = 1{,}471.$$

The exponential projection would be

$$\text{anti-ln}(\ln \hat{Y}_{10}) = \text{anti-ln}(a + b(10)) = \text{anti-ln}(6.028 + .147(10))$$

$$= \text{anti-ln}(7.498) = 1{,}803.$$

If we could not comfortably reject $H_0$ with either the linear or the nonlinear $F$ value, our projection would be

$$\hat{Y}_{10} = \bar{Y} = 855.$$

The corresponding projections for year 15 are

$$\text{(linear) } \hat{Y}_{15} = 2{,}031,$$

$$\text{(exponential) } \hat{Y}_{15} = 3{,}763, \text{ and}$$

$$\text{(no trend) } \hat{Y}_{15} = 855.$$

For planning purposes, it is clear that the projection of the past trend into, say, year 15 very significantly depends on which process is being projected. There should be strong subjective evidence or opinion that an exponential growth will continue into the future before making an exponential projection. For example, suppose the exponential trend had been the best fit. There might be strong opinion that the last eight years' exponential growth reflected the community's "catching up" with the use of cardiac care facilities following a period of limited access and knowledge, and now the community has caught up. This might lead us to make a linear projection (based perhaps on population growth of susceptible cardiac-age patients) even if the evidence was stronger for exponential growth in the past. Another option would be to project a use rate from past use rates in your community or, to avoid the "catching up" problem, use rates in similar communities and apply these projected use rates to the appropriate segment of your population, projected separately. The fact that another hospital in the area will open its own CCU unit should of course influence the projection. It cannot be stressed too often that the statistical techniques we have used establish only whether there has or has not been a *past* trend. The projection of future behavior should consider an established past trend together with subjective data or opinion of the likely future behavior of the process in question.

There are two reasons why none of the above forecasts for the year 10 or 15 will be *exactly* correct. The first is, of course, that the past trend may not continue into the future. For example, if the community population will not continue to grow at all, then we would likely be overestimating the level of $Y_{10}$ by using the linear or nonlinear trend, but underestimating $Y_{10}$ with $\hat{Y}_{10} = Y_8$, because of a likely increasing use rate for the CCU.

Even if the past trend that we choose does continue into the future, we will expect the actual values of $Y_t$ to lie off the projected trend line, just as they have in the past. This is because time ($t$) is only *one* factor explaining the behavior of $Y_t$, the other factors being "chance." If we make the assumption that these chance factors will influence the behavior of $Y_t$ in the future *as they have in the past*, then we can make the additional prediction that $\hat{Y}_{10}$ will fall within some confidence interval with $Y_{10}$ as its midpoint; i.e., $\bar{Y}_{10}$ is a random variable following a distribution with mean $\hat{Y}_{10}$. It is usually assumed that $\bar{Y}_{10}$ will follow the Student $t$ distribution, with $n - 2$ degrees of freedom, mean of $\hat{Y}_{10}$, and standard deviation

$$S_{t_p} = \sqrt{\left(\frac{\Sigma Y_t^2 - a \Sigma Y_t - b \Sigma t Y_t}{n - 2}\right)\left(\frac{n + 1}{n} + \frac{(t_p - \bar{t})^2}{\Sigma t^2 - n\bar{t}^2}\right)}$$

where $t_p$ is the $t$ of the projection (e.g., $t_p = 10$ or 15 in our above projection).

Thus we can construct a $(1 - \alpha)$ percent confidence interval for our estimate as

$$\hat{Y}_t - T_{\alpha/2} S_{t_p} \leq \text{estimate} \leq \hat{Y}_t + T_{\alpha/2} S_{t_p},$$

where $T_{\alpha/2}$ refers to the $\alpha/2$ percentile of the Student $t$ distribution. For example, to establish a 95 percent confidence interval ($\alpha/2 = .025$) for our linear projection for $Y_{10}$,

$$S_{t_p}^2 = \left[\frac{6,461,920 - (352.4)(6,848) - (111.9)(35,516)}{6}\right]$$
$$\cdot \left[\frac{9}{8} + \frac{(10 - 4.5)^2}{204 - (8)(4.5)^2}\right]$$

$$= \left(\frac{74{,}444.4}{6}\right)\left(1.125 + \frac{30.25}{42}\right) = (12{,}407.4)(1.845) = 22{,}891.65$$

$$S_{t_p} = \sqrt{22{,}891.65} = 151.3.$$

Since $T_{\alpha/2} = T_{.025} = 2.447$ for 6 degrees of freedom, our 95 percent confidence interval is

$$\hat{Y}_{10} = 1{,}471 \pm (2.447)(151.3)$$

or

$$1{,}101 \le \hat{Y}_{10} \le 1{,}841$$

—a rather wide range for planning purposes, reflecting again the likelihood of other factors (chance) having had a significant effect on the past behavior of $Y_t$.

It is important to remember that by using the confidence interval, we are assuming that (1) the past linear trend is going to continue into the future, *and* (2) the variation about that trend is going to continue as it has in the past.

Note that $S_{t_p}$ increases as $t_p$ increases, giving us wider and wider confidence intervals the farther we are from $\bar{t}$. The confidence interval lines for the projected linear trend bow outward, as shown in Figure 7.9.

## Multiple Regression

We have noted that there are factors other than time which might explain the past behavior of the dependent variable $Y$. We could include some of these factors explicitly by constructing the *multiple regression* (as opposed to simple regression) equation

$$\hat{Y} = a + b_1 X_1 + b_2 X_2 + b_3 X_3, \ldots, + b_n X_n,$$

where the $X_i$ are independent variables thought to explain the past behavior of $Y$.

Multiple regression is not often appropriate for making long-term forecasts of demand because the independent variables *themselves* are usually closely related to time; thus a simple regression model using time as the independent variable indirectly includes their effect. Consider our example above. CCU demand in the past could be hypothesized to be explainable in terms of growth in population (or a certain segment of it), growth in number of physicians on the hospital staff, and possibly the past temporal behavior of other factors.

*Figure 7.9*

*Confidence Interval Lines for Hypothesized Linear Trend*

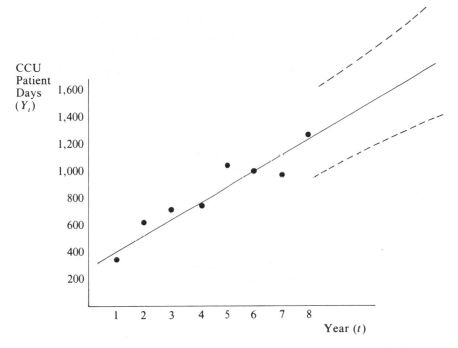

All of these factors may already be indirectly represented by $t$ in a simple regression.

Multiple regression is more useful for our purposes in estimating the demand for a *new* service in our community (state, etc.) by comparing our community to other communities that already offer the service in question. For example, a model to estimate the demand for inpatient days per year for a community without its own hospital (or with grossly inadequate facilities) might be proposed as

$$\hat{Y} = a + b_1 X_1 + b_2 X_2 + b_3 X_3 + b_4 X_4 + b_5 X_5,$$

where

$\hat{Y}$ = the estimated number of patient days demanded (per year),

$X_1$ = population,

$X_2$ = percent of population over 65 years of age,

$X_3$ = percent of population with insurance,

$X_4$ = percent of population in metropolitan area,

$X_5$ = number of physicans per 1,000 population,

and $a$, $b_1$, $b_2$, ..., $b_5$ are the multiple regression coefficients which minimize the sum of squared differences between $\hat{Y}$ and $Y$ (actual). Like simple regression, the coefficients will be derived from actual data; but instead of using data groups $(Y_t, t)$ from past years, the data groups $(Y, X_1, X_2, ..., X_5)$ will come from other communities that have sufficient facilities already. Analogous to simple regression, the two major assumptions underlying the model are:

1. the $X_i$ can explain the differences in $Y$ from community to community, and

2. the $X_i$ can estimate $Y$ in *our* community in the same way it explains it in others.

As before, we can test the first assumption statistically, but we can only use subjective judgment to evaluate the second one.

The first assumption is evaluated by the null hypothesis

$$H_{0_i}: b_i = 0 \text{ for all } i,$$

which is tested by an $F$ statistic with $k$ and $n - k - 1$ degrees of freedom, where $k$ is the number of independent variables and $n$ is the sample size. (In addition, there are individual tests for each independent variable: $H_{0_i}: b_i = 0$ (i.e., $X_i$ does not significantly add to the explanation of $Y$) which are tested by the Student $t$ statistic, $T_i$.) Finally, there is also the *coefficient of multiple determination—$R^2$*, the *coefficient of multiple regression—R*, and the ability to construct confidence intervals as in simple regression.

The calculation of the $a$, $b_i$, $F$, $T_i$, $R^2$ and $S$ for multiple regression equations is beyond the scope of this text and indeed (like simple regression) would seldom be done by hand, since computer programs for regression are widely available. However, the following cautions about the use of multiple regression for estimating should be made, after which we will work through the above example with actual data, and interpret the results.

## Selecting the Independent Variables to Be Included

There are several factors to consider here. Firstly, there must be reliable estimates of the *present* and *future* values of each of he independent variables $X_i$ in order to be able to substitute values for them into the estimated multiple regression equation to calculate $\hat{Y}$. This, of course, is no problem in simple regression, since the future behavior of $t$ is obvious.

Secondly, we must be careful not to include independent variables which are highly correlated with one another. If $X_1$ is highly correlated with $X_2$, then $X_1$ might be interpreted as a significant factor, and $X_2$ as an insignificant factor, in explaining the behavior of $Y$, or vice versa, or both $X_1$ and $X_2$ might be mildly significant in explaining the behavior of $Y$. There are two methods to guard against this hazard and both should be considered. The first is to inspect carefully the individual pair-wise correlations of the candidate independent variables before including them as independent variables. The second is to use a computer program that allows control over the order in which independent variables are included, or that automatically includes independent variables in the order of the strength of their individual correlation with $Y$ (step-wise regression).

Thirdly, a warning that applied to simple regression must also be made for multiple regression. The regression fit, no matter how strong, is based on the relationship of $Y$ to the $X_i$ in *other* situations. If there is good reason to believe that the relationship between $Y$ and the $X_i$ in "our" situation is significantly different from the "others," the multiple regression estimate must be discounted. Again, the regression estimate must be carefully tempered with available subjective data and opinion.

Finally, like simple regression, there is no causal relationship established by multiple regression. We cannot say that $Y$ is *caused* by $X_1$, $X_2$, ..., $X_n$, but only that the past behavior of $Y$ can to some extent be explained by $X_1$, $X_2$, ..., $X_n$.

Returning to our example, suppose the community health planner initially hypothesized the model

$$\hat{Y} = a + b_1 X_1 + b_2 X_2 + b_3 X_3 + b_4 X_4,$$

where

$Y$ = use rate,

$a$ = a constant,

$X_1$ = percent of population 65 and older,

$X_2$ = percent of population with insurance,

$X_3$ = median family income, and

$X_4$ = number of physicians per 100,000 population.

The planner obtains values of $Y$ and the $X_i$ from 40 communities similar to his own. To avoid including independent variables which are highly correlated with other independent variables, the first step is to generate (with the use of a commonly available computer program) the covariance matrix: Figure 7.10. We see that $X_2$, $X_3$, and $X_4$ are all highly intercorrelated, so that we should choose only one of the three for the final model. The choice is between $X_2$ and $X_4$ because they have the highest individual correlation with $Y$ (.29 and .25, respectively). The planner feels he is better able to establish *future* values of insurance ($X_2$) than physicians ($X_4$), so the model becomes

$$\hat{Y} = a + b_1 X_1 + b_2 X_2.$$

Again using the computer program, the line which best fits the data by the least squares criterion (closely analogous to simple regression) is

$$\hat{Y} = 639.04 + 142.05\, X_1 + 9.12\, X_2.$$

The $R^2$ of the regression (the proportion of the total variance in $Y$ explained by $X_1$ and $X_2$ together) is .68. The $F$ statistic, with $2$ and $40 - 2 - 1 = 37$ degrees of freedom for testing $H_0$, is 2.46. This is low for the test of $H_0$, since $F_{.05,\, 2,37}$ is 3.23. Thus we cannot reject the null hypothesis *with these data;* we should either use the

*Figure 7.10*

*Covariance Matrix*

| $X_1$ | 1 | | | | .68 |
|-------|------|------|------|------|------|
| $X_2$ | $-.24$ | 1 | | | .29 |
| $X_3$ | $-.32$ | .97 | 1 | | .12 |
| $X_4$ | $-.30$ | .99 | .98 | 1 | .25 |
| | $X_1$ | $X_2$ | $X_3$ | $X_4$ | $Y$ |

*average use rate* of the sample (817.4), or formulate a new model
and/or collect more data. Since we purposely kept our example
simple for explanation, it would seem likely that both a larger sample
and a model that considered more independent variables might give
better results. Indeed, multiple regression usually requires a substantial
sample size, especially if the number of independent variables is
large. Again, it is not our intention here to examine multiple regression
in any but a very cursory manner; the reader is referred to Freund
and Williams for a complete discussion.

## Concluding Remarks

1) It is often the case that demand can be viewed as the product
of two factors, each of which can be individually forecasted. For
example, the number of OB arrivals ($Y$) is equal to the population
of women 14–44 years old ($P$) times the fertility rate ($u$). The number
of births per 1,000 women 14–44 years old is thus

$$Y = uP/1,000.$$

It may be that high quality estimates of $P$ are already available from
other sources. In this case, the $u$ itself could be regressed on time
as

$$\hat{u}_t = a + bt$$

and then applied in the above equation to get $\hat{Y}_t$. Another reason
for considering individual projections of $P$ and $u$ is the case where
they are exhibiting different trends: say $P$ is growing exponentially
but $u$ is falling linearly. It may be possible to obtain two very good
fits for $P$ and $u$ separately, rather than one fit for

$$\hat{Y}_t = a + bt.$$

2) The farther back in time that data are included in the analysis,
the larger the sample; and if a trend does exist, generally the $F$
value will be more significant and the $R^2$ higher. On the other hand,
the farther back in time, the more difficult it is to make the assumption
that the future will behave as the past. For our simple regression
example (Figure 7.9), it may be significant that years 5, 6, and 7
show a downward trend when taken separately. If year 8 had been
in line with that trend, it might have been appropriate to base the
regression on the last four years only, since an apparent *change*
in the long term trend occurred in year 5. Because year 8 *did* "get
back in line" with years 1 through 4, we instead assumed that the

behavior of years 6 and 7 was due to chance. Again, all subjective data and opinion available should be considered in choosing how far back to include data.

3) There are very few instances where an actual analysis would be carried out by hand. The widely available computer programs (some for hand calculators) are quicker, less likely to include error, and, for all but the simplest cases, less expensive.

## 7.3 INTERMEDIATE-TERM AND SHORT-TERM FORECASTING

Figure 7.11 gives the demand for CCU patient days on a monthly basis for the past 4 years. Notice that there seem to be *two* temporal effects. One is the overall *long-term* decrease in years 5 through 7; another is an increase in year 8 that we described by regression in the preceding section. The other is a *seasonal* (month by month in this case) trend, or *cyclical* trend showing that, in general, $Y$ increases for the winter months and decreases in the summer months.

Often it is desirable to plan the supply of resources (especially manpower) to meet not only long-term changes but also the month by month changes in demand. What we will develop in this section is a technique called *monthly indices,* which will allow the estimate of demand for each year to be broken down into estimates of demand by month, based on the past seasonal trend of demand.

Table 7.5 gives an expansion of the data on which Figure 7.11 is based. Note again the apparent seasonal fluctuation.

Let $m$ index the twelve months of the year ($m = 1, 2, ..., 12$),
let $t$ index the years of the sample data ($t = 1, 2, ..., n$), and

*Table 7.5*

*CCU Patient Days per Month*

|  | J | F | M | A | M | J | J | A | S | O | N | D |
|---|---|---|---|---|---|---|---|---|---|---|---|---|
| Year 5 | 98 | 106 | 101 | 90 | 75 | 70 | 78 | 72 | 82 | 93 | 100 | 115 |
| Year 6 | 100 | 94 | 96 | 82 | 70 | 61 | 66 | 72 | 88 | 84 | 98 | 97 |
| Year 7 | 98 | 94 | 90 | 82 | 70 | 60 | 56 | 70 | 80 | 84 | 96 | 100 |
| Year 8 | 121 | 120 | 98 | 110 | 100 | 96 | 88 | 92 | 102 | 114 | 125 | 130 |
| Total | 417 | 414 | 385 | 364 | 315 | 287 | 288 | 306 | 352 | 375 | 419 | 442 |
| Average ($\bar{Y}_m$) | 104.3 | 103.5 | 96.3 | 91.0 | 78.8 | 71.8 | 72.0 | 76.5 | 88.0 | 93.8 | 104.8 | 110.5 |

Grand Mean $\bar{Y} = \sum_m \bar{Y}_m / 12 = 1,091 / 12 = 90.92$

$\bar{T} = \sum_m T_m / 12 = 4,364 / 12 = 363.7$

Figure 7.11

CCU Patient Days by Month

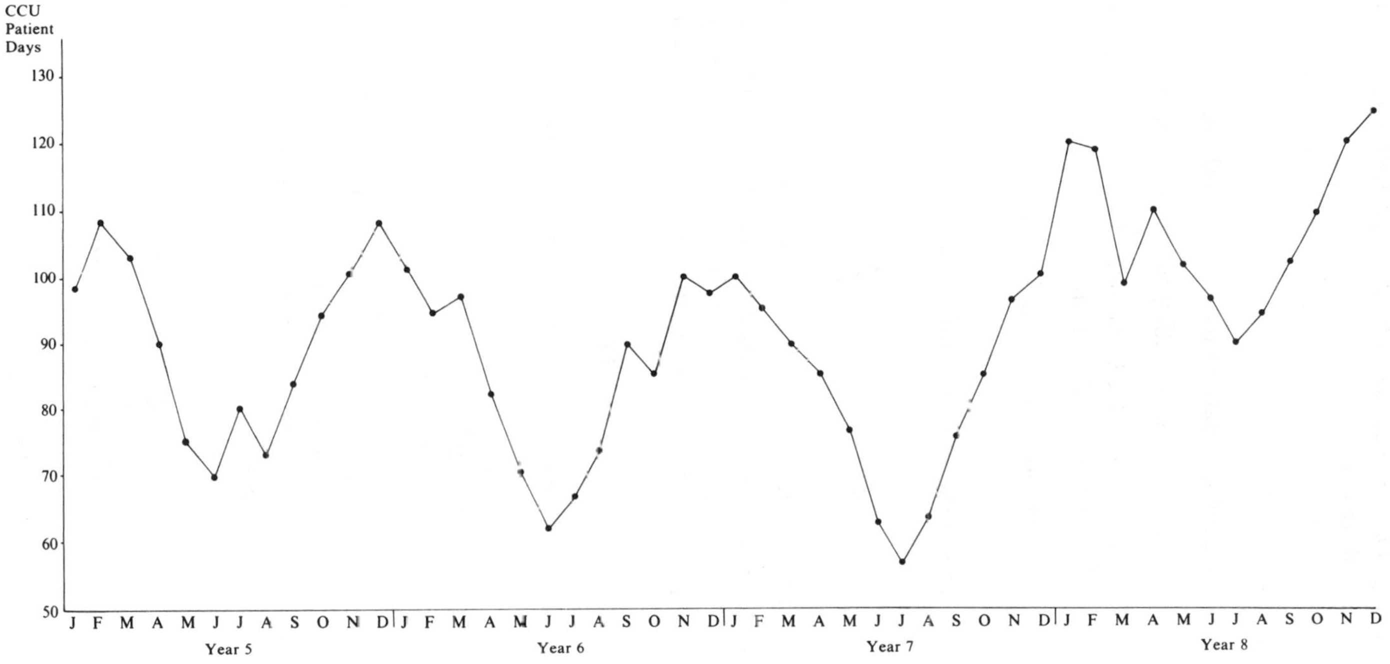

let $Y_{tm}$ be the number of CCU patient days in the $m$th month of year $t$.

Now define:

$T_m$ = total CCU patient days for month $m$,

$\bar{T}$ = average (over months) total days per month,

$\bar{Y}_m$ = the average CCU patient days for month $m$ using $n$ years = $\Sigma_t Y_{tm}/n$, and

$\bar{\bar{Y}}$ = the grand mean = $\Sigma_m \bar{Y}_m/12$.

Now we define the *monthly indices* as

$$I_m = \frac{\bar{Y}_m}{\bar{\bar{Y}}}.$$

Figure 7.12 gives the indices calculated from the data in Table 7.5. The indices can be interpreted as follows: In the past, month $m$ has on the average been $I_m \times 100$ percent of the typical month. For example, July has been 79 percent of the average month.

### Figure 7.12

*Monthly Indices for CCU Patient Days*

| JAN | FEB | MAR | APR | MAY | JUN | JUL | AUG | SEP | OCT | NOV | DEC |
|------|------|------|------|-----|-----|-----|-----|-----|------|------|------|
| 1.15 | 1.14 | 1.06 | 1.00 | .87 | .79 | .79 | .84 | .97 | 1.03 | 1.15 | 1.22 |

As in regression, there are many factors that might be used to explain the variation of the monthly averages, and again we divide them into two types: a seasonal trend (defined by the $I_m$) and everything else (called chance). We may test statistically the null hypothesis that *all* of the variation is due to chance, noted by

$$H_0: I_m = 1 \text{ for all } m,$$

which we will try to reject in favor of

$$H_A: I_m \neq 1 \text{ for at least one } m.$$

The evidence against $H_0$ is as follows: If $H_0$ is true, then the statistic

$$\chi^2 = \sum_m (T_m - \frac{\bar{T})^2}{\bar{T}}$$

will follow the chi square $(\chi^2)$ distribution with $m - 1$ degrees of freedom, where $m$ is the number of terms in the above equation ($m = 12$ in our case). (The $\chi^2$ test requires that *total* incidences be used as the term that varies—the $T_m$. It is incorrect to use averages—e.g., using $\bar{Y}_m$ would be incorrect.) Thus, if we find that the $\chi^2$ statistic for our data lies beyond the (say) 95th percentile of the $\chi^2$ distribution, we *reject $H_0$ with 95 percent confidence that $H_0$ is not true in this case.*

For our example,

$$\chi^2 = \frac{(417 - 363.7)^2}{363.7} + \frac{(414 - 363.7)^2}{363.7} + \ldots + \frac{(442 - 363.7)^2}{363.7}$$

$$= 89.62.$$

Since the 99.9th percentile of the $\chi^2_{11}$ (11 degrees of freedom) is 31.3, we may confidently reject $H_0$, and conclude that our indices do indeed explain a significant part of the past cyclical behavior of CCU patient days demanded.

**Making the Forecast**

To make monthly forecasts for the coming year using monthly indices, we first forecast the annual demand for year $t$ : $\hat{Y}_t$ (using, perhaps, linear regression). The "typical" *monthly* demand is $\hat{Y}_t / 12$. The estimated monthly demand adjusted for the seasonal effect is then

$$\hat{Y}_{tm} = I_m \hat{Y}_t / 12.$$

For example, if we use the linear regression for CCU bed demand for next year (year 9),

$$\hat{Y}_9 = 353.7 + 111.4(9) = 1,356.30,$$

$$\hat{Y}_9 / 12 = 113.03,$$

and Figure 7.13 gives the $\hat{Y}_{9m}$.

Suppose, in addition, the demand showed a significant day-of-week trend, specifically that weekdays were heavy and demand on weekends was very light. We may then need to adjust the $\hat{Y}_{tm}$ by the number of weekdays that fall in each month for the upcoming year. An approximation of this effect could be included by noting

*Figure 7.13*

*Predicted CCU Patient Days per Month for Year 9*

| JAN | FEB | MAR | APR | MAY | JUN | JUL | AUG | SEP | OCT | NOV | DEC |
|------|------|------|------|------|------|------|------|------|------|------|------|
| 130.0 | 128.9 | 119.8 | 113.0 | 98.3 | 89.3 | 89.3 | 94.9 | 109.6 | 116.4 | 113.9 | 137.9 |

that there are $52 \times 5 = 260$ weekdays in a year, or $260/12 = 21.7$ weekdays in the "typical" month for the coming year. Each $\hat{Y}_{tm}$ should now be multiplied by $W_m/21.7$, where $W_m$ is the number of weekdays in month $m$ for the upcoming year. (This is only an approximation since the $I_m$ already include the effect of the different number of days in the months).

The same process for developing and using monthly indices can be applied to day-of-week indices. Suppose data from the past 100 weeks show day-of-week totals (of 100 days) for CCU patient days as follows:

| Mon | Tues | Wed | Thur | Fri | Sat | Sun |
|------|------|------|------|------|------|------|
| 316 | 312 | 308 | 304 | 306 | 320 | 318 |

Since the expected demand under the null hypothesis

$H_0$: there is no day-of-week trend

is 312 (the average of the seven figures above), it does not look as if the data show a significant day-of-week effect. We can test $H_0$ with the $\chi^2$ test with the statistic

$$\chi^2 = \frac{(316 - 312)^2}{312} + \frac{(312 - 312)^2}{312} + \dots + \frac{(318 - 312)^2}{312} = .74,$$

which has $n - 1 = 6$ degrees of freedom ($n$ is the number of terms in $\chi^2$). (Note again that we are using *totals* in the $\chi^2$ test. It would be incorrect to use the average daily usage.) As expected, we cannot reject $H_0$ for the CCU example. It is, however, easy to think of many processes that would have significant day-of-week effect in hospitals, including radiology tests, laboratory tests, inpatient census on floors admitting elective patients, number of discharges, etc. The day-of-week indices, if significant, are calculated and applied in addition to the monthly indices (see Exercise 7.6 at the end of this chapter).

## Exponential Smoothing

It may be felt that only very recent information about the behavior of a process is relevant for making short-term forecasts. Specifically, each time a forecast is made, and then the forecast is compared with what actually happened and the error of the forecast observed, new information about the behavior of the process is learned. A method that formally incorporates this new information into the next period's forecast is called *exponential smoothing*.

Let $\hat{Y}_m$ = the forecasted value for month $m$,
let $Y_m$ = the actual value for month $m$, and
let $\alpha$ = a constant with a value between 0 and 1.

Exponential smoothing defines

$$\hat{Y}_{m+1} = \hat{Y}_m + \alpha(Y_m - \hat{Y}_m).$$

Thus, some portion ($\alpha$) of the error in last month's forecast is added to the forecast for last month to make a new forecast. The size of $\alpha$ depends on the situation. An $\alpha$ close to 0 means that a sequence of forecasts will react very slowly to errors, where an $\alpha$ close to .5 will cause recent errors to influence the next forecast strongly. Values of .1 and .2 are common for $\alpha$, but a better method for establishing the appropriate $\alpha$ for a particular situation is to try several values on past data and pick the one that "performs" best.

Consider the following example. Suppose we are currently in January ($m = 1$) and a forecast for February ($m = 2$) is required. Suppose further that the forecast for January was $\hat{Y}_1 = 127$ while the actual for January was $Y_1 = 148$. Finally, assume that $\alpha = .2$ has performed satisfactorily in the past. The forecast for February would be

$$\hat{Y}_2 = \hat{Y}_1 + \alpha(Y_1 - \hat{Y}_1)$$

$$= 127 + .2(148 - 127)$$

$$= 131.2.$$

Now suppose we later observe that $Y_2$ (actual) is 139. Our forecast for March could be

$$\hat{Y}_3 = 131.2 + .2(139 - 131.2)$$

$$= 132.76,$$

and so on month by month as the actual $Y_m$ are learned.

Note that this version of exponential smoothing does not include a cyclical effect. Thus where there is a strong cyclical effect, the indices method is likely to be superior to exponential smoothing of the form presented above. Other forms of exponential smoothing incorporate seasonal indices to create a method which uses both techniques. Still other forms use more than one month's error, weight recent errors more heavily than past errors, or have variable values of $\alpha$ depending on past errors. (The interested reader is referred to the references on exponential smoothing at the end of the chapter.)

## Markovian Forecasts

When a process is highly intercorrelated from time period to time period (especially short periods), it may be useful to use a method which bases the estimate of the next period *completely* on the preceding period.

> **Problem:** In order to plan to meet the need for nursing care services on a shift-by-shift basis, the number of patients of each of three levels of care must be forecast. Type I patients need little care, while Type III patients need a great deal of care. The state of each patient (i.e., his level) for the next shift is felt to depend most heavily on which state he was in during the preceding shift, and to depend very little on his state during shifts previous to the immediately preceding one.

The heart of the Markovian prediction method is the transition matrix—a matrix showing the probability of a patient changing from any one state to any other state in any *one* time period. For our example, let us define two additional states (other than I, II, and III) in which a patient might be. State A is the state of waiting for admission to the unit, where the admission will definitely take place during the next shift. State D is the state of being discharged. Now we can define the transition matrix of Figure 7.14 showing the probability of a patient's moving from one state to another in any 8-hour period. (For simplicity, assume that all changes occur exactly at the beginning of the shift. Since admission and discharge normally take place during the day shift only, it would be necessary to establish different transition matrices for each shift and perhaps for each day of the week. For our example, however, we will use only one matrix.)

To predict how many patients of each type will be present on the *next* shift, we first establish how many patients are in each state *this* shift. Suppose we know the following:

| State | Number |
|-------|--------|
| A | 8 |
| I | 16 |
| II | 22 |
| III | 7 |
| D | 2 |

To predict the number of patients in each state next shift, we multiply the *vector* of current status by the *transition matrix*. In general, we call the current status vector $C$, and the transition matrix $T$, and the predicted status vector $\hat{C}$, so that

$$\hat{C} = TC.$$

In our example

$$
\hat{C} = \begin{bmatrix}
0 & 0 & 0 & 0 & 0 \\
.60 & .80 & .20 & .05 & 0 \\
.30 & .07 & .70 & .24 & 0 \\
.10 & .03 & .05 & .60 & 0 \\
0 & .10 & .05 & .10 & 0
\end{bmatrix}
\begin{bmatrix}
8 \\
16 \\
22 \\
7 \\
0
\end{bmatrix}
$$

$$
= \begin{bmatrix}
(0)(8) + (0)(16) + (0)(22) + (0)(7) + (0)(0) \\
(.60)(8) + (.80)(16) + (.20)(22) + (.05)(7) + (0)(0) \\
(.30)(8) + (.07)(16) + (.70)(22) + (.24)(7) + (0)(0) \\
(.10)(8) + (.03)(16) + (.05)(22) + (.60)(7) + (0)(0) \\
(0)(8) + (.10)(16) + (.05)(22) + (.10)(7) + (0)(0)
\end{bmatrix}
$$

$$
= \begin{bmatrix}
0 \\
22.4 \\
20.7 \\
6.6 \\
3.4
\end{bmatrix}
$$

## Figure 7.14

### Transition Matrix

|                |     | A | Probability of Moving from State . . . | | | D |
|                |     |   | I | II | III | |
|----------------|-----|---|-----|-----|-----|---|
|                | A   | 0 | 0   | 0   | 0   | 0 |
| . . . to       | I   | .60 | .80 | .20 | .05 | 0 |
| State . . .    | II  | .30 | .07 | .70 | .25 | 0 |
|                | III | .10 | .03 | .05 | .60 | 0 |
|                | D   | 0 | .10 | .05 | .10 | 0 |

(There may be better information available on the number of discharges to expect. If so, this information should be substituted for the estimated 3.4 discharges and the other estimates should also be adjusted appropriately.) To predict the patients' status for the shift following the next shift, we first replace the first element of $\hat{C}$ with the number of admissions (let's say 2) that we predict will occur in the shift after next:

$$\begin{bmatrix} 2.0 \\ 22.4 \\ 20.7 \\ 6.6 \\ 3.4 \end{bmatrix}$$

Now to predict $\hat{\hat{C}}$ (the status of the shift after next):

$$\hat{\hat{C}} = T\hat{C},$$

and so on. Like all forecasts, the quality of the prediction can be expected to deteriorate as the prediction moves further into the future. For our problem, however, only an 8-hour estimate (or possibly a 16-hour estimate) is needed. If patients are observed to change states less frequently than every 8 hours, we may redefine the transition period as 24 hours and remeasure our transition probabilities.

The transition probabilities are measured from empirical experience of the process in the past. Thus element $t_{I,II}$—the probability of changing from State I to State II—could be set equal to the number of Type I patients observed changing to Type II, divided by the total number of Type I patients subject to change. An adequate sample would need to be taken to ensure that stable estimates of each element were established.

Markovian estimates might be applied to many situations where the process in question normally falls into different states and the result of the process in each state is of interest. For example, Markovian estimates have been used to predict the health status of entire communities through time. The interested reader is referred to the articles at the end of the chapter for further discussion.

## Forecasting the Distribution of a Process

Up to the present, we have been content to make *point forecasts,* i.e., to forecast the expected *mean* of a process. It is often desirable to be able to predict not only the mean but also the expected distribution about the mean. (We did in fact incorporate this notion to some extent in establishing confidence limits on regression estimates.)

> **Problem:** In line with our policy, we want to staff an outpatient clinic so that it experiences understaffing only 25 percent of the time. In other words, we want to staff the clinic at the 75th percentile of daily demand (measured in clinic visits). We want to establish estimates of the staff necessary to meet this policy each month of next year.

Let us suppose we have estimated from a regression that the number of visits next year will be 2,600. Applying monthly indices to this estimate (divided by 12), we determine that in March of next year we can expect 264 visits. Since March of next year has 22 weekdays (let us assume), we expect a *mean* of $264/22 - 12$ visits per weekday. But what *distribution* will daily visits follow? We must know this in order to establish the 75th percentile for determining necessary staff.

As we have done for our other forecasts, we will formulate two hypotheses, one we can test and one we cannot:

A. Daily visits have followed some recognizable distribution in the past, and

B. This *distribution* will continue into the future, even though its parameters (mean and standard deviation) may change.

We first examine data on the past behavior of daily visits to try to identify a recognizable distribution. Figure 7.15 gives the distribution of daily visits from March, April, and May of last year. (Here we have assumed that there is no difference between weekdays. This, of course, can be tested, and if we found such a difference, we would have to

*Figure 7.15*

*Actual Distribution of Daily Weekday*
*Visits for March and April*

Of the 66 Weekdays . . .

| |
|---|
| 8 had less than 5 visits |
| 5 had exactly 5 |
| 9 had exactly 6 |
| 10 had exactly 7 |
| 9 had exactly 8 |
| 7 had exactly 9 |
| 7 had exactly 10 |
| 4 had exactly 11 |
| 8 had more than 11 |

try to establish a distribution for each of the weekdays. This, however, would lead to substantially smaller sample sizes for the $\chi^2$ test, below.) The mean of the 66 days is 8. As a first estimate, we may want to try to establish that daily visits follow a Poisson process, with $\lambda = 8$. If the process had produced a Poisson distribution *exactly*, we would expect the results of Figure 7.16.

The relevant question in this case is, Do the actual data of Figure 7.15 truly follow the Poisson distribution with $\lambda = 8$, with the difference between Figure 7.15 and Figure 7.16 representing only random fluctuation; or do the data of Figure 7.15 follow some other distribution? If the actual data do follow the Poisson distribution with mean $\lambda = 8$, the $\chi^2$ goodness of fit statistic will follow the $\chi^2$ distribution with $n - k - 1$ degrees of freedom where $n$ is the number of terms in the $\chi^2$ statistic calculation (rows in Figure 7.17) and $k$ is the number of parameters being estimated in the hypothesized distribution (in our case Poisson, with one parameter)—see Section 5.2 for the $\chi^2$ goodness of fit test.

*Figure 7.16*

*Poisson Distribution of Daily Weekday Visits with $\lambda = 8$*

| Event $x$ | $f(x)$ of Poisson | . . . . times 66 Gives Expected Number ($E_i$) |
|---|---|---|
| Less than 5 visits | .10 | 6.6 |
| Exactly 5 visits | .09 | 5.95 |
| Exactly 6 visits | .12 | 7.9 |
| Exactly 7 visits | .14 | 8.4 |
| Exactly 8 visits | .14 | 8.4 |
| Exactly 9 visits | .12 | 7.9 |
| Exactly 10 visits | .10 | 6.6 |
| Exactly 11 visits | .07 | 4.6 |
| more than 11 visits | .13 | 8.6 |

## Figure 7.17

### Calculations Required to Obtain $\chi^2$

|  | $A_i$ | $E_i$ | $(A_i - E_i)^2$ | $(A_i - E_i)^2 / E_i$ |
|---|---|---|---|---|
| $i = 1$ | 8 | 6.60 | 1.96 | .30 |
| $i = 2$ | 5 | 5.95 | .90 | .15 |
| $i = 3$ | 9 | 7.90 | 1.21 | .15 |
| $i = 4$ | 10 | 8.40 | 2.56 | .30 |
| $i = 5$ | 9 | 8.40 | .36 | .04 |
| $i = 6$ | 7 | 7.90 | .81 | .10 |
| $i = 7$ | 7 | 6.60 | .16 | .02 |
| $i = 8$ | 12 | 13.20 | 1.44 | .11 |
|  |  |  |  | $\chi^2 = 1.19$ |

The goodness of fit test requires that the expected number of incidents $E_i$ be at least 5, so we must collapse the last class into the next to last (making one class of "more than 10 visits") to give us the analysis between columns $A_i$ and $E_i$ of Figure 7.17. This result (1.19) falls on the .025th percentile (that point at which .975 of the area is to the right) of the $\chi^2$ distribution with $8 - 1 - 1 = 6$ degrees of freedom (see Table III in Appendix). Thus we can say that, if the true process is Poisson with $\lambda = 8$, we could obtain data like these (i.e., data which deviated this much from the $E_i$) 97.5 percent of the time. We could therefore accept the hypothesis that the process is Poisson.

Suppose we now test other distributions against the actual data and end up accepting the Poisson as the most likely fit. To make the projection, we use whatever subjective or objective evidence we can find to evaluate the hypothesis that the process will continue to be Poisson in the future (at least next year), but with higher $\lambda$. We know from our regression and indices forecast that the mean number of daily visits for next March will be 12. So if we can accept the second hypothesis, our projection is that daily visits in March will be Poisson with $\lambda = 12$. This in turn allows us to project the distribution of daily visits in March (Figure 7.18) from a table of the Poisson distribution, and we see that the 75th percentile is 14 visits per day. So we staff on the basis of 14 daily patient visits.

Often a process is much too complex for us to predict its behavior by predicting only one distribution, since the process itself may be the result of several factors, some stochastic and some deterministic. The number of emergency turnaways from a hospital is one such example. Recall that we addressed the prediction of complex stochastic phenomena in Chapter 5.

*Figure 7.18*

*Poisson Distribution of Daily Weekday Visits for March if λ = 12*

| Event | Probability $f(x)$ | Cumulative Probability $F(x)$ |
|---|---|---|
| less than 10 visits | .35 | .35 |
| exactly 11 visits | .11 | .46 |
| exactly 12 visits | .11 | .57 |
| exactly 13 visits | .11 | .68 |
| exactly 14 visits | .09 | .77 |
| exactly 15 visits | .07 | .84 |
| exactly 16 visits | .05 | .89 |
| exactly 17 visits | .11 | 1.00 |

## Exercises

7.1 The concept of randomness implies that a random event is uncontrolled. Can you name a truly random event? Is there such a thing as a truly random event in hospital activities? Why would you treat an event as random for analytic purposes even though you knew it was not?

The following exercises involve forecasting over a relatively long-range period. To complete them you will need linear graph paper and semi-log graph paper. You may wish to use a computer routine to assist you in your calculations.

7.2 Plot the following data on linear and on semi-log paper and plot a visual trend line. Then calculate the linear regression equation manually. Compare your projections. Which would you accept as a forecast for years 10 and 15? What would be the approximate 95 percent confidence range?

| Year | Value |
|---|---|
| 1 | 5 |
| 2 | 7 |
| 3 | 11 |
| 4 | 9 |
| 5 | 10 |
| 6 | 11 |
| 7 | 14 |
| 8 | 15 |

Suppose this were a real process, such as the mean daily pediatric hospital discharges. If the average patient stayed 3 days, the average census for year 8 would be 45. If there were 50 beds available (and no hope for changing that), what would you accept as a forecast for years 10 and 15? What conclusions would you draw about the difference between your best calculated projection and your forecast?

7.3 The following data represent annual visits to the emergency room of a community hospital, 1964 to 1970. Plot these in linear and logarithmic form, and fit visual trend lines. Then prepare regression estimates. Select a forecast to 1975, and justify your selection in terms of $F$ values. Give the probability of an error of 10 percent or greater in either direction based on forecast selection.

| Year | Visits |
| --- | --- |
| 1964 | 18,112 |
| 1965 | 21,388 |
| 1966 | 22,834 |
| 1967 | 23,164 |
| 1968 | 25,374 |
| 1969 | 29,661 |
| 1970 | 32,632 |

7.4 The following data represent actual adult medical/surgical patient days in your hospital.

| Year | Patient Days |
| --- | --- |
| 1965 | 81,215 |
| 1966 | 79,985 |
| 1967 | 79,695 |
| 1968 | 81,158 |
| 1969 | 81,999 |
| 1970 | 82,575 |

What forecast do you recommend for 1975? What are the assumptions on which it is based? (Your answer should include the exploration of trends in the series, with such graphs and regression calculations as you feel necessary.)

7.5 You are the administrative assistant in a 287-bed hospital. The following data are from the adult MED/SURG service (218 beds) and show patient days since you opened in 1958 to the present (1964). Plot these on linear and on semi-log graph paper, and prepare visual and regression estimates through 1970. Select an estimate which you will recommend to the administrator as a forecast in terms of beds and personnel for 1970. What alternative forecast should be presented?

| Year | Patient Days |
|------|-------------|
| 1959 | 28,884 |
| 1960 | 32,298 |
| 1961 | 32,910 |
| 1962 | 33,648 |
| 1963 | 43,189 |
| 1964 | 60,737 |

The following data on emergency room visits have been compiled for Exercises 7.6 through 7.8.

DATA FOR CALCULATION OF MONTHLY SEASONAL INDICES FOR EMERGENCY
ROOM VISITS: OBSERVED NUMBER OF VISITS

| Month | 1961 | 1962 | 1963 | 1964 | 1965 | 1966 |
|-------|------|------|------|------|------|------|
| January | 197 | 288 | 351 | 464 | 589 | 834 |
| February | 188 | 285 | 372 | 439 | 588 | 952 |
| March | 255 | 329 | 424 | 463 | 667 | 785 |
| April | 210 | 325 | 424 | 430 | 656 | 701 |
| May | 276 | 305 | 411 | 462 | 633 | 731 |
| June | 304 | 366 | 521 | 495 | 588 | 786 |
| July | 432 | 506 | 732 | 695 | 1,178 | 1,112 |
| August | 502 | 450 | 688 | 618 | 1,029 | 1,105 |
| September | 353 | 359 | 511 | 517 | 840 | 814 |
| October | 292 | 284 | 465 | 540 | 732 | 848 |
| November | 222 | 296 | 466 | 474 | 780 | 774 |
| December | 261 | 319 | 408 | 495 | 875 | 842 |

EMERGENCY ROOM VISITS

| Day of Month | April 1967 | | May 1967 | |
|------|-----------|---------------|-----------|---------------|
| | Scheduled | Non-Scheduled | Scheduled | Non-Scheduled |
| 1 | 11 Sat | 25 | 8 Mon | 29 |
| 2 | 0 | 23 | 9 | 32 |
| 3 | 9 | 27 | 6 | 25 |
| 4 | 10 | 26 | 3 | 34 |

| | | | | |
|---|---|---|---|---|
| 5 | 13 | 31 | 9 | 22 |
| 6 | 9 | 24 | 3 | 24 |
| 7 | 11 | 22 | 0 | 12 |
| 8 | 12 Sat | 43 | 7 Mon | 29 |
| 9 | 0 | 18 | 7 | 20 |
| 10 | 13 | 31 | 6 | 29 |
| 11 | 17 | 29 | 9 | 33 |
| 12 | 5 | 35 | 12 | 31 |
| 13 | 7 | 27 | 0 | 22 |
| 14 | 7 | 29 | 0 | 15 |
| 15 | 5 Sat | 26 | 8 Mon | 23 |
| 16 | 0 | 17 | 9 | 24 |
| 17 | 18 | 33 | 5 | 26 |
| 18 | 20 | 37 | 8 | 32 |
| 19 | 10 | 35 | 5 | 23 |
| 20 | 9 | 30 | 2 | 26 |
| 21 | 6 | 34 | 0 | 19 |
| 22 | 7 Sat | 31 | 8 Mon | 30 |
| 23 | 0 | 22 | 2 | 33 |
| 24 | 16 | 33 | 2 | 33 |
| 25 | 11 | 30 | 3 | 19 |
| 26 | 4 | 26 | 9 | 24 |
| 27 | 6 | 26 | 5 | 24 |
| 28 | 15 | 43 | 0 | 20 |
| 29 | 9 Sat | 27 | 7 Mon | 27 |
| 30 | 0 | 14 | 3 | 18 |
| 31 | — | — | 6 | 33 |

7.6 Develop and test:

Monthly demand index

Day-of-week demand index

Frequency distribution for nonscheduled visits (test for conformity to Poisson)

7.7 Construct a forecasting model for daily estimates for a given month.

7.8 Based on your knowledge of the process, estimate the probabilities of daily visits exceeding 110% and 120% of the expected value. What level of daily visits is exceeded only one day in 20? Suppose you were to staff the emergency room sufficiently to accommodate demand 19 out of 20 days. What would you expect the efficiency of utilization of that staff to be?

7.9 The following data on output of major surgery, minor surgery, anesthesia, and blood bank are to be used to forecast for a five-year interval. Check the individual time series relationships on these, and if they do not yield satisfactory values, develop the correlation matrix between the variables. You may wish to include the sum of major and minor surgery as an additional variable. Develop reasonable equations for estimating as many as possible of these variables using multiple regression. Indicate how this could be used to forecast demand. (This problem requires a computer regression program.)

SURGERY

| Year | Major | Minor | Anesthesia | Blood |
|------|-------|-------|------------|-------|
| 1964 | 1,837 | 3,618 | 6,961 | 8,856 |
| 1965 | 1,969 | 3,891 | 7,333 | 10,223 |
| 1966 | 2,038 | 3,780 | 7,145 | 10,477 |
| 1967 | 1,931 | 3,608 | 6,893 | 9,796 |
| 1968 | 2,064 | 3,730 | 7,037 | 9,349 |
| 1969 | 2,085 | 3,712 | 7,071 | 10,113 |
| 1970 | 2,316 | 4,084 | 7,882 | 11,733 |

7.10 Your boss has asked if you would assist the Head Laboratory Technologist in preparing her *monthly* budget for 1977. After several days of concentrated effort, you have finally accumulated the following data on past demand:

| Year | Number of Lab Tests (x 1,000) |
|------|-------------------------------|
| 1968 | 48 |
| 1969 | 77 |
| 1970 | 84 |
| 1971 | 88 |
| 1972 | 120 |
| 1973 | 113 |
| 1974 | 110 |
| 1975 | 142 |

NUMBER OF LAB TESTS (x 1,000)

|     | 1972 | 1973 | 1974 | 1975 | Total |
|-----|------|------|------|------|-------|
| JAN | 10.8 | 11.0 | 10.8 | 13.1 | 45.7 |
| FEB | 11.6 | 10.3 | 10.4 | 13.0 | 45.3 |
| MAR | 11.1 | 10.5 | 10.0 | 10.9 | 42.5 |
| APR | 10.0 | 10.2 | 9.2 | 12.0 | 41.4 |

| | | | | | |
|------|------|------|------|------|------|
| MAY | 8.5 | 8.0 | 8.0 | 11.0 | 35.5 |
| JUNE | 8.0 | 7.1 | 7.0 | 10.7 | 32.8 |
| JULY | 8.8 | 7.5 | 6.6 | 9.9 | 32.8 |
| AUG | 8.2 | 8.1 | 8.0 | 10.2 | 34.5 |
| SEPT | 9.2 | 9.7 | 9.0 | 11.2 | 39.1 |
| OCT | 10.3 | 9.3 | 9.4 | 12.4 | 41.4 |
| NOV | 11.0 | 10.7 | 10.6 | 13.6 | 45.9 |
| DEC | 12.5 | 10.6 | 11.0 | 14.0 | 48.1 |
| TOTAL | 120.0 | 113.0 | 110.0 | 142.0 | 485.0 |

You have eagerly awaited this moment to apply your recently acquired quantitative skills. After two days of hunting for that quantitative specialist Holloway said you would get to manage, your suspicions are confirmed: Holloway was really trying to make *you* a quantitative specialist. With renewed conviction you begin analyzing the data, hoping that the Lab Technologist won't laugh you out of her office and your boss won't decide you're as crazy as Holloway.

a. Plot yearly data—what do you see?

b. Calculate $a$ and $b$—interpret.

c. Calculate residuals, plot residuals—interpret.

d. Calculate $F$; test $H_0$: $b = 0$—interpret.

e. Calculate $R^2$—interpret.

f. Calculate 95% confidence interval—interpret.

g. Calculate monthly indices—interpret.

h. Forecast next six months.

7.11 Baker hospital is a 400-bed community hospital located on the edge of a large (3 million population) city, which is served by several other hospitals, one of which is within a mile of Baker. Baker currently (January 1975) employs 4 full-time radiologists to do inpatient and outpatient exams, and has 8 fully equipped examining rooms. Up until 1968, there were only 2 radiologists using only 4 rooms. The third radiologist was added in January 1968 when the additional 4 rooms were opened. Many new outpatient procedures were also begun at that time. The fourth radiologist was added in January 1970 when 90 new medical and surgical beds were added to the hospital. Inpatient occupancy, which had been 92% on the medical and surgical units before the expansion, rose back up to 92% within 9 months.

Baker now needs to consider an additional expansion of its

# X-ray Exams by Month at Baker (All Data Is × 100)

## INPATIENT (× 100)

| Year | Total for Year | JAN | FEB | MAR | APR | MAY | JUN | JUL | AUG | SEP | OCT | NOV | DEC |
|---|---|---|---|---|---|---|---|---|---|---|---|---|---|
| 1964 | 143 | | | | —MISSING— | | | | | | | | |
| 1965 | 151 | | | | —MISSING— | | | | | | | | |
| 1966 | 170 | | | | —MISSING— | | | | | | | | |
| 1967 | 189 | 17 | 14 | 18 | 19 | 15 | 18 | 13 | 15 | 13 | 18 | 16 | 12 |
| 1968 | 188 | | | | —MISSING— | | | | | | | | |
| 1969 | 204 | | | | —MISSING— | | | | | | | | |
| 1970 | 270 | 24 | 22 | 26 | 25 | 23 | 24 | 21 | 20 | 23 | 23 | 22 | 17 |
| 1971 | 300 | 27 | 24 | 27 | 24 | 24 | 30 | 24 | 24 | 23 | 27 | 24 | 22 |
| 1972 | 301 | 26 | 25 | 26 | 27 | 25 | 28 | 22 | 25 | 25 | 27 | 26 | 19 |
| 1973 | 303 | 28 | 23 | 30 | 26 | 25 | 27 | 22 | 24 | 27 | 25 | 26 | 20 |
| 1974 | 311 | 27 | 25 | 29 | 28 | 26 | 28 | 24 | 26 | 27 | 27 | 26 | 18 |

## OUTPATIENT (× 100)

| Year | Total for Year | JAN | FEB | MAR | APR | MAY | JUN | JUL | AUG | SEP | OCT | NOV | DEC |
|---|---|---|---|---|---|---|---|---|---|---|---|---|---|
| 1964 | 86 | | | | —MISSING— | | | | | | | | |
| 1965 | 104 | | | | —MISSING— | | | | | | | | |
| 1966 | 106 | | | | —MISSING— | | | | | | | | |
| 1967 | 129 | | | | —MISSING— | | | | | | | | |
| 1968 | 210 | | | | —MISSING— | | | | | | | | |
| 1969 | 269 | 28 | 24 | 23 | 23 | 23 | 24 | 20 | 18 | 17 | 28 | 24 | 17 |
| 1970 | 260 | | | | —MISSING— | | | | | | | | |
| 1971 | 271 | 29 | 20 | 27 | 25 | 25 | 27 | 20 | 20 | 17 | 26 | 19 | 16 |
| 1972 | 290 | 28 | 26 | 30 | 24 | 24 | 28 | 21 | 22 | 24 | 30 | 20 | 13 |
| 1973 | 308 | 29 | 27 | 26 | 27 | 26 | 27 | 25 | 24 | 23 | 29 | 23 | 22 |
| 1974 | 340 | 34 | 28 | 30 | 28 | 28 | 30 | 25 | 27 | 26 | 31 | 27 | 26 |

radiology facilities, as its present facilities have begun to be severely taxed during 1974. Baker believes it should plan its radiology facilities for the next 10 years.

Tables detailing the number of X-ray exams by month at Baker for both inpatients and outpatients appear on the next page. Refer to them in working out the following problems.

a. Describe how you would go about preparing a forecast for the number of radiology exams that will be demanded at Baker in 1980 and 1985. Be explicit about what you will do with particular data and why.

b. Make the forecast for 1980 and 1985. What assumptions do your forecasts imply?

c. What statements of confidence can you make about the forecasts? What assumptions do these imply?

d. Prepare monthly forecasts for 1980 and 1985. What assumptions do these forecasts imply?

e. Baker learns that a group of 6 radiologists in town (including the head of Baker's radiology department) may build a 4-room facility to do outpatient work. Discuss exactly how you would include this information in your forecast for Baker. Make the necessary assumptions so that you can demonstrate your modifications with actual numbers.

f. What additional information would aid your forecast? How would you get it and how much do you think it would cost? Would the additional information be cost-effective?

## Additional Reading

*Technique*

Draper, N. R. and Smith, H. *Applied Regression Analysis.* New York: John Wiley and Sons, 1966.

Freund, J. E. and Williams, F. J. *Elementary Business Statistics.* Englewood Cliffs, N.J.: Prentice-Hall, Inc., 1972.

Parsons, R. *Statistical Analysis: A Decision-Making Approach.* New York: Harper and Row, 1974.

[*Markovian Prediction*] Wagner, H. M. *Principles of Operations Research with Applications to Managerial Decisions.* Englewood Cliffs, N.J.: Prentice-Hall, Inc., 1969.

[*Exponential Smoothing*] Brown, R. G. *Statistical Forecasting for Inventory Control.* New York: McGraw-Hill, 1959.

*Applications*

[*Markovian*] Bithell, J. F. "A Class of Discrete-Time Models for the Study of Hospital Admissions Systems." *Operations Research,* January/February 1969, p. 48.

[*Markovian*] Bush, J. W., Chen, M. M. and Zaremba, J. "Estimating Health Service Outcomes Using a Markov Equilibrium Analysis of Disease Development." *American Journal of Public Health* 61 (December 1971): 2362–2375.

[*Regression, Seasonal Indices, and Exponential Smoothing*] Heda, Shyam. "Manpower Budgeting." In *Cost Control in Hospitals,* edited by John R. Griffith, Walton M. Hancock, and Fred C. Munson. Ann Arbor, Michigan: Health Administration Press, 1976.

[*Markovian*] Kolesar, P. "A Markovian Model for Hospital Admission Scheduling." *Management Science,* February 1970, p. B-384.

# 8

# Computer-Based Information Systems

## 8.1 Introduction

The past 25 years have seen dramatic progress in two areas which, alone and in combination, offer health care managers a new perspective on decision making and control. The first is the field of decision theory, which has driven the empirical and theoretical development of models of human decision making in organizations, and the role of information in those processes. The second is a technological development: the explosion in information and the means to process it rapidly and accurately. Advances in the computer's capacity and abilities are documented almost daily in the media.

Advances in these fields support the computerization of the information systems that, in theory, are to support the operations, management, and planning of health care delivery. Whether they succeed in application depends on the understanding and interest of many parties. An organization's investment in a computer-based information system is significant in terms of the resources, both monetary and nonmonetary, which may be expended on it. The focus of this chapter will be the organizational issues and technical concepts which deserve the health care administrator's attention if resource allocation is to be effective and efficient.

## 8.2 Example: Admissions Scheduling

Admissions scheduling in a hospital requires the collection, processing, and transmission of massive quantities of information, often in a very short time. Meeting the needs of patients, providers, and staff in placing or discharging patients appropriately is a crucial function of a well-run facility. In many hospitals, these needs are being supported by computer systems.

One or more persons (often known as reservation coordinators), usually in an admitting department, coordinate the functions of several persons and offices. Nurses or ward clerks from the nursing units supply census information, including anticipated discharges or transfers from the unit at varying points of time. Personnel from physicians' offices call with patients' names and expected date and reason for admission, providing the coordinator with clues about nursing unit and operating room needs. The emergency room staff notify the coordinator of the immediate need for placement of urgent care patients. The account personnel in the business office notify the coordinator if a patient has been previously admitted and therefore has an existing account identifier. Housekeeping staff need to be notified when vacated rooms need cleaning in preparation for the next admission. Laboratory and radiology staff need notice of patients requiring preadmission testing. Efficient control over these data inputs and outputs ensures that patients requiring emergent admissions are placed swiftly and appropriately and that those with elective admissions are scheduled when the hospital's census and staff can accommodate them.

A computer-based information system can be designed to collect information at the point of its generation, store it, organize it for the reservation coordinator and other potential users, and display or print it in a manner that supports decision making. Throughout this chapter, the admission scheduling or reservation coordination function will be used to illustrate the role and components of an information system.

## 8.3 DATA REPRESENTATION

One commonality between the computer and the rest of the world is that communication is based on symbols. All languages are systems of symbols. In computers, information is represented through the use of binary notation, which relies on only two symbols, 0 and 1. A series of these binary digits, or *bits,* can be used to represent numbers, letters, or other symbols as needed. Combinations of bits (usually eight) are referred to as *bytes,* which, in general, are the minimum number of bits needed to represent a character or a very small number. Some number of bytes constitutes a *word,* which can represent a large number, and—as in other languages—is the basic unit of "conversation" for a computer. The number of bytes per word varies by computer manufacturer. For instance, IBM 370 machines combine four 8-bit bytes to form a word (a "32-bit machine"). Most desk-top (or personal) computers are 8-bit or 16-bit machines. Words of this size are then transferred one at a time to and from storage. Each word, or in some cases byte, has a unique address which tells the computer where the data is located in storage.

## Data Bases

The combination of words or bytes constitutes an *item* (or *field*) of information, or an "attribute," such as age, name, or sex, of an "entity": a client, an employer, or a patient awaiting admission. Groups of items form a *record*; a set of records constitutes a *file* (see Figure 8.1). In some types of computerized data processing, one or more files of records exist for each application. In this system, the same data item may be stored in many places. While this may provide wanted redundancy, it might also cause confusion: an item may be updated in one place but not in others. For example, a patient's admitting diagnosis may appear in the admission scheduling data base, just as it does in the accounting and medical records data bases; but an update in medical records may not occur automatically in accounting unless the data bases are somehow shared. Ad hoc queries are also

*Figure 8.1*

*Data Representation and Organization*

| | |
|---|---|
| bit | 0 or 1 (or "on" or "off," "yes" or "no") |
| byte | 8 bits (usually) |
| word | 4 bytes (typically, for mainframe computers) |
| item (or field) | One or more words (usually), such as patient's medical record number (one or two words), name (several words), age (one word or perhaps a half word), total bill (one word) |
| record | Several items (or fields) that go together logically, such as a patient's medical record number, name, address, age, sex, diagnosis, admitting physician, total charges, insurance coverage code, etc. This might be called a discharge record (typically containing over 100 items). |
| file | A group of records, such as all discharge records from the month of April for a hospital |
| data base | A group of files (typically), such as the discharge file above, plus an insurance coverage file. Each record of the insurance coverage file would contain fields showing how hospital costs are to be divided up between patient and insurance. This file would be keyed to the discharge file by the "insurance coverage code" field. |

difficult in such a file system since, unless the files are restructured, information cannot easily be produced in a way that was not originally intended. A seemingly small change in one file can impact many files in the same system, and changes are expensive. Given the dynamic nature of most information needs in an organization, such system modification can absorb the majority of a data-processing budget.

A *data base* is a collection of data, usually a collection of files, which is shared by several users and used for several applications. One of the main objectives of a data base system is to control redundancy by having programs and data insulated from the effects of changes to either. Programs can be changed and data reorganized without causing the other to change or reorganize. This independence of the data is especially important in a data-intensive organization such as a health care institution, where there are multiple users and uses of the data, and many ad hoc requests. A data base should make it easier to respond to these unique needs, but only if data have been structured appropriately and logically. This structuring can be complex enough to warrant an organization's using several data bases rather than just one.

The logical and physical structure of a data base is chosen to accurately represent the organization's unique data relationships in the most efficient manner the computer is capable of. The proper choice determines the accessibility of the data, the applications that can be performed, the size of the system needed, and the maintenance time and costs.

The simplest structure is that of a list, in which all data units are independent and can be ordered or not ordered. This form allows access to any piece of data, and random retrieval is often quicker than in the more complex structures. More common, however, is the hierarchical or tree-like arrangement of data items. In this case, data are dependent on other data items and are ordered in subordinate levels. Each unit has a single "owner" which may own one or more units. Tree-like arrangements are often used to represent data relationships in which there are repeating fields or multiple data items for one entity. For example, an HMO markets to and serves multiple employers who have multiple employee groups, each of which receives different premium rates. Each of the employees within each group is enrolled in the HMO and has multiple visit records. Figure 8.2 presents a diagrammatic illustration of this example. This method of structuring data and files is convenient since many of the data relationships commonly needed can be organized in such a fashion.

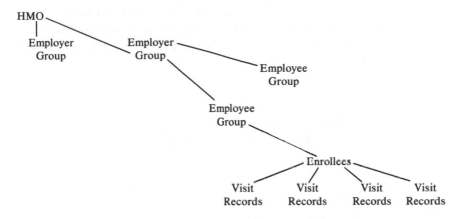

*Figure 8.2*

*Hierarchial Data Base Structure*

A network-type data structure permits the user to access the data in several ways, thus, it is complex but flexible. Data units are dependent as in the tree structure, but owners can have multiple units and units can have multiple owners. For instance, the HMO may be said to "own" provider records, patient records, visit records, and payer records; providers may be said to "own" patient records, and lab and X-ray records; patient records may be said to "own" visit records, lab and X-ray records, and payer records. In each case the owners exhibit some "control" over those data in that they are responsible for its content. Figure 8.3 illustrates this structure.

*Figure 8.3*

*Network Data Base Structure*

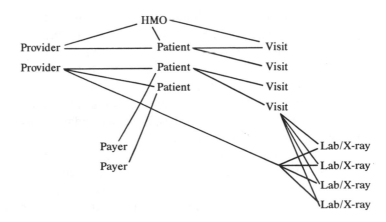

The physical data structure to support this type of organization is complex and therefore more difficult to develop.

For existing admission scheduling systems, the data base design most commonly mirrors the hierarchical relationships of the data elements, with the admitting physician owning the patient records, which in turn own the treatment records, which in turn own lab, X-ray, and other ancillary service records (Figure 8.4).

*Figure 8.4*

*Hierarchical Data Base Design for Admission Scheduling System*

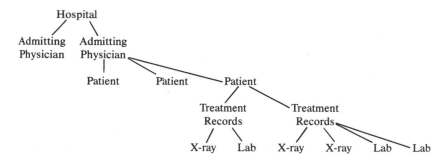

The logical structure of the data base must represent the fundamental operations and relationships of the organization. Which data base design is selected and how it is implemented depend in part on the computer system chosen. Understanding some of the fundamentals of the machine and how it operates is necessary to evaluate intelligently the many alternatives.

## Hardware

Computers have traditionally been viewed as consisting of two parts: the hardware, the parts which can be "touched"; and the software, the instructions to the computer, known as programs. Advances in both components have tended to blur the distinction between them, as will be evident in the description which follows.

Computer hardware has typically consisted of four functional units: a central processing unit (CPU), secondary storage facilities, input units, and output devices.

The central processing unit is the key component in the computer. It controls the entire system, and contains an arithmetic/logic unit, a control section, and a primary (or main) storage unit. The arithmetic/logic unit performs the four basic arithmetic functions, compares numbers, determines whether two characters are the same, and moves and shifts data. The control section of the CPU performs no actual processing operations on the data, but rather controls the input and output devices, and directs, fetches, and schedules operations called for in the program stored in the main memory unit. This main storage unit for data and programs is under the direction of the control unit and is the working memory for the arithmetic/logic section. This storage unit has been equated with an electronic storage cabinet, each bin holding data or instructions identified by an "address" that allows the control section to locate it. The size, or capacity, of this unit determines the amount of data and number of programs available for rapid but costly access and retrieval. The "size" of a machine is typically stated in terms of the size of this main storage.

Commonly, more data storage is needed than is available in main memory. In this case, secondary storage units are added in the form of punched cards, magnetic tapes, magnetic disks, or bubble storage units. These types of auxiliary storage devices represent the ways storage can be accomplished: (1) mechanically, by a notch or lack of a notch in a punch card; or (2) magnetically, by the charge (or polarization) or the lack of it, as in magnetic tapes, disks, or bubbles.

The development of virtual storage technology (VM) has made the limitations of main storage less significant. When a system has VM, addresses in the auxiliary storage can be accessed as if they existed in the main storage unit.

Capacity of a storage mechanism, the speed with which data are accessed, cost per unit of storage, and reliability vary by method of storage. In general, the cost per unit of storage is proportional to access time: the faster the access, the higher the cost. The CPU and primary memory may operate at speeds of less than 100 nanoseconds (1/10,000,000 of a second), while secondary storage devices operate at access speeds 10,000 or so times slower, although still in the millisecond (1/1,000 of a second) range. Magnetic tape is one of the oldest forms of storage, and is now used mainly for secondary storage. It uses serial or sequential access, which is slow, since the tape must be searched until the designated item is reached. It is particularly slow when compared to the random access devices such as disks or bubbles. Disks record data on tracks on a plate which revolves around a spindle. The newest type of storage device is the bubble, the result of the combined efforts of material scientists and electronic systems designers. Magnetic "domains"—which is what the bubbles are—have been studied for some time, but their use in computer technology had been unexplored until 1966, when Bell Laboratories discovered that they could be manipulated to transfer and store data. The microscopic magnetized volumes are placed on a film or "chip" of different but uniform polarity. The presence of a bubble represents a "1" and the absence a "0," the binary digits used in the computer. Data are transferred to and from the bubble memory systems by bubble generators, which create a bubble when a current is passed through; and by readers, which detect the presence or absence of bubbles.

At present, disks are the most common form of secondary storage device because of their speed of access, relatively low cost, and reliability. However, tapes will continue to be useful as low-cost backup storage devices, and bubble technology will soon advance to the point at which its costs will be competitive with those of disks.

Input and output devices permit the introduction of the data in a format the machine can use, and the return of information which has been processed by the computer in a form legible to the user. Input devices include, among others, magnetic tape units, card reader-punchers, and video display terminals. Output devices include printers, point-of-purchase terminals, teletypes, and video display terminals. Note that terminals can be used for both functions, and are classified according to their ability to perform the functions of the main computer: (1) "dumb," if they only accept or transmit data to or from the CPU; (2) "semismart," if they perform data transfer but have some short-term memory as well; and (3) "smart" or "intelligent," if they perform a considerable amount of computing and have enough memory to perform many operations without accessing the CPU.

One common arrangement for the computer machinery used in admission scheduling is illustrated in Figure 8.5. In this example, a main CPU in the admitting department interfaces with a disk storage unit and a nearby printer. Semismart terminals in the admitting office, nursing stations, housekeeping office, and business office act as input and output devices. Section 8.5 will explore the different computing patterns possible for the scheduling system.

### Software

The software of a computer is the programs that make up its operations. These include *system programs,* which give the computer instructions on how to operate, and *user programs*, which are interpreted by the system program.

*Application programs* are those programs designed for a particular organizational function or operation, such as hospital admission scheduling, billing, statistical analysis for marketing, HMO member

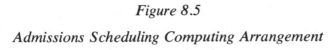

*Figure 8.5*

*Admissions Scheduling Computing Arrangement*

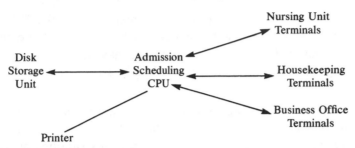

management, or data base management. The application program interacts with the system via a user language. Members of the organization's staff can design a program unique to the need, or a prepackaged program written by a vendor can be purchased or leased. Designing and programming are labor-intensive and therefore costly, which makes prepackaged programs attractive. On the other hand, the vendor often designs packages for wide distribution or generalizable functions. A package that is too general for a manager's specific needs can be costly in terms of efficiency of execution and input time.

Both system and user programs are "written" in computer *languages,* a group of statements that instruct the computer what to do. System programs are always written in *low-level languages,* because of the need for flexibility and speed. User programs are written in less flexible and slower *high-level languages,* because they more closely approximate common language, are easier to change once written, and are more "portable" from computer to computer. (High-level programs are translated or "compiled" into very low-level languages before they are run.)

Many of the high-level user languages on which application programs are based are familiar to the modern administrator:

—FORTRAN (Formula Translation), a language designed for mathematical use, especially by scientists and engineers

—BASIC (Beginners' All-Purpose Symbolic Instruction Code), a language that is easy to learn and use; used for solving numeric and business problems, usually in nontechnical applications

—APL (A Programming Language), a general language that resembles mathematical notation

—COBOL (Common Business-Oriented Language), a language designed for commercial business applications which uses English-like formats

—PASCAL (named in honor of Blaise Pascal, the French philosopher and mathematician who developed the first mechanical adding machine), an easy-to-learn, increasingly popular language with a highly structured format

The choice of language depends on the application, the hardware, the skills of the user, the costs, and the computer's operating system. The *operating system* (OS) is a collection of instructions provided by the manufacturer of the hardware to assist and in part to control the computer's processing—tasks once done by a computer operator. The OS is responsible for instruction to the control portion of the CPU: selecting jobs to run, notifying the operator when the controller has lost functioning, accepting and retrieving data from the input and output devices. Operating systems are processor-specific, but one OS may be designed for use with many different machines. An example of this is Bell Laboratories' UNIX operating system, which can operate on some processors manufactured by both IBM and DEC (Digital Equipment Corporation). Representing organizational relationships with a data base that can be managed by software on a reliable machine is only part of the information system. To allow communication between sites of activity, whether within the same building or across the globe, teleprocessing must be provided.

## 8.4 DATA COMMUNICATIONS

Basically, telecommunications systems include a sender, a message, communications channels, and a receiver. The sending and receiving unit can be a terminal linked with a "modem," a device that converts the pulse form understood by the computer to a wave form for transmission. The communication channel is the path over which the message must flow, most commonly telephone lines, cables, microwaves, or satellite equipment. Channel capacity depends on the range of frequencies which can be sent down the channel: the broader the range or band width of frequencies, measured in cycles (of a particular wave) per second, the higher the capacity and the higher the quality of the signal.

When discussing the speed of transmission, or capacity, the common unit of measurement is bits per second (bps). If the number of bits per character is known, then characters per second can be calculated. The term *baud* is often used to refer to the transmission speed, when in actuality it is the signaling speed (per second) of the channel. If the signaling speed is one bit or the absence of one bit, then it is the same as the transmission speed and baud rate is equivalent to bps. However, for most new transmitters, one baud equals two or three bps; for the sake of clarity, therefore, transmission speed should be expressed in bits per second rather than baud rate.

Although microwave transmitters and receivers are growing in prevalence, the most common communication channel for computers today is still the telephone line, which can transmit at rates ranging from 300 bps, the speed of most terminals, to 9600 bps, sufficient to drive a high-speed impact printer. The choice of communication channels is based on costs, data volume, and urgency of the data. The make-buy analysis used in an earlier chapter can apply to the decision on communication media—for instance, whether to "dedicate" a telephone line for the computer (say, lease it from a telephone company) or use the existing lines in the organization and public dial-up facilities. The greater the volume and urgency of the data, the more likely it is that leasing will be the most cost-effective solution. Even with leased lines, however, dial-up facilities can be used as backup or auxiliary transmitters.

## 8.5 COMPUTING PATTERNS

Developments in communication and processor technology have made it possible to construct the basis of an information system from a series of processors and peripheral devices connected by communication links. Distributed processing, as this is called, is based on old concepts of division of labor and specialization and has been made economically feasible through the development of *mini-* and *microprocessors.*

Miniprocessors were made possible by the development of a fabrication process known as *large-scale integration* (LSI) and *very large-scale integration* (VLSI), in which thousands of components are placed on a small silicon chip. Further developments led to the "supermini" which had the power of the old mainframes but was the size of a refrigerator. Released in 1971 was the first *microprocessor,* a one-chip central processing unit less than an eighth of an inch square and capable of handling four bits at a time. Since that time hundreds of designs of microprocessor chips have been developed, each more powerful than the one before, each capable of doing any number of tasks. The *microcomputers,* which are built around them, are increasingly found in all areas of health care.

The hospital admission scheduling system often uses a large mainframe computer that controls terminals in several sites, printers, and one or more data storage units. However, another system based on the mini- and/or microprocessors can be used to accomplish the same tasks, often at lower costs and with greater system expandability.

The minicomputer or microcomputer *networks,* as they are often called, distribute functions to minicomputers (or microcomputers) throughout the hospital. One minicomputer is used to control the other processors: its sole function is to distribute commands to these other processors. Thus, for example, an admission scheduling minicomputer in the admissions scheduling unit would communicate with this controlling minicomputer, the terminals in the relevant units, and printers located nearby. The admissions scheduling CPU would operate only within its "minisystem" of terminals, and would switch to the main controlling CPU only when data were needed by another minisystem outside of admissions scheduling, such as radiology or laboratory (Figure 8.6).

## *Figure 8.6*

### *Admission Scheduling—Minicomputer Network*

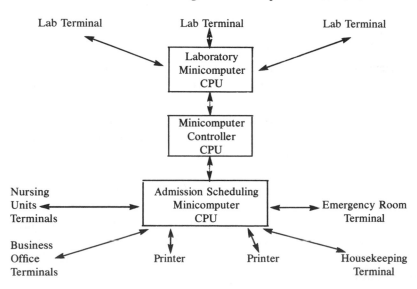

A true "system" design is seen in a minicomputer-based, distributed processing system. In this type of computing pattern, several minicomputers or processors handle the load of the entire hospital, not just admission scheduling (Figure 8.7). The software distributes

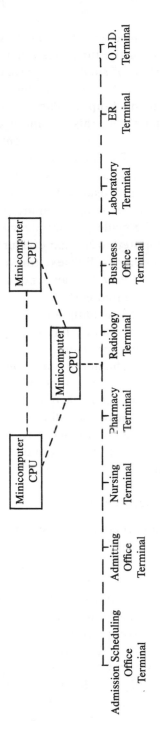

*Figure 8.7*

*Distributed System Network*

or directs the transactions to the CPU available at that moment. Each CPU can do all of the functions required by any unit in the hospital. The attractiveness of such an approach lies in its cost, often less than that of one large CPU, and even more in its reliability, which is due to the constant back-up available through all the CPUs. While the philosophy underlying this advanced design is well established, the software is still in its late developmental phase.

The variety of equipment has expanded the market for "plug-compatible" equipment manufacturers. These firms manufacture hardware that can be used with the hardware and software of another manufacturer. An existing computer-based information system in a clinic can thus be made compatible with a hospital's computer system even if the computers were manufactured by different companies. The decision of whether to link existing systems, replace equipment, or do all processing centrally can, once again, be subjected to the make-buy analyses presented earlier.

In addition to providing a hospital's main information-processing activity, the "stand-alone" microcomputer is increasingly being used for special purpose application, especially in finance, planning, nursing, and research. The nurse scheduling system described in Chapter 6 is now operating on stand-alone microcomputers in many nursing offices, and many finance departments are using microcomputers to perform budgeting, control, and financial analysis functions. While these microcomputers perform most of their tasks independently, they may also communicate with the hospital's main information-processing activity as needed.

## Back-up and Recovery

Back-up and recovery of data are functions that are often forgotten in the design of information systems. There are several reasons for having a back-up of the data base and a system for recovering an earlier form of the data base. Erroneous data may be entered into the data base either through a program bug or an otherwise unknown source; or the system may shut down as the result of some natural calamity or relatively minor system problem. In either case, having "dumped" or copied the data base on a periodic basis, while expensive, would have provided a copy of the data base as it existed prior to the error or disaster. Keeping an ongoing log of data base modifications from the time of the dump also makes accurate reconstruction more probable. While both techniques require time and can incur substantial costs depending on the size of the data base and the numbers of users, they are necessary to insure the integrity of the system.

## Security

Because computer-based information systems are often a shared resource, data related to sensitive operations are vulnerable to damage or infiltration. Protection techniques can be designed, such as passwords or password matrices, which are easy to implement but ineffective if not guarded; audit logs, which monitor data base activity; or methods for testing a "canned" portion of data against the data base to detect changes. As systems grow, the opportunities for security breaches also grow; if sensitive data must be kept in a widely accessible data base, then experts in data security should be consulted.

## 8.6 Implementation

In 1975 Henry Lucas published a model of information systems in the context of organizations. This model, as well as others which followed, emphasized that the mechanical component is only part of the information system. The models and their empirical support show that user attitudes and perceptions of systems determine in large part the extent of use and satisfaction with the system. It has also been shown that strong management support of the activities surrounding design, implementation, and maintenance increases the acceptance and technical quality of a computer-based information system.

The role of the administration in actions surrounding development of an information system can be significant. The potential impact on individuals, jobs, and relationships, which has been documented by several researchers, must be appreciated by the administrator if she is to be effective. Computers are seen by some as communication obstacles that interfere with personal contact and cause dependence on a machine. Those who see information as power view installation of a computer system as a challenge to the existing power structure. Those who have experience with older data systems may discredit their value in decision making, because the older system provided either too much data or the wrong kind. Those in data-handling positions may fear that the change will increase their work loads or eliminate their usefulness and thus their jobs.

While management and decision-making styles vary, those who have experienced the organizational traumas and successes that are possible when an information system is implemented have several recommendations. The first involves definition of the organization itself. The decision makers must jointly determine the goals of the organization, the decision processes which support the viability of that organization, and the environment in which it must survive. Once this has been decided and specified, the second recommendation is that a plan be formulated, preferably by a steering committee of potential users, management, and members of the data-processing or information services department if one exists. In hospitals or HMOs, this committee should include at a minimum persons from administration, service delivery, medical staff, and medical records. This group's responsibility and authority will also vary but may be very broad, as evidenced by the recommended tasks:

—define objectives of the project

—examine existing and budgeted resources (monetary and nonmonetary)

—prioritize and schedule design system, with the aid of experts

—evaluate computer options

—implement and train

—evaluate impact on the organization

—assess ideas for expansion and modification

Some authors recommend that a formal strategic information system plan be written, updated, and modified as the organization's needs and desires change. This has been especially important in guaranteeing that objectives are met and adequate resources are allocated throughout the life of the project. It is apparent that an ad hoc committee established only at the conception of a project would not be able to meet the long-term needs of a successful information system implementation.

One tool that has proven useful for outlining many of the tasks facing the committee is the information flow chart. The technique underlying the chart can aid the manager, designer, and user (ideally one and the same) in defining, presenting, and reviewing the problem, by documenting the information exchange and "flow" within and between organizations before and/or after computerization or any other change in operations. The lack of standardization in the process of flow charting stems from its widespread adaptation in many settings for many different needs. The technique involves using symbols to represent how decisions are made; how forms are used; and who communicates what information to whom, when, and how. Most processes can be charted using only the symbols shown in Figure 8.8.

## Figure 8.8

### Flow Charting Symbols

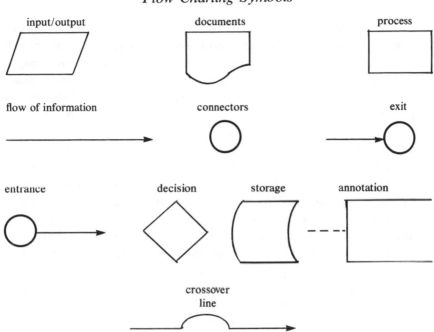

Templates are available with those and other more specific symbols. Although there are no real guidelines as to exactly how they should be used, there are some conventions which ease the execution and improve the product:

1. Make certain the project objective is clearly specified.

2. Note title, date, and author on each page.

3. Start with a high level of aggregation and work down to more detail or to subsystems. Chart the major communications flows first and minor flows second.

4. Start at the top of the page and work down; go from left to right.

5. Don't clutter a page; use page connectors to continue a complex flow. Keep crossover or intersecting lines to a minimum.

6. Use the symbols consistently.

7. Write only within the symbols, minimizing words. Use
the annotation symbol when more description is necessary.

Administrators might use the charts to identify characteristics of
the communications within the organization: for example, is there duplication of effort or unnecessary paperwork? System designers might
use charts to clarify the data relationships which must be understood
to design an accurate and useful data base. Both may find the charts
helpful in identifying areas within the organization which may require
special attention during the project.

Figure 8.9 illustrates the use of flow charting in identifying a set
of procedures done manually for patients who come to the hospital in
advance of the day of admission for laboratory and radiologic testing
(preadmission testing). This set of procedures and others related to
admission scheduling are examined through flow charting prior to
computer system design to ensure that all necessary activities are
accommodated in the design and unnecessary or redundant activities
are eliminated. The sample flow chart follows a patient and the accompanying forms from the registration desk to the service units,
business office, and data processing departments. Not all activities,
such as the laboratory notifying the admission scheduling clerk that
the preadmission tests have been completed, can be entered on one
page; therefore, details of the procedures in each of the departments
appear on different pages of the flow chart report, as indicated by the
connector symbols within which the page is noted. The flow chart
provides an overview of the number and type of documents utilized
as well as the procedures the patient must undergo on entry to the
facility. Review of the flow charts should help the computer system
designers in decisions about placement of terminals, choice of software, number of printers needed, as well as overall data base design
issues.

Flow charting is only one method of collecting and presenting
data about the project. Structured or unstructured observation of processes within an organization can reveal crucial interactions and decision points. Interviews with individuals who may in some way be
affected by the system, including administrators, providers, technicians, receptionists, and sometimes patients, can guide all stages of
development and implementation. Using members of the committee
to conduct the observations and interviews provides informal education of staff members and valuable feedback to the committee, as well
as data relevant to the design.

*Figure 8.9*

*Example Flow Chart of Preadmission Testing Arrival*

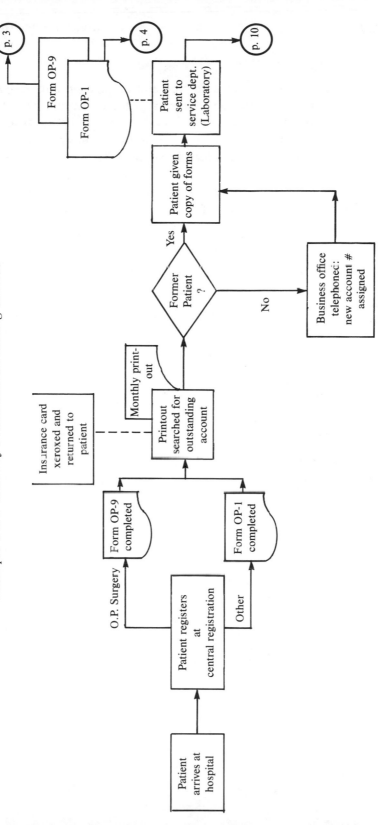

## Evaluating Alternatives

Once data have been collected and the appropriate design objectives have been formalized, the committee is faced with a task that seems to some to be impossible. Choosing the computer is an integral part of the design; but even given a particular design, there are multiple options for the machinery to support it. Here is where detailed specification of the project's objectives is once again critical. If the objectives are clear, then criteria on which to judge their satisfaction can be formulated and an informed choice can be made.

*Figure 8.10*

*Criteria for Consideration in Selection of a System*

Technical

       System capacity
       System expandability
       User friendliness
       Security of data
       Speed of performance
       Accuracy of output
       Ability to meet ad hoc requests
       Report-generating capability
       Maintenance record of company
       Accessibility of "trouble shooters"
       Reliability of equipment
       Weight, size of machine (space requirements)
       Performance of certain functions

Economic

       Initial cost of equipment
       Communication costs
       Maintenance costs
       Personnel costs (development, training, use)
       Duplication of resources
       Modification or expansion costs
       Risks and costs of obsolescence

Psychological

       Satisfaction of users
       Organizational changes required
       Interface ability
       Continuity of performance

While many attributes of computer systems can be examined (see Figure 8.10), some, such as satisfaction of users or technical security, are more difficult to measure than others. Many technical measures can be obtained from equipment or package vendors who have design specifications available. Evaluation of other performance attributes is best obtained from other organizations with operational experience with a system. If users desire specific report functions such as "expenditures to date" vs. "premiums paid to date" for employer groups within an HMO, or length of stay for patients receiving preadmission testing vs. those who did not, then the system should be investigated to insure that these special functions are possible. Involving the project team and other members of the organization in investigating and assessing the adequacy of each alternative increases the probability of making a satisfactory decision.

## Evaluating Organizational Impact

Managers become involved in computerization because they believe their organization will benefit. But much computerization has taken place with little heed to the actual gains or losses to the organization *as a system*. This can hinder an organization's ability to understand its own needs, to adapt to internal and external pressures, and to expand appropriately. An evaluation of the impact of the information system on the organization and its members should begin before installation of any equipment, and should extend throughout the life of the system. This evaluation should be based on the already specified objectives of the system, and some measurable criteria that provide a comprehensive but sensitive view of the impact at several levels of the organization.

The project team can use many of the tools developed during the design phase to supplement the information derived from the formal evaluation. Interviews and observations conducted prior to implementation can be viewed as baseline measures, and data on the same opinions, operations, etc., can be collected again at various times during and after installation of the computer system. Many of the measures will require new forms or aggregation of data already collected for another purpose. Examples of measures amenable to fairly simple collection methods appear in Table 8.1. Administrators often find that monitoring for the evaluation provides opportunities to assess the functioning of many aspects of the organization not usually examined so carefully.

*Table 8.1*

*Suggested Measures for Various Evaluative Criteria*

| Criterion | Measures |
|---|---|
| Impact on financial viability | Occupancy rates by department<br>Lengths of stay<br>Preadmission testing revenues |
| Impact on service delivery | Time and motion studies in admitting<br>Satisfaction of patients<br>Access time to records |
| Impact on organizational satisfaction | Satisfaction scales<br>Employee turnover rates per department<br>Number of employee complaints<br>Number of requests for transfer per department<br>Number of employees using system |
| System's technical performance | System down time (time inaccessible because of system failure)<br>Maintenance and repair costs<br>Error rates per function<br>Training time<br>Time to generate particular reports |
| Impact on patient health | Appropriateness of tests and outcomes of care, monitored by use of tracer diagnoses<br>Patient accessibility to facility |

## 8.7 CONCLUSIONS

Successful implementation of a computer-based information system relies as much on organizational sensitivity as it does on information-processing technology. If information systems are to make a positive contribution to strategic planning and operations, the administrators must know how to utilize the technology to meet the organization's objectives.

### Exercises

8.1 Prepare a PERT chart of the implementation of an information system for a rural acute care hospital with 75 inpatient beds and an emergency room.

8.2 As an assistant to the administrator, you have been given the responsibility to investigate computer alternatives for a new information system for the stand-alone surgical center. Prepare a two-page report supporting your recommendation to use microcomputers rather than minicomputers.

8.3 Detail the advantages and disadvantages of using distributive processing in your multisite prepaid physician group practice.

8.4 Using an actual health care setting with which you are familiar, prepare a flow chart for the information flow within a service unit, such as laboratory, admitting, patient registration, or billing. Verify your charting with the manager of the unit.

8.5 Medicare has decided to adjust its reimbursement by a regional case-mix index applied to each hospital. Detail the components of and necessary data relationships in a data base designed to accommodate that decision.

8.6 What are the trade-offs in buying a vendor-designed, prepackaged program rather than having the data-processing department design the package?

8.7 Present the techniques you would use to convince top management that the present hospital computer system needs replacement.

8.8 Prepare a flow chart of an activity in your department, such as course scheduling or admissions. Who might use this information and how?

## Additional Reading

Austin, Charles J. and Greene, Barry G. "Hospital Information Systems: A Current Perspective." *Inquiry* 15 (1978): 95–112.

Bohl, Marilyn. *Information Processing.* Chicago: Science Research Associates, 1980.

Chapin, N. "Flowcharting with the ANSI Standard: A Tutorial." *Computing Surveys* 2, no. 2 (June 1970): 89–110.

Gorry, G. Anthony and Scott Morton, M. S. "A Framework for Management Information Systems." *Sloan Management Review,* Fall 1971, pp. 21–36.

Kroenke, David. *Database Processing.* Chicago: Science Research Associates, 1977.

Leavitt, H. J. and Whisler, T. L. "Management in the 1980's." *Harvard Business Review,* November–December 1958, pp. 41–48.

Lucas, Henry C., Jr. *Information Systems Concepts for Management.* New York: McGraw-Hill Book Company, 1982.

Lucas, Henry C., Jr. *Why Information Systems Fail.* New York: Columbia University Press, 1975.

Martin, James. *An End-User's Guide to Data Base*. Englewood Cliffs, N.J.: Prentice-Hall, 1981.

Murdick, Robert G. *MIS: Concepts and Design*. Englewood Cliffs, N.J.: Prentice-Hall, 1980.

Rochester, J. B. (ed.). *Perspectives on Information Management*. New York: John Wiley and Sons, 1982.

Rogers, J. L., Haring, O. M., Wortman, P. M., Watson, R. A. and Goetz, J. P. "Medical Information Systems: Assessing the Impact in the Areas of Hypertension, Obesity and Renal Disease." *Medical Care* 20, no. 1 (January 1982): 63–74.

Steinwachs, D. M., Fahey, M., Horky, R., Perkel, S. and Tower, D. "MIS Requirements for Managing a Hospital under 'Per Case' Reimbursement." *Institute of Electrical and Electronics Engineers*, March 1979, pp. 122–129.

Whisler, T. L. *Information Technology and Organizational Change*. Belmont, Cal.: Wadsworth Publishers, 1973.

# 9

# Measurement

## 9.1 INTRODUCTION

In previous chapters, we demonstrated the need for measuring quality of care, aversion as a factor in scheduling nurses, cost of nursing assignments, seriousness of shortages, adequate access, and need for primary care. We also illustrated the use of such measures as time between arrivals, service time, number of arrivals, nursing hours, number of nurses, number of turned-away patients, and number of cancellations. In the examples of Part II we assumed that methods to make these measurements were available. We now return to the questions of how measurements can be made, how new measurement instruments can be constructed, and how the administrator can evaluate a measurement when considering it for use in decision making and control.

Before discussing the criteria for evaluating a measure, we will examine two types of measurement rules—*counting rules* and *scaling rules.* Counting rules are the more straightforward. They simply require us to count the number of times we observe an event. If we cannot afford to count *every* patient, patient day, nurse, bed, turned-away patient, or cancelled appointment, sampling strategies are available to count *part* of the population and infer from the sample what the count would have been if we had counted the entire population. We will discuss one such sampling scheme, work sampling, in detail.

Scaling rules are not well known by administrators or indeed by many quantitative staff specialists. Yet measurements of quality, aversion, subjective cost, seriousness of shortages, adequate access, or need require some sort of scaling rule, or psychological measurement technique, even if it is implicit. Often, scaling rules simply need to be made explicit in order to construct a measurement instrument. At other times, completely new measures need to be constructed. Counting rules are called the *frequentistic* approach, and scaling rules, the *subjective* approach. Scaling rules differ from counting rules since they require a person to assign a number based on his beliefs, values, attitudes, or other subjective psychological attributes. Other examples of subjective measurements are personnel satisfaction, patient satisfaction, and urgency of service. Satisfaction, urgency, quality, aversion, seriousness, adequacy, and need are based on value judgments that can often be quantified (or "scaled," if we use the psychologists' term).

As we shall see in Part IV, being able to use scaling rules has several advantages for controlling systems.

1. Observations of systems can be described in finer detail. If administrators want to detect small changes in the nursing unit from one month to the next, a scaling rule for assigning a number to the nursing unit's quality will provide finer distinctions than qualitative assessments alone.

2. Scaling rules provide the basis for making measures of performance explicit. Explicit measures of performance often enhance communication, allowing the nursing unit a more complete understanding of how its quality is being judged. Telling head nurses that their units are delivering "poor quality" does not communicate very useful information, whereas specifying the scaling rule will make it clear how "poor quality" was defined and measured.

3. Scaling rules can also reduce the time required by highly-trained professionals to make measurements. Nurses or physicians may have to make judgments about the quality of nursing or medical care, and a scaling rule predicting their judgments will often enable less expensive personnel to make these observations (either directly or from medical records). Even if the scaling rule requires nurses or physicians to make observations, the rule will save time by directing their observations and will make the observations more consistent.

The criteria for evaluating a measure to decide whether to use it in decision making and control are the same regardless of whether the measure is based on counting or scaling. In the final section of this chapter we shall use a combination of counting and scaling to construct a quality measure of nursing care and then apply the evaluation criteria to this measure.

## 9.2 MEASUREMENTS BY COUNTING

Four steps are involved in constructing a counted measurement:

1. An unambiguous rule for counting needs to be developed,

2. A time during the year to make the count needs to be selected,

3. The sample size needs to be determined if less than a 100 percent sample is going to be taken, and

4. The timing of the sample observations needs to be selected.

The measurements made for the OB merger decision are summarized in Tables 9.1 and 9.2. Every measurement listed in Table 9.1 is a counted measurement. Column 3 specifies the rule to measure the attribute in Column 1 for the system in Column 2: count people, hospitals, beds, OB physicians, filled beds, dollars, or births. The resulting measurement is in Column 4. Table 9.2 lists additional measurements made when the OB merger decision was revisited in Chapter 5 (Figures 5.8 to 5.13), again presenting counted measurements—minutes, hours, or days. For interarrival times, the hours from one patient's arrival to the next patient's arrival are counted. For service times, the number of hours the patient is in the labor and delivery beds and the number of days in the postpartum beds are counted.

Once an unambiguous rule has been developed, the next step requires choosing the time interval(s) in which to make the count. As reported in Chapter 5, the measurements in Table 9.2 were made in January, April, July, and October of the study year. Why not all months, and why those particular four months? Limiting the count to four months was a practical decision since the cost of extending the count to additional months was not thought to be worth the possible additional statistical accuracy. Every third month was used to account for potential seasonal differences (Chapter 7). Thus these time intervals were chosen to get a representative sample of interarrival times and service times throughout the year, while minimizing the cost of data collection.

The third and fourth steps are choosing the number and timing of observations (counts) to be made within the time interval chosen.

## Table 9.1

### Measurements Made for the OB Merger Decision from Chapter 2

| Attribute (1) | System (2) | Rule (3) | Number (4) | Unit (5) |
|---|---|---|---|---|
| 1. Size | Balham | Count people | 60,000 | People |
| 2. Accessibility | Balham Health Service | Count hospitals | 2 | Acute hospitals |
| 3. Availability | Balham Health Service | Count beds | 500 | Beds in acute hospitals |
| 4. Size | Hospital A labor room | Count beds | 4 | Labor beds |
| 5. Size | Hospital A delivery room | Count beds | 3 | Delivery beds |
| 6. Size | Hospital A postpartum unit | Count beds | 36 | Postpartum beds |
| 7. Size | Hospital B labor room | Count beds | 3 | Labor beds |
| 8. Size | Hospital B delivery room | Count beds | 3 | Delivery beds |
| 9. Size | Hospital B postpartum unit | Count beds | 30 | Postpartum beds |
| 10. Availability | Balham Health Service | Count physicians | 14 | OB physicians |
| 11. Utilization | Hospital A or B postpartum unit | Count filled beds each day for one year, divide by 365, divide that by number of postpartum beds. | 40 | % OB occupancy |
| 12. Utilization | Hospital A or B | Same as above for OB unit | 70 | % hospital occupancy |

| No. | Measure | Location | Method | Value | Description |
|---|---|---|---|---|---|
| 13. | Degree of under-serving | Hospital A or B labor room | Count patients | 0 | Patients arriving to find all labor beds filled |
| 14. | Degree of under-serving | Hospital A or B delivery room | Count patients | 0 | Patients arriving to find all delivery beds filled |
| 15. | Degree of under-serving | Hospital A or B postpartum suite | Count patients | 0 | Patients arriving to find all postpartum beds filled |
| 16. | Construction cost today | Hospital A or B OB unit | Count dollars | * | Cost for construction |
| 17. | Equipment cost today | Hospital A or B OB unit | Count dollars | * | Cost for equipment |
| 18. | Staff cost today | Hospital A or B | Count payroll dollars | * | Cost for staff |
| 19. | OB demand | Balham Health Service | Count births | 2,300 | Births last year |
| 20. | Quality | Hospital A OB unit | Count births | 1,090 | Births last year |
| 21. | Quality | Hospital B OB unit | Count births | 1,210 | Births last year |
| 22. | OB physician satisfaction | Balham | Count complaining physicians | 8 | Complaining OB physicians |

*These measurements were not reported

# Table 9.2

## Additional Measurements for OB Merger Decision from Chapter 5

| | Attribute | System | Rule | Number | Unit |
|---|---|---|---|---|---|
| 1. | Distribution of interarrival times | OB unit | Count the number of patients who arrive 0.0 to .50 hours after the preceding patient | 112 | patients |
| | | | Count the number of patients who arrive .51 to 1.00 hours after the preceding patient | 60 | patients |
| | | | 1.01 to 1.50 hours | 56 | patients |
| | | | 1.51 to 2.00 hours | 54 | patients |
| | | | 2.01 to 2.50 hours | 41 | patients |
| | | | (etc.: see Figure 5.8) | | |
| 2. | Distribution of service times | Labor beds | Count the number of patients who remain in labor bed from 0.0 to .50 hours | 76 | patients |
| | | | .51 to 1.00 hours | 57 | patients |
| | | | 1.01 to 1.50 hours | 35 | patients |
| | | | 1.51 to 2.00 hours | 25 | patients |
| | | | 2.01 to 2.51 hours | 34 | patients |
| | | | (etc.: see Figure 5.9) | | |
| 3. | Average waiting time | Labor beds | Count minutes between when each patient arrives and when placed in labor bed—calculate average | 0 | average number of minutes |
| 4. | Distribution of service times | Delivery beds | Count the number of patients who remain in delivery bed from 0.0 to .17 hours | 28 | patients |
| | | | .18 to .33 hours | 43 | patients |
| | | | .34 to .50 | 130 | patients |
| | | | .51 to .67 | 148 | patients |
| | | | .68 to .83 | 124 | patients |
| | | | (etc.: see Figure 5.10) | | |
| 5. | Average waiting time | Delivery beds | Count minutes between when each patient arrives and when placed in bed—calculate average | 0 | average number of minutes |
| 6. | Distribution of service times | Postpartum beds | Count the number of patients who remain in postpartum bed from 0.0–1.00 days | 0 | patients |
| | | | 1.01 to 2.00 days | 24 | patients |
| | | | 2.01 to 3.00 days | 232 | patients |
| | | | 3.01 to 4.00 days | 224 | patients |
| | | | 4.01 to 5.00 days | 70 | patients |
| | | | (etc.: see Figure 5.13) | | |
| 7. | Average waiting time | Postpartum beds | Count minutes between when each patient arrives and when placed in postpartum bed—calculate average | 0 | average number of minutes |

Since the OB study made counts on the entire population of 588 OB patients arriving during the above four months, these steps cannot be illustrated. They will be discussed further under work sampling below.

A clever and relatively inexpensive way of counting minutes between arrivals and minutes for service in an outpatient setting, in contrast to the OB example where inpatient logs are used, is to use a punch clock (for punching time in and out of work). One could be purchased or rented for each station (receptionist, examining room, laboratory, X-ray room, etc.). Arriving patients are given time cards that they take with them to each station. The cards are punched when the patients arrive and depart from each station. Each punch clock has its own identifying number punched next to the times on the cards. The punch cards are then coded for a computer tally of times between arrivals to clinic (the difference between the first times punched on sequential time cards), service times at each station (the difference between time punched on arrival and time punched on departure), and waiting times for each station (the difference between time punched on departure from one station and time punched on arrival to next station). In addition, the cards show the flow of patients from one station to the next.

This method requires one or two people to explain the process to clinic personnel, to set the punch clocks in position one day, and to return in two weeks (or whatever time interval is decided upon) to collect the raw data. It is useful because several different clinics could be studied at the same time.

## Work Sampling

**Problem:** In order to establish the number of Registered Nurse, Practical Nurse, and Nurse's Aide positions to fund for a nursing unit (the staffing decision), the time required to perform each of a set of task categories must be measured. The number of positions and the mix of skill levels is established so that the time needed by each appropriate skill level is available to carry out the tasks. At the same time, the salary and "lost quality costs" are to be minimized.* How can the time required on each unit be measured?

---

*For readers who are familiar with the linear programming formulation of the staffing decision in section 6.6, the problem is to measure $B_j$—the total number of full-time equivalent positions required to perform task category $j$.

## Table 9.3

### Definitions of Task Categories Used by Wolfe and Young

#### Highly Technical Tasks

This category includes all personnel procedures that require advanced knowledge, understanding of principles underlying procedures, and the exercising of judgment. Procedures which fall into this category are:

1. Use of complicated apparatus including hypothermia units, suction machines, heat lamps, inhalators, peritoneal dialysis, parenteral fluids, tube feedings, oxygen equipment, alternating pressure pads, artificial kidney, tidal drainage, respirators.

2. Therapeutic procedures such as irrigations, medications, injections, dressings, sterile compresses, sterile application of heat and cold, alcohol sponge bath, tracheotomy care, catheterization, bladder treatments.

#### Less Highly Technical Tasks

This category includes all nursing procedures that can be performed with on-the-job training. Procedures which fall into this category are:

1. Admission, discharge, transfer.

2. Isolation procedures.

3. Personal care of patient including bed baths, shampoo, oral hygiene, skin care, backrubs, positioning patient, providing for elimination, serving meals, etc.

4. Therapeutic procedures including application of heat and cold, sitz baths, enemas, temperature, pulse, respirations, and application of binders.

5. Use of equipment for patient comfort, including making occupied beds, special beds while occupied, bed boards, Bradford frames, patient lifter, wheelchair, stretcher.

6. Assisting with diagnostic procedures including collection of specimens, preparation for radiological studies, preoperative care, preparation for examinations.

7. Signal detection including observing patients for obvious changes, answering patient calls or requests, general communication with patient.

8. Assisting in care of the dead.

#### Evaluation of Patient Needs and Assignment

This category includes personal interviews with patients, receiving reports from other personnel about patient, conferences with physicians and other health personnel, analysis of total information on patients, determination of objectives for patients, evaluation of staff capabilities, and making the necessary assignments. This would also include planning and assignments for other shifts and adjusting the care plan and assignments.

#### Supervising and Teaching

This includes all contacts with patients or other personnel primarily for the purpose of guiding patient care or imparting information. This includes periodic checking of work done by other personnel, the teaching of new techniques to other personnel, and the giving of information to patients as to how to care for themselves when they leave the hospital.

#### Tasks Preparatory to Highly Technical Tasks

This category includes all activities associated with the performance of Highly Technical Tasks that are done away from the patient. This would include preparation of equipment for sterile purposes, acid tests, specific gravity tests, and preparation of medications.

### Tasks Preparatory to Less Highly Technical Tasks

This category includes all activities associated with the performance of Less Highly Technical Tasks that are done away from the patient. This would include filling and measuring fluids, gathering and disposing of linen and equipment, clinic tests, etc.

### Clerical Tasks Directly Related to Patient

This category includes all tasks of recording on worksheets all information concerning the patient, such as temperature, pulse, and respiration, intake and output, height and weight, preoperative check list, listing of valuables, personal belongings.

### Clerical Tasks Less Directly Related to Patient

This category includes record-keeping such as weight sheet; transcribing work sheets; copying doctors' orders and medicine tickets; preparing records for admission and discharge; provision of patient services such as receiving visitors and new patients, sorting and distributing mail, flowers, and patients' gifts; fulfilling patient requests for all unit services; and provision of telephone services including answering calls, taking messages, giving information, making calls for patients and staff, and making calls to obtain services.

### Medical Record Notation

This category includes pertinent notations in the medical record concerning all treatment and observations, reports for nursing administration, personnel evaluation, referral forms, requisitions and audits for narcotics, critical conversation in person or on telephone pertaining to patients, to visitors, physicians, or other departments.

### Housekeeping

This category includes all tasks which are performed primarily for the purpose of keeping the unit and equipment clean and in good order. This would include making unoccupied beds, cleaning and keeping patients' immediate environment neat, and cleaning equipment.

### Escorting and Emergency Errands

This category includes all productive tasks off the nursing unit except for formal meetings, such as head nurses' meetings, nursing aide programs, etc. This includes accompanying the patient anywhere in the hospital and going to other units to deliver or pick up messages, supplies, or equipment.

### Maintenance, Checking, and Ordering of Supplies and Equipment

This category includes all activities that are primarily for the purpose of seeing that all supplies and equipment are in stock and in good condition—for example, ordering drugs and other items, checking inventories to see that standards are maintained, checking equipment to see that it is in good order, arranging for repair of damaged equipment.

SOURCE: Wolfe, H. and Young J. "Staffing the Nursing Unit, Part II: The Multiple Assignment Technique," *Nursing Research* vol. 14, no. 4, Fall 1965.

Work sampling (random observations) is an alternative to continuous observation by punch clock or an observer with a stopwatch. If continuous observation is thought of as looking at a motion picture, random observation can be thought of as looking at only a sample of frames (time instants) randomly selected from the film. The random observations are made often enough that statistical inferences can be made about what the continuous observations would have been.

Work sampling was used by Wolfe and Young to obtain the hours spent by a nursing unit on the day shift for each of the task categories described in Table 9.3. The results are shown in Table 9.4. The unit averaged 12 self-care, 11 intermediate-care, and 3 intensive-care patients. Naturally, these time estimates would change as the mix of patients changed.

To count the number of hours spent on each task category, the following steps are required. First, clearly define each task category to ensure that the same observations would be made by anyone viewing them (to illustrate, the definitions used by Wolfe and Young are in Table 9.3, and the distinction between self-care, intermediate-care, and high-care patients for task categories 1–6 are in Table 9.5).

Second, determine when the observations will be made. Wolfe and Young made observations on fifteen days spread over a two month period. It is hoped that those two weeks adequately represented the

*Table 9.4*

*Hours Needed by One Nursing Unit to Perform Each Task Category on the Day Shift*

| Task Type | Description | Time (hours) Required |
|:---:|---|:---:|
| 1 | Highly technical tasks made on high-care patients | 2.0 |
| 2 | Highly technical tasks made on intermediate-care patients | 2.0 |
| 3 | Highly technical tasks made on self-care patients | .5 |
| 4 | Less highly technical tasks made on high-care patients | 3.5 |
| 5 | Less highly technical tasks made on intermediate-care patients | 5.0 |
| 6 | Less highly technical tasks made on self-care patients | 3.0 |
| 7 | Evaluation of patient need and assignment | 11.5 |
| 8 | Supervising and teaching | 1.5 |
| 9 | Tasks preparatory to highly technical tasks | 5.0 |
| 10 | Tasks preparatory to less highly technical tasks | 12.0 |
| 11 | Clerical tasks directly related to patient | 3.0 |
| 12 | Clerical tasks less directly related to patient | 7.0 |
| 13 | Medical record notation | 2.0 |
| 14 | Housekeeping | 4.5 |
| 15 | Escorting and emergency errands | 5.0 |
| 16 | Maintenance, checking, ordering | 1.5 |
| 17 | Other (nonproductive and personal) | 10.0 |
| | Total | 82.0 |

SOURCE: Wolfe, H. *A Multiple Assignment Model for Staffing Nursing Units.* Ph.D. dissertation, Johns Hopkins University, 1964.

## Table 9.5

## Characteristics of Patients in Dependency Categories

Category I. Self-care

Any of the following combinations checked
(a) Ambulatory, or up in chair—self (without assistance)
   Feeding self, or requires food cut
   Bathing in bathroom, or at bedside—partial self
   (can bathe self except for back and perhaps extremities)
(b) Ambulatory—with assistance
   Up in chair—self
   Bathing in bathroom, or at bedside—partial self
(c) As in (a and b) with
   Vision inadequate
   Oxygen therapy
   I. V. feeding
   but no two of these factors simultaneously

Category II. Partial- or intermediate-care

Any of the following combinations checked
(a) Ambulatory—with assistance
   Bathing in bathroom, or at bedside—partial self
   Feeding—complete assistance (except I.V. feeding)
   Vision inadequate ⎫
   Oxygen therapy  ⎭ optional (does not affect classification under these conditions)
(b) Up in chair—self
   Bathing at bedside—complete assistance
   Feeding self, or requires food cut or I.V. feeding
   Oxygen therapy   ⎫
   Vision inadequate ⎭ optional
(c) As in (b) with the following changes
   Up in chair with assistance
   Bath at bedside
(d) Up in chair with assistance
   Bath at bedside—partial self
   Feeding—complete assistance
   Vision inadequate ⎫
   Oxygen therapy   ⎭ optional
(e) Bath at bedside
   Feeding—self, or requires food cut, or I.V. feeding
   Vision inadequate ⎫
   Oxygen therapy   ⎭ optional
(f) Requiring special care by necessity (patient has continuous nursing assistance to the
   extent that meal relief must be provided for the special duty nurse)

NOTE: Any patient who otherwise falls into Categories I or II, but who is under suction
therapy or is in isolation, incontinent (including wound drainage necessitating change
of bed linen), or markedly emotionally disturbed (needs almost constant observation,
in single room, creates disturbance) will de dropped to the next category.

Category III. Intensive or "total" care

All combinations not previously mentioned.

SOURCE: Wolfe, H. and Young, J. P. "Staffing the Nursing Unit, Part I: Controlled Variable
Staffing." *Nursing Research*, vol. 14, no. 3, (Summer, 1965).

remainder of the year. They would not be representative if the seasonal variation in census was not accounted for, if the absenteeism rate was especially high, or if a holiday occurred on one of the days.

Third, determine the number of observations that should be made. The more observations, the closer we come to making continuous observations—but the more expensive they are to make; the fewer observations, the less confidence we have in inferring what the continuous observations would have been—but the less expensive they are to make. Some introductory industrial engineering texts (Barnes, for example) provide tables for determining the number of observations needed in order to maintain different confidence levels for the inferences we are making. Wolfe and Young made 5,631 observations in the fifteen days.

Once the number of observations is determined, the fourth step is to develop a scheme to insure that their timing is random. During an 8-hour shift, each of the 480 ($8 \times 60$) minutes must have an equal chance of being observed. A random number table (Table 5.9) can be used to select the time *instants* to begin a tour through the nursing unit to make the needed number of observations. Each tour results in several observations since each staff member would be observed separately.

Once the observations are made, divide the number of times each task was observed by the total number of observations made. This is then an estimate of the frequency with which we would expect to observe these tasks being performed if we had made continuous observations. Therefore, we can multiply this frequency by the total number of nursing hours (which is eight times the number of RNs plus LPNs plus AIDEs) to get an estimate of the number of hours required for each task.

Consider an example. Assume Task 1 was observed 49 times out of 2,000 observations made and that there were 82 hours of nursing time on the observed unit. An estimate of the number of hours spent for Task 1 is, therefore,

$$\text{Hours for Task 1} = \frac{49}{2,000} \times 82 \text{ total nursing hours per shift}$$

$$= 2.00 \text{ hours per shift.}$$

Continuous observation in this application would have been expensive and difficult, requiring observers to follow the ten or eleven RNs, LPNs and AIDEs continuously. Determining when one task stopped and the next one started would also have been very difficult. On the other hand, the accuracy of the times determined for each task using work sampling depends on the personnel being observed, the time interval selected for collecting data, the absence of unusual events, and the sample size.

Consider another example. As the assistant administrator, you have been designated project director responsible for a massive interviewing of a random sample of your hospital's market area in order to collect data relevant to a needs assessment. The 25 interviewers have been hired to conduct the 1,500 interviews, but need training. The instrument has been designed and pretested; it has 100 questions to be asked of the head of household. In the training sessions, you stress the importance of contacting every person sampled so that the interview can be completed and the high response rate can preclude claims of nonrespondent bias leveled against the hospital's earlier projects. You also stress the need to ask *every* question in the instrument.

While you are fairly confident that you have conveyed the importance of completing every interview, it is necessary to sample a portion of the interviewers' work to insure the validity and reliability of responses. In the cases which are selected for review, your associate will recontact the respondent and re-ask certain questions. Determining the number of interviews to check and the number of questions which need re-asking involves formulating a sampling without replacement problem, modeled well by the hypergeometric distribution.

## Hypergeometric Distribution

A population consists of two types of objects of differing colors, say, black and white. The drawings of a sample size of $n$ are made *without* replacement. The number of black objects in the sample, $X$, is the random variable of interest. (If the sampling were done *with* replacement, the $X$ would be distributed binomially.) The frequency distribution of $X$ is described by

$$fX(u) = \frac{\binom{M}{u}\binom{N-M}{n-u}}{\binom{N}{n}}$$

where

$u = 0, 1, \ldots, n,$

$M$ = number of black objects in the population,

$N$ = total number of objects in the population,

$N - M$ = number of white objects in the population, and

$n$ = number of objects drawn as a sample, without replacement.

For a random variable with a hypergeometric distribution, the expected value is $np$ and the variance is $[(N - n) / (N - 1)]\, np\, (1 - p)$, where $p = M/N$.

Assume the completed interviews consist of truly completed ($T$) and falsely completed ($F$) interviews (no interview took place but an instrument was completed by the interviewer and submitted); our population is thus described by $N = F + T$. We wish to sample from $N$ in order to detect the existence of $F$s in the population. This sample will be the number of verifications our associate will do, represented by $V$. $X$ is the number of falsified interviews out of $V$ verifications, or the number of falsified interviews drawn by our *sample*. It is possible to calculate the probability of $X$ falsified interviews detected by $V$ verifications, using the following formula:

$$\frac{F!\; V!\; (N - F)!\; (N - V)!}{X!\; (F - X)!\; (V - X)!\; N!\; (N - F - V + X)!}.$$

To simplify, we assume $X = 0$ or that the sample drew no falsified interviews, in which case the

$$p\left(\frac{not \text{ detecting a falsification}}{F \text{ falsified interviews and } V \text{ verifications}}\right) = \frac{(N - F)!\; (N - V)!}{N!\; (N - F - V)!}$$

To reiterate, a lot of size $N$ containing $F$ "defectives" is submitted for inspection. A sample of size $V$ is drawn without replacement and the lot is accepted if the number of defectives found in the sample is less than or equal to $X$. The probability of accepting the lot is given by $p\,(N, V, F, X)$.

Applying the distribution to our example requires some initial assumptions in order to arrive at a workable number of validations.

The assumptions include a range of probable falsification rates; this range can be determined by meetings with project staff and is based on the difficulty of conducting the interview and expected respondent problems.

Any probability can be considered acceptable; but for this example, it is decided that a 95 percent probability of detecting a falsified interview would be the lowest acceptable limit for the validation rate determination.

Given these assumptions and our original scenario, there are 1500 respondents (assuming 100 percent response rate), 25 interviewers, and 60 interviews/interviewer.

$N = 60$

$X = 0$

$p_o$ = probability of no falsified interview or of missing a falsified interview in $V$ verifications given $F$ falsified interviews/interviewer

A matrix can be created:

| $V$ \ $F$ | 5 | 10 | 20 | 30 |
|---|---|---|---|---|
| | | $p_o$ | | |
| 5 | .637 | .389 | .120 | .026 |
| 7 | .525 | .259 | .048 | .005 |
| 10 | .388 | .140 | .011 | .000 |

Assuming that if the interviews were to be falsified, at least one third or more of them per interviewer would be falsified, the associate would have to validate at least 7 out of 60 interviews done by each interviewer for a valuation rate of 11 percent and a confidence of at least 95.2 percent of detection.

A matrix can be created to determine how many questions per interview would need to be validated.

| $V$ \ $F$ | 5 | 10 | 15 | 30 | 50 |
|---|---|---|---|---|---|
| $N = 100$ | | $p_o$ | | $X = o$ | |
| 3 | .85 | .72 | .61 | .33 | .12 |
| 5 | .77 | .58 | .43 | .16 | .02 |
| 7 | .69 | .46 | .30 | .07 | .01 |
| 10 | .58 | .33 | .18 | .02 | .00 |

If you and your associate believed it likely that entire sections of the interview, amounting to one-third or more, would be omitted or falsified, then validating 7 questions out of 100 would achieve a 93 percent confidence or probability of detection.

Tables are available which permit calculation of $p_o$ without using the formula provided here. The technique provides statistical justification of the necessary efforts to insure quality control in projects. It has been applied to any number of work sampling situations in which the population size is relatively small. In cases where $N$ is very large relative to $n$ (or $V$, in our example), then for all practical purposes we are sampling *with* replacement, and $X$ can be described by the binomial distribution.

Although counting may often be most accurate, there are situations in which it is less accurate than scaling. If, in the above example, nursing procedures were changing, the counted measurements would not represent the future. If, for some reason, the work sampling procedure were poorly administered or simply too difficult to administer, the counted measurements might not be accurate or might be too expensive to obtain. If we wanted to know how long tasks would take if quality care were provided, rather than simply describing how long it takes, then counted measurements may not result in adequate estimates. We are then forced to turn to measurements by scaling—to measurements relying on subjective judgment.

## 9.3 MEASUREMENTS BY SCALING

**Problem:** Since labor, delivery, and postpartum beds already existed in the OB units in Balham, the service times could be counted as described in Section 9.2. But recall from Section 5.2 that the OB physicians wanted to establish beds for the patients' recovery after delivery before being transferred to postpartum beds. How long will patients be in these beds? How can we measure the service time for recovery beds when there is nothing to count?

This type of measurement problem occurs often enough that administrators should be aware of methods for obtaining subjective probabilities—for example, probabilities of the time in recovery beds. The frequentistic probabilities in Table 9.2 would not be appropriate to use if it was anticipated that service times were going to change, or if it was felt that, in making time measurements, the times were recorded incorrectly, or observers were poorly trained in knowing what to measure, or a substantial number of patients were missed in the count. A recount may delay the project or increase expenses beyond the budget.

There are a great many methods for scaling subjective estimates, and each has its own advantages and disadvantages. The approach we will take is to illustrate several methods that can easily be adapted to other uses. There is no general method of scaling.

## Scaling Subjective Probabilities

Subjective probabilities are obtained by asking persons directly how likely it is that an event will occur and by assigning numbers between 0 and 1.0 to the event's probability. A "0" is assigned to events that will not happen for certain, a "1.0" to events that will happen for certain, and a ".50" to events that are as likely to happen as not to happen. Other numbers between 0 and 1.0 are assigned to indicate the degree to which events will (or will not) happen.

What may be surprising is that people often can give accurate subjective estimates of existing frequentistic probabilities. Just as one would not expect frequentistic probabilities to be accurate without trained observers and without an unambiguous counting rule, one cannot expect subjective probabilities to be accurate without trained estimators and a rule for scaling subjective probabilities that reduces estimators' bias (their overestimates or underestimates of frequentistic probabilities).

To illustrate the process of scaling subjective probabilities, consider obtaining the probabilities that OB patients will remain in recovery beds for 0–1 hours, 1–2 hours, 2–3 hours, 3–4 hours, 4–5 hours, 5–6 hours, and 6–7 hours. As with frequentistic probabilities of the service time in labor, delivery, and postpartum beds, we have made time a discrete variable by breaking it into intervals. Assume we have discussed this with the OB physicians, who believe the probability that a patient will stay longer than 7 hours is equal to zero. We will start by obtaining the subjective probabilities from one OB physician.

The dialogue between the decision analyst and OB physician might go as follows:*

---

*The methods and format in this section were adapted from Huber (1974).

ANALYST:            Which of these time intervals is least likely to occur?

OB PHYSICIAN:       Well, I'd say it is least likely that the time in the recovery bed will exceed 6 hours, so I'll say 6–7 hours.

ANALYST:            Okay, now how likely is 6–7 hours? What probability would you assign it?

OB PHYSICIAN:       Oh, about 2 percent, about 1 patient out of every 50.

ANALYST:            Now, holding aside for the moment that 6–7 hours has a probability of .02, which of the remaining time intervals is least likely and what do you think its probability is?

OB PHYSICIAN:       Well, it's hard to say. I think 0–1 hours is unlikely as well. I would say its probability is 2 percent also.

ANALYST:            Keeping out 0–1 and 6–7 hours, which is now least likely?

OB PHYSICIAN:       5–6 hours is not very likely either. I would guess its probability is the same as the other two.

ANALYST:            Keeping out 0–1, 5–6, and 6–7 hours, which is now least likely?

OB PHYSICIAN:       4–5 hours, then 3–4 hours, and then I would guess 1–2 and 2–3 hours are equally likely.

ANALYST:            What probabilities would you assign—keeping out each one you've assigned a number to?

OB PHYSICIAN:       Well, I would say 3 out of every 50 patients will stay 4–5 hours, probably 9 out of 50 would stay 3–4, and the rest would stay either 1–2 or 2–3 hours.

At this point it is helpful to review the estimates with the OB physician. When he sees all of his estimates together, he may want to change them. Does he still believe 0–1, 5–6, and 6–7 hours are equally likely? Are 1–2 and 2–3 hours equally likely?

The results are as follows:

| | |
|---|---|
| 0–1 hours | .02 |
| 1–2 | .35 |
| 2–3 | .35 |
| 3–4 | .18 |
| 4–5 | .06 |
| 5–6 | .02 |
| 6–7 | .02 |
| | 1.00 |

Note that these estimates are now in a form that can be used directly in the simulation in Section 5.2.

When subjective probabilities have been obtained where there are frequentistic probabilities with which to compare, two types of biases have been observed. The first is called the *overconfidence bias*. It can occur if, for example, the OB physician is asked to make his best guess of the most likely time interval, and then to assign probabilities. The OB physician would in effect be asked to estimate the probability that his most likely guess was correct, and people tend to assign probabilities to this guess that are too high. This bias can be reduced by training the OB physician and by starting with the least likely time interval.

The second bias is called the *extreme-value bias*. People tend to overestimate low probabilities and underestimate high probabilities. One explanation for this is that people remember the exceptions and tend to overestimate their low probabilities. Since the probabilities still have to add up to 1.0, an underestimate of the high probabilities results, compensating for the overestimation. This bias, which occurs more often with people unfamiliar with the content area being judged than with experts, can be partly overcome by using people familiar with the use of recovery beds, for example. In our case, it would be appropriate to use OB physicians with experience in treating patients in the recovery phase.

In addition, the extreme-value bias can be overcome by a scaling method based on estimating the odds that an event will occur rather than directly estimating the probability. The dialogue for this method might go like this:

ANALYST:     Please rank order the events, from the most likely to the least likely.

OB PHYSICIAN:        1–2, 2–3, 3–4, 5–6, 0–1, and 6–7.

ANALYST:             Okay, how many times more likely is it that 1–2 hours will occur than 2–3? What are the odds in favor of 1–2 compared to 2–3?

OB PHYSICIAN:        About equal, 1 to 1.

ANALYST:             What are the odds in favor of 1–2 compared to 3–4?

OB PHYSICIAN:        About 2 to 1.

ANALYST:             What are the odds in favor of 1–2 compared to 4–5?

OB PHYSICIAN:        It is 6 times more likely that 1–2 will occur than 4–5.

ANALYST:             What are the odds in favor of 1–2 compared to 5–6?

OB PHYSICIAN:        The last three intervals, 5–6, 0–1, and 6–7 are all about the same. Maybe 1–2 is 16 times more likely than these.

Again, the analyst should review the estimates with the physician. Does the physician feel 2–3 hours is also twice as likely as 3–4 hours, and that 3–4 hours is 3 times more likely than 4–5 hours?

The results of the dialogue are as follows:

| | Most Likely |
|---|---|
| 1–2 hours | |
| 2–3 | 1–1 |
| 3–4 | 2–1 |
| 4–5 | 6–1 |
| 5–6 | 16–1 |
| 0–1 | 16–1 |
| 6–7 | 16–1 |

To transform these odds estimates to probability estimates, the analyst assigns an arbitrary probability to the most likely event, 1–2 hours. Say .50 is assigned. Then the odds are used to generate the other probabilities, which would be

| | |
|---|---|
| 1–2 hours | .50 |
| 2–3 | .50 |
| 3–4 | .25 |
| 4–5 | .08 |
| 5–6 | .03 |
| 0–1 | .03 |
| 6–7 | .03 |
| | 1.42 |

If the odds in favor of 1–2 hours over 3–4 hours are 2 to 1, the probability of 3–4 hours should be half the probability of 1–2 hours. If the probability of 1–2 hours is arbitrarily .50, the probability of 3–4 hours must be .25. These "arbitrary" probabilities are totaled to get 1.42, and this total is divided into each so the sum is 1.00, as follows:

| | | |
|---|---|---|
| 1–2 | .50/1.42 = | .35 |
| 2–3 | .50/1.42 = | .35 |
| 3–4 | .25/1.42 = | .18 |
| 4–5 | .08/1.42 = | .06 |
| 5–6 | .03/1.42 = | .02 |
| 0–1 | .03/1.42 = | .02 |
| 6–7 | .03/1.42 = | .02 |
| | | 1.00 |

As suggested above, to overcome both the overconfidence bias and the extreme-value bias, training the estimators is necessary. The estimators should be aware of probability (what the numbers between 0 and 1.0 mean), frequentistic probabilities, subjective probabilities, and odds if that method is used. Methods of training have been developed using examples, charts, discussions, etc., but they are outside the scope of this book (see the Ludke reference).

Another way to improve subjective probabilities (have them come closer to frequentistic probabilities, if known) is to obtain and combine estimates from more than one expert. The preferred way to combine estimates is first to obtain separate estimates from each expert, then simultaneously disclose all estimates to all experts for a discussion of the reasoning behind the estimates, reobtain their separate estimates, and finally to calculate the average of the second estimates. Consensus is not required. Somehow the estimate–talk–re-estimate sequence results in more accurate estimates than either making one estimate without talking or making one estimate after talking. (This method is common to the nominal group technique to be discussed later in Section 9.6.)

## Scaling Preferences

**Problem:** Reconsider the nurse-staffing decision. We have discussed work sampling to measure the time required to perform 16 task categories. However, LPNs and AIDEs cannot perform some tasks, and can perform other tasks only at a "cost" of a possible loss of patient-care quality. Let $C_y$ denote the cost of lost quality due to having a nurse of skill class $i$ ($i = 1$ for RN, 2 for LPN, and 3 for AIDE) perform task category $j$ for one hour. How can we measure $C_y$?

The first decision the administrator must make is *who* will scale the $C_{ij}$. Before considering that question, let's examine one method for scaling $C_{ij}$, assuming the scaling is being done by the nurse who usually assigns nursing personnel to tasks. To make the problem more realistic, assume five skill classes—head nurse ($i = 1$), staff nurse ($i = 2$), licensed practical nurse ($i = 3$), nurses aides ($i = 4$), and ward clerk ($i = 5$).

The dialogue between the decision analyst and the nurse might go like this:

ANALYST:    Consider the first category, "highly technical tasks performed for high care patients." From the standpoint of quality, and without regard for differences in salary, which class of nursing personnel would you prefer to have perform these tasks?

NURSE:    The staff nurses, since head nurses will probably be too busy to do a good job.

ANALYST:    But if no staff nurses were available?

NURSE:    Well, then head nurses, of course.

ANALYST:    If they were both unavailable, which class?

NURSE:    The LPNs. But under no circumstance would I have aides or ward clerks even attempt these tasks.

ANALYST:    Okay, now just looking at staff RNs and head nurses, how much increase in your daily nursing budget would you be willing to pay to have staff nurses perform these tasks rather than head nurses?

NURSE: Well, from a quality standpoint, I really don't care. I wouldn't pay anything.

ANALYST: Okay, now if it were between staff nurses and LPNs, how much would you be willing to pay over and above the LPN's salary for a staff nurse rather than an LPN to do this work?

NURSE: For how long is she going to do the task?

ANALYST: Let's say one hour.

NURSE: Well, not more than $2: that's the difference between the hourly wage, and I wouldn't have to pay more than the difference in the hourly rate for staff nurses and LPNs because I know I can get a staff nurse for that, so . . .

ANALYST: Wait—let's suppose there are no more staff nurses looking for positions at your hospital and there aren't likely to be any more. But you do know of some highly qualified nurses who might come in if the salary were high enough. How much above an LPN's salary would you offer these nurses to try to get them to come in?

NURSE: Well, I guess I'd pay about $3 an hour above the LPNs' hourly rate, even though the present difference is only $2.

ANALYST: Okay, how about aides. How much above the hourly wage of an aide would you pay to have a staff nurse rather than an aide do the task for an hour?

NURSE: Almost anything. In fact, I wouldn't let an aide do it under any circumstances—I'd do it myself. And the same goes for a ward clerk.

ANALYST: Okay, now consider the second category of tasks . . . (continue the above dialogue for each of the sixteen categories).

At this point, the analyst can assign this nurse's estimates of the costs of lost quality. $C_{21}$ is arbitrarily assigned zero, because the highest quality is obtained, in her opinion, when staff nurses ($i = 2$) perform Category 1 tasks ($j = 1$). Zero cost is arbitrary since nurse specialists could conceivably be even better, but that category was not included. $C_{11}$, the cost of lost quality to have a head nurse ($i = 1$) perform task category 1 ($j = 1$) rather than the staff nurse, is also zero. $C_{31}$, the cost of lost quality by having the LPN ($i = 3$) perform task category 1 ($j = 1$), rather than the staff nurse, is \$3 for one hour. $C_{41}$ and $C_{51}$ would be assigned infinity ($\infty$), implying that "I wouldn't let an aide (or ward clerk) do it under any circumstances." Even though the nurse would not say how much she would be willing to pay, her statement implies that she would pay anything ("I'd do it myself") to avoid having aides and ward clerks perform these tasks. If the nurse has difficulty making a single-cost assignment, a high and low estimate could be obtained, and the mathematical programming formulation in Section 6.6 solved twice.

Table 9.6 shows the results obtained for all task categories by Wolfe in 1964. Ten persons participated, five with nursing backgrounds and five with administrative backgrounds. The values in Table 9.6 are obtained by averaging their cost assignments.

In this problem, *who* should be asked how much they would be willing to pay? Head nurses? Physicians? Patients? Blue Cross? Medicare Program Administrators? Medicaid Program Administrators? Congress? You can always start with the person making the nursing assignments now. But at some point, the service payer—usually a third party—gets involved. Administrators then have to consider the trade-off between their willingness to pay for what nurses may consider quality, and the third-party payer's willingness to pay.

One objection to using this method is that, when asking patients or hospitals about their willingness to pay, the answer depends on how much money they have. Patients or hospitals with little money will not be willing to pay as much as wealthy patients or wealthy hospitals.

If dollars (salary) are to be added to cost of lost quality (preferences), preferences and salary must be scaled in the same units. The scale of preference is sometimes called *utility,* and the units of measurement are called *utiles.* The term utility was once used to refer to values meeting a specific set of axioms. The term utility is now used more widely, and it often refers to measurements of satisfaction, desirability, aversion, worth, or value obtained using any of the many psychological scaling methods (see Hayes for other scaling methods).

## Table 9.6

### Willingness to Pay per 8-Hour Day to Avoid Having Skill Class Perform Task Category
#### (Compared to Most Preferred Skill Class)

| Task Type | Description | Head Nurse | Staff RN | LPN | AIDE | Ward Clerk |
|---|---|---|---|---|---|---|
| 1 | Highly technical tasks made on high-care patients | 0 | 0 | 7.40 | ∞ | ∞ |
| 2 | Highly technical tasks made on intermediate-care patients | 0 | 0 | 3.10 | ∞ | ∞ |
| 3 | Highly technical tasks made on self-care patients | 0 | 0 | 2.00 | ∞ | ∞ |
| 4 | Less highly technical tasks made on high-care patients | 0 | 0 | 3.00 | 9.80 | ∞ |
| 5 | Less highly technical tasks made on intermediate-care patients | 0 | 0 | 0 | 2.20 | ∞ |
| 6 | Less highly technical tasks made on self-care patients | .10 | .10 | 0 | .10 | ∞ |
| 7 | Evaluation of patient need and assignment | 0 | 0 | 0 | 9.20 | 0 |
| 8 | Supervising and teaching | 0 | 7.00 | 16.60 | ∞ | ∞ |
| 9 | Tasks preparatory to highly technical tasks | .20 | 0 | 4.00 | ∞ | ∞ |
| 10 | Tasks preparatory to less highly technical tasks | 0 | 0 | 0 | .50 | 18.10 |
| 11 | Clerical tasks directly related to patient | 0 | 0 | 0 | .20 | 12.40 |
| 12 | Clerical tasks less directly related to patient | 1.20 | 1.20 | 1.20 | 12.20 | 0.00 |
| 13 | Medical record notation | 0 | 5.00 | 13.00 | ∞ | ∞ |
| 14 | Housekeeping | 0 | 4.90 | 13.20 | ∞ | ∞ |
| 15 | Escorting and emergency errands | 0 | 0 | 0 | 0 | 15.40 |
| 16 | Maintenance, checking, ordering | 0 | 0 | .50 | 2.00 | 10.30 |

SOURCE: Wolfe, H. A Multiple Assignment Model for Staffing Nursing Units, Ph.D. dissertation, Johns Hopkins University, 1964.

**Problem:** Consider the method discussed in Section 6.6 to obtain nurses' aversions to various schedules. There were eight patterns of work stretches and days off that could show up in a nurse's schedule:

1. a single day on,
2. a single day off,
3. a stretch of 6 days without a 3 day weekend,
4. a stretch of 7 days without a 3 day weekend,
5. a stretch of 8 days without a 3 day weekend,
6. a stretch of 6 days with a 3 day weekend,
7. a stretch of 7 days with a 3 day weekend, and
8. a stretch of 8 days with a 3 day weekend.

The linear programming formulation used $c_{ij}$, nurse $i$'s aversion to working the $j$th schedule, where each schedule includes some combination of the above patterns. How can the $c_{ij}$ be measured? (Note that $c_{ij}$ has a different meaning here than in the preceding example.)

Each nurse was asked to scale her aversion to working each pattern. To force her to make trade-offs between these eight patterns, she was limited to 50 points (it could have just as easily been 100 points, or 50 dollars) to distribute among the patterns.

The dialogue between the decision analyst and nurse might go like this:

ANALYST:     Rank order the patterns from the one you least prefer or have most aversion to, to the one you most prefer or have least aversion to.

NURSE:       I least prefer a stretch of 8 days without a 3 day weekend. Next, I dislike single days on; they break up my free time too much. Then, I dislike a stretch of 7 days without a 3 day weekend, then a single day off, then a stretch of 6 days without a 3 day weekend, and finally the last three—8 days, 7 days, and 6 days, with a 3 day weekend. I don't mind working 6 or 7 days in a row if I know I'll have a 3 day weekend.

ANALYST:     Okay, you have 50 points to allocate to these eight patterns. If you assign all 50 to a stretch of 8 days without a 3 day weekend, and 0 to all the others, this means you really feel strongly about not working that stretch. If you assign 6 or 7 points to all eight patterns, this means you are indifferent between them—one is just as bad or as good as another.

NURSE:      Okay, I'll give half the points to the 8 day stretch without a 3 day weekend and spread the other 25 evenly among the seven remaining patterns.

The analyst should review the nurse's assignments to make sure she really feels this way.

In this case, the issue of *whom* to ask to assign aversion points is more apparent. The scheduling method allows for asking the person most affected, the nurse, for her aversion to various schedules. But *without* the scheduling system, the nurse scheduler in the central office would implicitly be assigning aversion points for every nurse. It only makes sense that nurses themselves should input their preferences.

Other examples of scaled measurements discussed in previous chapters include the seriousness of the nursing shortage and the desirability of extra nursing hours. These are generally scaled, rather than simply counted, since a shortage of two nurses is much more than twice as serious as a shortage of one nurse, or having two extra nurses is much less than twice as desirable as having one extra nurse. The scaling approach is similar to the one used above.

We will illustrate the combination of counted and scaled measurement for quality nursing care in Section 9.6.

## 9.4 LEVELS OF MEASUREMENT

Before examining how administrators should decide whether or not a measurement is useful, it is important to realize that not all numbers assigned according to a rule can be used in the mathematical models in previous chapters. For example, if the nurse who assigned the cost of lost quality above had rank-ordered her preferences instead, the numbers assigned (1 for staff nurse, 2 for head nurse, 3 for LPN, 4 for aides, and 5 for ward clerks) could not be used in the linear program formulated in Chapter 6. If, in a planning region with 10 OB units, those having more than 2,500 births per year were assigned a quality score of 3, those having 1,500 to 2,500 births per year were assigned a 2, and those below 1,500 births per year were assigned a 1, it would not be correct to say that the average quality was 2.2 for the 10 units. Administrators need to know what to look for in a measurement before using it in the models or calculating statistics.

In most cases, whether measurements can be used in models or to calculate averages and standard deviations depends on the rule used to assign the number. The possible empirical operations in a measurement rule are:

1. determining whether an attribute of one system is equal to the attribute of another system;

2. determining whether one system possesses *more or less* of an attribute than another;

3. determining *how much more or less* of an attribute one system possesses compared to another system; and

4. determining whether an attribute has an *absolute zero* quantity.

Each operation, in combination with the ones above it, corresponds to a specific type of scale—nominal, ordinal, interval, or ratio, respectively, which we will now discuss individually.

**Nominal Scale**

The measurement rule for the first empirical operation is stated thus: if the attribute of one system is equal to the attribute of another, assign the same number to each system; if the attributes are not equal, assign different numbers. The International Classification of Diseases, Adapted (ICDA) uses this rule to classify diseases. If two diseases are the same, they are assigned the same number. If they are not the same, they are assigned different numbers. The same scheme can be used to classify patients. Knowing the ICDA code number assigned to two patients, we know whether they have been classified as having the same disease or different diseases. The scale resulting from applying this rule is called a *nominal scale.*

Other common nominal scales are football-player numbers, patient ID numbers, nursing unit numbers, social security numbers, and student ID numbers. In the previous section we assigned numbers 1 to 16 to the task categories for nurses—a nominal scale. Numbers on the nominal scale are used only to identify or classify systems or activities; words could be used as well. However, we assign numbers for easier identification and classification.

Some argue that the nominal scale should not be considered measurement. We have described it because it illustrates the application of a rule in the assignment of numbers. The number does *not* represent the *quantity* of an attribute, since it is simply used as a label. Because it is used this way·so frequently in health service systems (for labeling patients, employees, diseases, nursing units, etc.), we feel it is important to understand this scale compared to the other scales.

The only mathematics we can perform on this scale without changing its meaning is simply substituting or interchanging numbers. One patient's ID number could be interchanged with another's, and as long as all documents reflect the change, the numbers' purpose could be achieved just as well—simply being patient labels.

The descriptive statistics and charts that can be used with the nominal scale are (1) the number of cases (number of observations in work sampling), (2) the mode or most frequently occurring number when more than one observation is assigned the same number, (3) a bar chart, and (4) chi-squared and other nonparametric statistics (see Siegel).

## Ordinal Scale

If, in addition to assigning numbers to label a system, the numbers indicate which system has more or less of one attribute compared to another system, the numbers are on an *ordinal scale*. For example, if we assign a 3 to a patient requiring an acute facility, a 2 to a patient requiring a skilled nursing facility, a 1 to a patient requiring a home health agency, and a 0 to a patient requiring none of these, then the numbers tell us which patients require more or less intensive service compared to other patients. We are rank-ordering the facilities based on their intensity and amount of service, and classifying patients using these numbers according to the intensity of services they require.

Two examples of an ordinal scale were given above: rank-ordered preferences for skill levels, and OB units' quality, measured by assigning numbers 3, 2, or 1. As another example of an ordinal scale, nursing directors could rank-order nursing units based on their judgment of the quality of nursing care provided—3 West, first; 2 East, second; 4 East, third; etc. An administrator's rank-ordering of applicants for an open assistant administrator position would also be on the ordinal scale.

The ordinal scale's significance is what it does *not* tell us—*how much* more or less of an attribute a system possesses compared to other systems. The difference in the quantity of an attribute between two systems is unknown; we only know the rank order. We do not know from our number assignments above how much more intensive the services are in an acute facility than in a skilled nursing facility, or how much greater the quality of nursing care is in one OB unit compared to another.

With numbers on an ordinal scale, the statistics that can be calculated include those for the nominal scale plus the median and percentile (for example, percent of OB units assigned less than a 3). We cannot technically calculate either averages or standard deviations, since their calculation requires that the difference between numbers reflects the difference in the quantity of an attribute. For example, what would it mean to say that the average of the numbers assigned to patients indicating the intensity of service they required was 2.8? The 3, 2, 1, and 0 were only rank-ordered labels for acute, SNF, home health, and none of these. The numbers do not indicate the difference in intensity between one facility and another; therefore, we cannot report that "the average intensity of service for patients in a hospital is 2.8." If we do make this report, we are assuming that the difference between the intensity of care in an acute facility and an SNF is the same (one unit) as between a SNF and home health care.

## Interval Scale

If the *difference* between the numbers assigned to systems on an ordinal scale is meaningful, the ordinal scale becomes an *interval scale.* The empirical operation required for interval scaling, in addition to nominal and ordinal scale operations, is the assignment of numbers so that the difference between numbers reflects the difference between the quantity of an attribute possessed by each system. Most people associate *measurement* with this characteristic. Almost all the usual statistics can be calculated: e.g., average, standard deviation, and product-moment correlation coefficient.

The classic example of an interval scale is the measurement of temperature on the Fahrenheit or Centigrade scales. Equal intervals of temperature are scaled off by noting equal volumes of the expansion of mercury. An important step to developing an interval scale is the establishment of an *arbitrary* zero point. Zero on the Fahrenheit (F) and Centigrade (C) scales is arbitrarily assigned; the intervals between numbers are not arbitrary. The number on one scale can be transformed to a number on the other by the formula $F = (9/5)C + 32$. Adding a constant 32 to the number on one scale, and changing the size of the unit of measurement (by 9/5) still keeps the scale an interval scale.

Dates on a calendar can be transformed to dates on another calendar in the same way. Time did not begin 1,984 years before this text. The zero was conveniently and, some might say, arbitrarily assigned.

## Ratio Scale

The *ratio scale* is similar to the interval scale except it has a natural zero—zero distance, zero time, or zero patients. The important thing to recognize is that ratio scale zeros are not the same as zero degrees temperature on the Fahrenheit or Centigrade scale or the zeros on some scales of quality of nursing care. The ratio scale enables us to report that there are twice as many patients this month compared to last month (the ratio of patients this month to patients last month is 2). This comparison cannot be done on an interval scale. 60° F is not twice as hot as 30° F.

The apparently subtle difference between an interval scale and a ratio scale may not be important for administrators to understand since interval scales without absolute zeros are as useful as ratio scales for most decision making. We rarely need to know the *absolute* quality of nursing care (the difference between the quality on a nursing unit and 0 quality). Usually we need to know the difference in quality between two nursing units or between two points in time for one nursing unit. For capital decision making, we need to know the difference between costs and benefits for two alternatives, not the *absolute* cost or benefit of one alternative. These measurements are analogous to measuring temperature on the Fahrenheit scale. However, logarithmic transformations of the type in Chapter 7 can only be made to measurements on a ratio scale.

The most common ratio scale is the number scale which we use to *count* dollars, patients, minutes, days, etc. So when we discussed measurement by counting, the results were on a ratio scale. Like the interval scale, units of the ratio scale can be multiplied by a constant. Unlike the interval scale, the ratio scale's zero point has meaning so that a constant cannot be added to the numbers on the scale without changing the meaning. All statistics may be calculated for ratio scale measurements.

If there is a set of rules for assigning numbers to systems, we know we are concerned with measurement. In order to make sure we are using the measurement appropriately in models and statistical analyses, we then have to determine the kind of measurement and therefore the kind of scale. In most cases, we can determine scale type by the rules themselves (rules for assigning ICDA codes, rank-ordering nursing units, etc.). When the rules do not reveal the kind of scale, we ask, In what ways can we transform a measurement's values and still have it serve all the functions previously fulfilled? Without changing the type of scale, we can change the size of the unit (from hours to days, for example) on all four types of scales by multiplying their numbers by a constant. If we can add a constant to the measurements (i.e., establish a new zero point), the scale is *not* ratio. If we can square the measurements and still use them as originally intended, the scale is *not* interval. Finally, if we can interchange any two numbers, we know it is not ordinal. Therefore, the scale must be nominal.

Before calculating statistics, the administrator must be aware of the limitations caused by the rule for assigning numbers and of the steps (or assumptions) required to change the rule so the necessary statistics can be calculated.

## 9.5 RELIABILITY AND VALIDITY OF MEASURES

Because scaling is such a simple tool for quantifying what might otherwise be nonquantifiable, knowing how to decide whether or not a measurement is useful is very important. Any unambiguous rule for assigning numbers constitutes a legitimate measure, so administrators must decide which measures are useful and which are not.

In our experience, administrators accept measurements based on counting more readily than measurements based on scaling, even though this is not always wise. Consider the counted measurement of births per year to measure *quality* of an OB unit, or the counted measurements of hospital admissions per year and lengths of stay per admission to measure *need* for hospital beds. Neither counting nor scaling necessarily leads to a useful measure. On the other hand, as with scaling, these counted measurements may be useful enough, so let's examine how to determine usefulness.

Before accepting a measurement as useful, two questions must be asked: (1) Is the measurement reliable? and (2) Is the measurement valid?

### Reliability

Reliability is the extent to which a number assigned to a system can be repeated. If the measurement rule were applied again, would the same person or different people get the same number?

> **Problem:** When counting the frequency with which the 16 categories of nursing tasks were performed, would the same count be obtained if the first observer made another count several weeks later, or if other observers made the count at the same time using a different set of random numbers to set the time to make observations?

If not, the frequency distribution is not useful. The measurement would be terribly confusing and unreliable if different numbers were obtained each time the count is made.

To test reliability, the count must be repeated—either at another time by the same observer or at the same time by other observers—and the results compared. The $\chi^2$ test can be used to test the degree of agreement between the frequency distributions over the 16 categories (nominal scale) obtained at different times or by different observers. The measurement is considered reliable if the differences are not statistically significant.

If the frequency distributions are significantly different, we might further train the observer, describe the counting rules more explicitly, improve the recording instrument, increase the number of observations, or use some combination of these steps. We would then have to retest reliability to be sure the measurements benefited from these efforts.

When scaling either subjective probabilities or preferences, would the first estimator assign the same numbers if he repeated the scaling procedure several weeks later, or would several estimators assign the same numbers when they perform the scaling procedure simultaneously? We would repeat the scaling procedures, either at another time with the same estimator, or at the same time with other estimators, to test reliability. Degree of agreement between numbers assigned at different times or by different observers can be calculated, using the correlation coefficient or some other measure of association depending on the level of measurement. The higher the correlation coefficient, the greater the reliability.

For example, if the OB physician who scaled the subjective probability that patients require $i$ hours in an OB recovery bed was asked to repeat the scaling procedure six weeks later, the results might be as follows:

| $i$ | Hours | First time | Second time |
|-----|-------|------------|-------------|
| 1 | 0–1 | .02 | .06 |
| 2 | 1–2 | .35 | .40 |
| 3 | 2–3 | .35 | .27 |
| 4 | 3–4 | .18 | .12 |
| 5 | 4–5 | .06 | .10 |
| 6 | 5–6 | .02 | .01 |
| 7 | 6–7 | .02 | .04 |
|   |     | 1.00 | 1.00 |

If we let

$P_{i1}$   be the probability of $i$ hours assigned by the OB physician the first time, and

$P_{i2}$   be the probability of $i$ hours assigned the second time,

then the correlation coefficient is calculated as follows (note that this is the same equation as in Chapter 7):

$$r = \frac{n(\Sigma P_{i1} P_{i2}) - (\Sigma P_{i1})(\Sigma P_{i2})}{\sqrt{[n(\Sigma P_{i1}^{2}) - (\Sigma P_{i1})^{2}]\,[n(\Sigma P_{i2}^{2}) - (\Sigma P_{i2})^{2}]}}$$

where $n$ is the number of time periods. The calculation is most easily made using the table:

| $i$ | $P_{i1}$ | $P_{i1}^{2}$ | $P_{i2}$ | $P_{i2}^{2}$ | $P_{i1} P_{i2}$ |
|-----|----------|--------------|----------|--------------|-----------------|
| 1 | .02 | .0004 | .06 | .0036 | .0012 |
| 2 | .35 | .1225 | .40 | .1600 | .1400 |
| 3 | .35 | .1225 | .27 | .0729 | .0945 |
| 4 | .18 | .0324 | .12 | .0144 | .0216 |
| 5 | .06 | .0036 | .10 | .0100 | .0060 |
| 6 | .02 | .0004 | .01 | .0001 | .0002 |
| 7 | .02 | .0004 | .04 | .0016 | .0008 |
| Totals | 1.00 | .2822 | 1.00 | .2626 | .2643 |

Then

$$r = \frac{7(.2643) - (1.00)(1.00)}{\sqrt{[7(.2822) - (1.00)^{2}]\,[7(.2626) - (1.00)^{2}]}}$$

$$= \frac{.8501}{\sqrt{.8176}} = .94$$

This provides a measure of reliability of the assignments made by this physician.

If the correlation coefficient is not close to 1 (say below .80), we decide the measurement is unreliable. We might further train the estimators to apply the scaling method, describe the scaling method more explicitly, change the scaling method, or discuss with the estimators the reasons for disagreements. We would then retest the reliability before using the measurement. As part of the measurement rule, we may include obtaining numbers from several estimators and calculating the average, thereby hoping to increase the reliability of the numbers (the average estimate may be more reliable than that of any one estimator's).

## Validity

Just being able to repeat the assignment of a number by counting or by scaling is not sufficient for the measurement to be useful. In addition, it must be valid.

A measurement is *valid* to the extent it can be used for what it was intended. Counted measurements are often valid because they are intended to measure quantity (size, time, distance, demand, frequency); counting is the accepted measurement rule for quantity.

However, counting is also sometimes used to measure quality. For example, counting births per year is one way to measure quality of OB units. We need a way to test the validity of such a measurement. In addition, we need ways to test the validity of measurements by scaling, since scaling is generally a less accepted measurement rule.

### Predictive Validity

For our purposes, there are two ways to use measurements and therefore two different approaches to testing validity. Measurements can be used either to *predict* the attribute of interest or to represent the *content* of the attribute. An example might best illustrate the difference.

> **Problem:** Assume, for the moment, there is one measurement that you agree measures *the* quality of an OB unit (we will italicize *the* when we refer to this particular measure). It captures everything that you think of as "quality" OB service. Assume someone proposes that to measure quality of OB units, we should count the number of births in a year. If that number is 2,000 or more, the unit provides high-quality OB services; if that number is less than 2,000 the unit provides low-quality OB services. Assume that using

2,000 births is significantly less time-consuming than using *the* measure of quality OB service. Is counting births, and setting 2,000 as the standard, a valid measure of quality?

Since we have *the* measure of quality OB service, we can compare it to the 2,000 births per year rule. The 2,000 births per year rule is an attempt to *predict the* measure of quality OB service. We therefore test 2,000 births per year for *predictive validity.*

Testing the *predictive validity* of a measurement is straightforward. To test the 2,000 births per year rule, all we need to do is count the number of births per year in a sample of OB units, apply *the* measure of quality OB service, and see if those units with 2,000 or more births per year have higher quality than those with fewer than 2,000 births per year. If they do, we say that the 2,000 births per year rule has predictive validity and is a valid measure of quality.

It is unlikely there will be a clean split between high-quality and low-quality OB service at 2,000 births per year. So we would have to calculate the average and standard deviation of *the* measure of quality OB service for those above 2,000 and those below 2,000. We would then test whether there was a statistically significant difference in the quality of OB service above and below 2,000 births per year. If there were, we would say the 2,000 births per year rule has predictive validity and is a valid measure.

If there is not a statistically significant difference, we could look for the number of births (perhaps 1,500) that separates OB units into high and low quality by *the* measure of quality OB service. And as a further step, we could determine the correlation between births per year and *the* measure. The higher the correlation coefficient, the more valid the births per year rule for predicting the quality of OB service. If the correlation is close to zero, births per year is not a valid measure of quality of OB service.

Likewise, to test the predictive validity of subjectively scaled probabilities given by OB physicians for the service time in recovery beds, all we need to do is count the minutes patients stay in recovery beds (in another hospital perhaps), count the number of patients who stay from 0–1 hour, 1–2 hours, 2–3 hours, 3–4 hours, 4–5 hours, 5–6 hours, and 6–7 hours, divide the number of patients in each time interval by the total number of patients observed, and compare this relative frequency—called frequentistic probability—to the subjective probabilities given by OB physicians. The Kolmogorov–Smirnov one-sample nonparametric test (see Siegel) can then be used to test the degree of agreement between the frequentistic and subjective probabilities. If they are not significantly different, we say that these subjective probabilities have predictive validity.

Naturally, obtaining both frequentistic and subjective probabilities is not always possible, or it may involve unnecessary duplication. Therefore, we might rely on past comparisons of the two and obtain subjective probabilities using a method that has resulted in greater predictive validity.

As another example, counting patient days per 1,000 population may be a valid measure of bed need. To test this measure, assume we have *the* measure of bed need. We would then apply this measure of bed need to a sample of communities, count the patient days per 1,000, and calculate the correlation. The higher the correlation, the more valid is patient days per 1,000 as a measure of bed need.

Frequently, measures used for prediction are confused with *the* measure they are meant to predict. Some people will discuss births per year, subjective estimates of frequentistic probabilities of service time, and inpatient days as if they were *the* measure of OB quality, *the* frequentistic probabilities of service times, or *the* measure of bed need. As an example, it may be suggested that to improve the quality of OB service, a unit should deliver more than 2,000 babies. Since 2,000 births per year is simply a predictor of quality, it does not follow that increasing births per year will improve quality. (Why not?)

Content Validity

When *the* measure is known, testing predictive validity is straightforward. But what about the validity of *the* measure of quality OB service, *the* measure of bed need, or *the* frequentistic probability of recovery stay before we have recovery beds in our facility? In this case, there is no measure to predict—these are *the* measures we want. Validity of *the* measure depends primarily upon how adequately *the* measure captures the *content* (behaviors) of quality OB service, bed need, and service time in recovery beds.

There is no single test that can be performed to establish *content validity*. Let's see why not. We could construct a measure of quality OB service that includes what *you* would have included in such a measure. We could ask a group of other people (you can pick them) and they could agree that the measure includes what they would have included in such a measure. We could perform a test and find that there is a statistically significant difference (in the right direction) between infant mortality rates in OB units high on the measure of quality and those low on the measure. Furthermore, we could improve the low quality OB units to change the measure to high quality, and find that the infant mortality rate goes down. We could also notice that when several OB units' quality decreased at one point, the infant mortality rate went up.

This is an impressive quality measure indeed. But the above tests only provide circumstantial evidence, even if this evidence is sufficient for *you* to decide this measure of quality OB service is useful. The above tests do not prove the measure is useful, however, since (1) the observed correlation between the quality measure and infant mortality could be spurious—it could be that uncomplicated deliveries happen to occur in the OB units high on the quality measure and vice versa, (2) the change in infant mortality rates might not have been caused by improvements or deterioration in quality— perhaps a disease complicated the deliveries, and (3) you and all the people you picked could agree on the measurement of quality OB service, but the measure could still be useless for improving or controlling quality.

We do not mean to imply that the above tests should not be done. In fact, they provide evidence that the measurement of quality OB service is probably useful. We have purposely stacked the above description to give you examples of the best tests that can be performed for content validity. We have also given reasons showing why these tests are not enough; the reasons illustrate arguments for not consider- ing the measure of quality OB service valid. These arguments can always be given; it is impossible to control for every intervening variable (uncomplicated deliveries, diseases, etc.). Therefore, rather than test the validity of such measures, we must ensure content validity by the way we construct the measures. The validity of a measure of quality OB service, bed need, accessibility, etc., is judged by the procedures used to construct the measures and by how well the procedures are carried out. If most potential users of the measure, or at least most administrators responsible for using them, agree that the procedures are sound and well carried out, the measure has a high degree of content validity.

Validity is not determined by testing a measure's "truthfulness." Imagine trying to test "truth." We could compare OB physicians' estimates of the frequency that patients will stay in recovery beds 0–1 hours, 1–2 hours, etc. with the truth—the actual frequency. But subjective probabilities are valuable precisely because we don't know the "truth." We are willing to use subjective probabilities because they are useful.

But administrators should not accept *just any* subjective probabilities. They should accept those subjective probabilities with reduced overconfidence and extreme-value biases. Section 9.3 discussed the methods (scaling, training, and experts) for overcoming these biases. Validity for subjective probabilities, like any other measurements, must depend on how the measurement rule was constructed and how well it was carried out.

Likewise, there is no truth to test when scaling preferences for each skill class performing certain tasks or for patterns of days on and days off in a nursing schedule. If administrators agree that the procedures for obtaining these preferences were sound, we have obtained valid measures of preference.

## 9.6 CONSTRUCTION OF A PERFORMANCE MEASURE

The importance of the plan for constructing performance measures should now be apparent. Validity is not simply tested after the measure has been developed. Validity is ensured by proper construction of the measure. The basic plan for constructing performance measures requires the following steps:

1. Decide the objectives of the system whose performance is being measured.

2. Identify the system's attributes, which define the system's objectives.

3. Develop the *counting* scheme for observing these attributes.

4. *Scale* the preference for various counts or the relative importance of each attribute for achieving the objectives.

5. Calculate a score for the system using the numbers obtained in 4.

6. Test the score's reliability.

7. Obtain evidence for the score's content validity.

At times these steps are implicit or even ignored. But without explicitly constructing performance measures in this way, administrators have no assurance the measure has content validity.

Our primary concern is not that administrators be aware of the availability of performance measures in hospitals, clinics, nursing homes, skilled nursing facilities, or admitting, dietary, or housekeeping departments. Nor are we concerned that they know these measures' shortcomings. With increasing pressure from external agencies to measure performance, or at least to make desired performance explicit, we are concerned that administrators know how to construct performance measures, and know what to expect from staff specialists who assist them. If administrators can respond to external pressures for new performance measures, they may facilitate changes necessary to overcome the shortcomings of currently available measures.

Likewise, we are not concerned with data sources for performance measures. The data sources ought not to constrain a measurement's construction any more than they constrain a model's construction. Once the measurement *is* constructed, costs and benefits associated with data collection can be considered in the same way as with data collection for models. It is possible that a measurement using available data is as reliable and valid as a measurement using currently unavailable data. Tests for predictive validity would have to be done to demonstrate this.

Consider the following example to illustrate the steps required to construct a performance measure.

> **Problem:** In order to control the quality of nursing care for each hospital unit, the administrator wants a measurement that can be used for tracking the quality of nursing care each month. How can such a measure be constructed?

Step 1: Decide Objectives

In Chapter 1 we discussed how the systems approach requires subsystems' objectives to serve the objectives of the parent system. When measuring performance on one system's objectives we assume the parent system's objectives will also be met if we meet the subsystem's objectives. Table 9.7 illustrates typical nursing care system objectives.* Objectives were defined for two subsystems— patients and nursing unit.

One way to visualize this table is as a pyramid diagram of

*Table 9.7*

*Nursing Objectives Used by Haussmann,
Hegyvary, and Newman*

---

1.0 The Plan of Nursing Care is Formulated.
    1.1 The condition of the patient is assessed on admission.
    1.2 Data relevant to hospital care are ascertained on admission.

---

*This example is taken from work done by Haussmann and Newman at the Medicus Corporation, and by Hegyvary at Rush College of Nursing, both in Chicago.

1.3 The current condition of the patient is assessed.
1.4 The written plan of nursing care is formulated.
1.5 The plan of nursing care is coordinated with the medical plan of care.

2.0 The Physical Needs of the Patient Are Attended.
2.1 The patient is protected from accident and injury.
2.2 The need for physical comfort and rest is attended.
2.3 The need for physical hygiene is attended.
2.4 The need for a supply of oxygen is attended.
2.5 The need for activity is attended.
2.6 The need for nutrition and fluid balance is attended.
2.7 The need for elimination is attended.
2.8 The need for skin care is attended.
2.9 The patient is protected from infection.

3.0 The Nonphysical (Psychological, Emotional, Mental, Social) Needs of the Patient Are Attended.
3.1 The patient is oriented to hospital facilities on admission.
3.2 The patient is extended social courtesy by the nursing staff.
3.3 The patient's privacy and civil rights are honored.
3.4 The need for psychological-emotional well-being is attended.
3.5 The patient is taught measures of health maintenance and illness prevention.
3.6 The patient's family is included in the nursing care process.

4.0 Achievement of Nursing Care Objectives Is Evaluated.
4.1 Records document the care provided for the patient.
4.2 The patient's response to therapy is evaluated.

5.0 Unit Procedures Are Followed for the Protection of All Patients.
5.1 Isolation and decontamination procedures are followed.
5.2 The unit is prepared for emergency situations.

6.0 The Delivery of Nursing Care is Facilitated by Administrative and Managerial Services.
6.1 Nursing reporting follows prescribed standards.
6.2 Nursing management is provided.
6.3 Clerical services are provided.
6.4 Environmental and support services are provided.

Source. Haussmann, R. K. D., Hegyvary, S. T., and Newman, J. F. *A Methodology for Monitoring Quality of Nursing Care.* DHEW Publication (HRA)76–25, January 1974.

*Figure 9.1*

*Pyramid Diagram of Nursing Objectives*

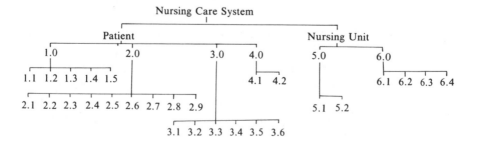

objectives and subobjectives (shown in Figure 9.1). Each pyramid level is a system, with subsystems under it and a parent system above it. The pyramid diagram is a useful tool for visualizing how the subsystems' objectives interrelate.

Because the nursing care system is organized differently from hospital to hospital, administrators may want to modify Haussmann's list of objectives. The important point is that the objectives and pyramid diagram provide the framework for measuring nursing care quality. In addition, the framework may suggest objectives not considered part of nursing care by individual institutions. In that case, performance on these objectives can still be measured, then separated from the nursing quality score.

## Step 2: Identify Attributes

What attributes of the nursing care system define the objectives? That is, what system behaviors will be observed to measure performance on the objectives? For the performance measure to be valid, these attributes must represent the content believed by administrators to define the objectives.

As a first step, the attributes used in previous performance measures can be examined and matched to the list of objectives. Some attributes will match the objectives. Some attributes will be so far removed fom the objectives that no one will believe they were ever really used. Some objectives will have no attributes matched to them; we can assume these objectives were not included in prior performance measures. When Haussmann, Hegyvary, and Newman did this for the objectives in Table 9.7, they discovered that somewhat fewer than 200 attributes could be matched to the 28 objectives. The unmatchable attributes were too general, not measurable, or not relevant to nursing care. For example, in the study by Haussmann, Hegyvary, and Newman (see Additional Reading), two unmatchable attributes were, Are pertinent recurring activities charted? and Are appropriate measures used for effective communication?

On the other hand, they found very few attributes from prior studies related to direct care provided to patients. Therefore, additional attributes, such as, Are respiratory rate and quality recorded? needed to be generated so they would describe patient-related objectives. Other examples are given in Table 9.8. Haussmann, Hegyvary, and Newman learned that almost all attributes would apply across age groups and types of nursing service (medical, surgical, and pediatric). However, the attributes did not apply equally to self-care, interme-

## Table 9.8

## Example of Attributes Defining Objectives

Questions To Be Answered From Recorded Patient Information

1. Is the patient contacted by the nursing staff 15 minutes after arrival on the unit?

   (To Patient: When you first arrived on the unit, how long was it before someone on the nursing staff came to see you?

   If patient cannot be questioned, ask family.)

2. Does the nurse interview the patient for assessment of problems within two hours of admission?

   (Look at chart for evidence that assessment was made. May ask patient, When you were admitted, did a nurse come to talk with you about your illness or about any special problems?

   How long after you were admitted did the nurse talk with you?

   Pursue for time only if evidence is present that assessment was made.)

3. Is the patient's dependence on prosthetic devices recorded at time of admission?

   (E.g., dentures, glasses or contact lenses, hearing aids, orthopedic shoes or braces, artificial limbs or eyes. Any devices used for ADL. May include dependence on cosmetic devices, such as wigs.)

4. Are the patient's elimination patterns recorded on admission?

   (Prior to hospital stay)

5. Is the patient's perception of his illness recorded on admission?

   (Refers to responses probably elicited by question, Can you tell me something about your illness? or What is the reason you are in the hospital? Acceptable if patient states diagnosis.)

6. Does the nursing plan specify long-range goals of care?

7. Does the nursing plan indicate nursing participation in diagnostic procedures?

   (See if diagnostic procedure is scheduled. If no nursing plan exists, ask nurse, Is there any special nursing care for Mr._____ in regard to his test?

   Probe: How is special care related to the procedure assigned?)

SOURCE: Haussman, *et al. A Methodology for Monitoring Quality of Nursing Care.* DHEW Publication (HRA)76–25, January 1974.

diate-care, and intensive-care patients. Therefore, the attributes differed between these groups of patients. The authors ended up with approximately 220 attributes; each of the 28 subobjectives had between 8 and 12 attributes.

How can new attributes for defining an objective be generated? For content validity, this task is probably best left to the nurse managers whose performance is to be judged. Obtaining head nurses' agreement that the quality measure was well constructed will be easier if they participate in its construction. Administrative and medical staff members may also want to participate in this task.

This means a small group (7 to 9 members) will generate the

attributes defining these objectives. This group could proceed using at least three techniques—brainstorming, nominal group, or delphi. For example, the task before the group could be to generate a list of attributes defining Objective 4.1: Records document the care provided for the patient.

*Brainstorming* is the most common method. A group using this method would meet, discuss the task, and record attributes, while the group leader would attempt to have members withhold judgment while attributes were being developed. The group would then eliminate duplication and attempt agreement on which attributes to use.

The *nominal group* technique forces the group to a certain structure. The task is first specified, then the attributes are generated and written independently and silently by each group member for ten minutes. Ten minutes allows people time to think of attributes that do not immediately come to mind. Members alternately present one attribute on their lists to the recorder until all attributes have been presented. The recorder lists and numbers each attribute on a flipchart or blackboard. Attributes are then discussed one at a time and duplications eliminated. Each member of the group separately rank-orders the attributes. If there are too many attributes, the most important seven (seven is the common number used in psychological literature) are rank-ordered instead. Each member would assign each attribute a score, giving the first-ranked attribute 7 points, the second 6 points, the third 5 points, etc. The overall score for an attribute is obtained by adding these scores. The group would then discuss the overall ranking and decide on a cut-off point. The attributes ranked below the cut-off point would not be used.

The *delphi* technique is similar to the nominal group technique except that the group never meets, and therefore never formally discusses the attributes among themselves. After members generate their lists of attributes, they submit their lists to one person who summarizes the responses and returns the summary to the members. Members then rank-order the attributes on the summary list and give their rankings to one person who scores the attributes as for the nominal technique. This rank order is returned and members are asked to identify a cut-off point.

Experiments done to compare these three group processes have shown that the nominal group technique produces the most attributes. The delphi technique's advantage is that the group never has to meet. Both the nominal and the delphi techniques tend to be superior to brainstorming for generating attributes because they force the group to withhold judgment while the attributes are being generated, and they eliminate status differentials between members—physicians and nurses, for example, could participate equally in the attributes' generation.

Step 3: Develop a Counting Scheme

The strategy for observing nursing care on a unit and then calculating a score for each attribute is in principle identical to a work sampling strategy (Section 9.2), except that attributes would replace tasks. Observations are randomly timed, across all shifts, for randomly selected patients, with a resulting mix of patient classes (self, intermediate, intensive). Attributes are observed at time instants as either Have occurred, or Have not occurred, or There is no information. The relative frequency of the attribute's *occurring* is calculated. The closer the relative frequency is to 100 percent, the more the objective with which it is associated is considered to be met.

Haussmann, Hegyvary, and Newman apply work sampling in the following way. Approximately 220 attributes are associated with the 28 subobjectives. About 170 relate to objectives specific to patients, and 50 relate to objectives specific to the nursing unit. To keep the observation process manageable, they select 56 patient-specific and 30 unit-specific attributes, and have a worksheet generated by computer. Every subobjective is represented, but the attributes are randomly selected within subobjectives.

This is a clever way to randomize the timing of attributes' observations so the nursing personnel being observed are not aware of which attributes are being examined. Although we want nursing personnel to modify their behavior to obtain more favorable readings, we do not want this modification only during observation. Recall from the discussion of work sampling that the observations are made randomly to represent what would be observed if continuous observations were made. If nurses modify their behavior on specific attributes only when being observed, we cannot infer that the results would be the same if continuous observations were made.

Each month twenty trips to each unit are made to observe the randomly selected attributes. Eleven are made on the weekday day shift; seven are made on the weekday evening or night shifts; one is made on a Saturday; and one is made on a Sunday. In this way, most observations are made when nursing care is most intense (weekday shifts), with some observations taking place at other times.

Within these general guidelines, observations are randomly distributed across days of the month and times of day. Specific patients are randomly selected from the unit census just prior to the observations. The patients' dependency classifications (self, intermediate, intensive) are determined and attributes appropriate to their classification are randomly selected. The computer generates the worksheet. As with work sampling in general, the attributes must be clearly described with explanations and guidelines for their application (see Table 9.8). Completed worksheets are keypunched and results accumulated by unit for each month. Quality indices are calculated for the 28 subobjectives by obtaining the ratio of positive responses for each attribute within the subobjective to the total possible responses for the attributes used that month. This is the same calculation made in work sampling studies to determine the percent of times a task was observed. If the ratio is 80 percent, management can infer that about 80 percent of the time the attribute would have been positive, and quality achieved.

To obtain the overall quality index for a unit meeting an objective, Haussmann, Hegyvary, and Newman simply averaged the subobjective scores.

Step 4: Scale Preference and Relative Importance

It may be that nurse managers feel that 100 percent positive responses for an attribute is not too different from 95 percent (5 percent difference); whereas, they may consider the differences between 90 percent positive responses and 85 percent positive responses—still only a 5 percent difference—more significant. An extension of the three authors' method, therefore, would be to have nursing supervisors scale their preferences for the various percentages of positive responses and use those scaled values as the quality index.

For example, a graph could be presented to each nursing supervisor for each attribute. Use Is the patient contacted within 15 minutes after arrival on the unit? as the example. The dialogue would go like this.

ANALYST:     Select that percent of positive responses that is most desirable.

NURSE:       Naturally, 100 percent.

ANALYST:     Okay, mark an X at that point on the graph.

NURSE:       Most desirable   1.0|            X

             Least desirable    0 |         100%

ANALYST: Select that percent of positive responses that is least desirable.

NURSE: Naturally, 0 percent.

ANALYST: Okay, mark an X at that point on the graph.

NURSE: Most desirable 1.0 │ X

Least desirable 0 ┼───── 100%

ANALYST: Now, starting with the most desirable percent, draw a line to reflect the desirability of the remaining percents. If you are indifferent between 100 percent and 99 percent, draw a straight horizontal line along 1.0. As you are no longer indifferent, but feel the percents are becoming less desirable, draw the line away from the top of the graph. You may want to go to the least preferred level and work your way back.

NURSE: Most desirable 1.0 │ X

Least desirable 0 ┼──── 50 ──── 100%

ANALYST: Okay, now notice that you feel 50 percent compliance is just as undesirable as 0 percent. Is that true?

NURSE: Yes, I think so. If we only do it half the time, why do it at all? Perhaps the attribute should be modified so we can achieve it. From the standpoint of quality, 50 percent on this attribute is just as bad as 0 percent.

The analyst should further discuss with the nurse the implications of the line that has been drawn.

After obtaining these scaled measurements from a group of nurses, the results could be pooled by averaging the lines at discrete points from 100 percent to 0 percent. To obtain the scaled index for an attribute, the scaled value (0.0 to 1.0) would be read off the graphs for whatever percent of positive responses was observed. On the above graph, 50 percent would be 0.0. (Notice that if scaling is not done, it is assumed that desirability is a straight line from 1.0 at 100% to 0.0 at 0%.) The quality index for a unit's meeting its objective could then be calculated by averaging these scaled values.

Finally, it may be that nurse managers do not feel that all attributes or subobjectives are equally important. For example, contacting the patient within 15 minutes after arrival on the unit may not be as important as making sure the patient's dependence on prosthetic devices is recorded upon admission, or vice versa. The relative importance of the attributes or subobjectives could be scaled, and a weighted average calculated.* This also would be an extension of Haussman, Hegyvary, and Newman's method. The scaling method used could be the same as the one described earlier for scaling aversion points for days on and days off.

As an example, the Commission on Administrative Services in Hospitals (CASH) has scaled the relative importance of objectives in its measurement of quality nursing care as follows:

| | |
|---|---|
| 1. General | 15 |
| 2. Patient welfare and safety | 15 |
| 3. Patient comfort | 15 |
| 4. Patient room | 05 |
| 5. Patient chart | 15 |
| 6. Nursing care plan | 15 |
| 7. Nursing unit | 05 |
| 8. Ward medical management | 10 |
| 9. Ward building management | 05 |

Both scaling procedures could be used in a nominal group or delphi process.

Step 5: Calculate Overall Score

To calculate the overall score, use the relationship

$$Q = \sum_{i=1}^{n} W_i U_i(I),$$

where

$Q$   is the overall score for one unit in one month,

$W_i$   is the relative importance of subobjective $i$,

---

*Haussmann, et al. found that weighting the importance of subobjective scores resulted in perfect rank order correlation with equal weighting of subobjective scores. Weighting would be unnecessary in their case.

$U_i(I)$   is the desirability of $I$ percent positive responses on subobjective $i$, and

$n$   is the total number of subobjectives.

If $W_i$ is not scaled, it is equal to $1/n$, or the average of the $U_i(I)$. The relationship then becomes

$$Q = \frac{\sum_{i=1}^{n} U_i(I)}{n}.$$

If, in addition, the $U_i$ are not scaled, then $U_i(I) = I_i$ and the relationship becomes

$$Q = \frac{\sum_{i=1}^{n} I_i}{n},$$

where $I_i$ has a subscript to refer to subobjective $i$ for which it was calculated. (Haussmann, Hegyvary, and Newman used the last formula.)

## Step 6: Test Reliability

So far we have discussed one measurement of quality nursing care and two possible extensions—scaling desirability of the percentage of compliance and scaling the relative importance of attributes and subobjectives. Our original question remains: Is the measurement, or its extensions, reliable and valid? We must apply the measurement or its extensions to real nursing units to determine usefulness.

The first test is for reliability. If the measurement is not reliable, we need not test it for validity. If declared unreliable, it is also invalid. A test for reliability is straightforward. Send at least two observers to each nursing unit with a worksheet, calculate the resulting scores, and compare their scores. An adequate sample size is required (determined by using statistics and good judgment), so it may be necessary to repeat the observations during several months. Reliability is determined by calculating the correlation coefficient between the scores assigned by each observer for all units. The higher the correlation coefficient, the greater the reliability. The same test could be performed to evaluate the reliability of the scaled desirability values for percent compliance and relative importance. However, if several persons' scaled values are averaged, and everyone agrees on the average value, these scaled values simply become constants in the formula. Before agreeing to a measurement, regardless of how it was constructed, an administrator should examine reliability test results.

Step 7: Obtain Evidence of Content Validity

The measure we have been describing is intended to measure, not predict, quality of nursing care. Administrators, therefore, need assurance that the observed attributes (behaviors) represent the content of quality nursing care.

The first question then is, How were the attributes established? Answer—see Steps 1 and 2.

The second question is, How will the nursing units be observed? Answer—see Step 3.

The third question is, How will the observations be combined into a score? Answer—see Steps 4 and 5.

The fourth question is, Will two people get the same answer? Answer—see Step 6.

Now, if administrators find that the attributes were not carefully developed or that the plan for making observations will not produce a representative sample of nursing care, or that the method for combining the scores of the attributes or subobjectives does not reflect their preferences or importance ratings, or that two people cannot agree on what they have observed on the unit, then the administrators can justifiably declare the measurement invalid.

If, on the other hand, the answers to these questions follow the steps described above, the measurement *may* be useful for measuring quality nursing care, and therefore *may* have content validity. A measurement has a high degree of content validity if most administrators who might use the measure agree that the plan (Steps 1 through 5) was sound and well carried out. Additional evidence that the measurement would be useful is obtained by actually applying it in a pilot test. Any commitment to use the measurement should be delayed until after it has been tested. For example, say we order a five-month pilot test. To evaluate the measure we would consider the following:

1. Do the nurses generally agree it captures the content of their profession and what their jobs should be? If the answer is no, can the reason be explained and is

the reason justified? Can the measure be modified to overcome the nurses' objections? If modified, is the measure still reliable?

2. Try another measure of quality nursing care—the CASH method (reference in Additional Reading), for example. Are the results comparable? If not, is there an explanation? With which do you agree?

3. There are usually intuitive judgments about the quality of various units. Does the measure of quality nursing care agree with your intuitive hunches? If not, is there an explanation? After examining the difference, do you agree with the measurement or with your intuitions?

4. If over the five-month test period the measurement of quality changes, is there a reasonable explanation for the change? In such a pilot study, Haussmann, Hegyvary, and Newman found a decrease in the measurement, which the manager believed was due to nurses' transferring to a new hospital and the remaining nurses' low morale. If the measurement increases, can the increase be explained by a change in the mix of RNs, LPNs, and AIDEs (larger percent of RNs, for example)? On the other hand, has the measurement remained the same even though nursing unit changes during the test period should have clearly improved quality? One study at the University of Iowa found that neither introducing larger nursing staffs nor establishing better in-service training programs changed their measure of quality.

5. If medical complication rates, or patient–family complaint rates, or physician complaint rates are calculated, do they decrease with increased quality scores or increase with decreased quality scores? If not, is there an acceptable explanation?

We reemphasize that none of these five kinds of circumstantial evidence can prove the measure is valid. Take the Iowa study, for example. The measure could still be valid because more nurses and better in-service training may not affect quality of care. An argument like this can be leveled at every piece of evidence discussed above. It eventually comes back to the administrators' agreeing that a particular measurement of quality nursing care is useful for their purposes.

**Exercises**

9.1 A nurse reallocation system is being developed in your hospital
that will attempt to assign a float pool of nurses among the
7 units on each shift in such a way that the sum of the "seriousness
of nursing shortage" over the 7 units is minimized. There are
three types of nurses: RNs, LPNs and AIDEs. The system will
work as follows. About two hours before the beginning of each
shift, the head nurse will examine

   1. the number of patients, and their mix, that will require
      care on the upcoming shift, and
   2. the number of RNs, LPNs and AIDEs scheduled to be
      on that shift.

She will then use her judgment to quantify what the seriousness
of shortage would be if

   —she got no more nurses,
   —she got one RN from the float pool,
   —she got one LPN from the float pool,
   —she got one AIDE from the float pool,
   —she had to give up one RN,
   —she had to give up one LPN, or
   —she had to give up one AIDE.

This quantified measure of the seriousness of shortage for each
of the 7 situations on each of the 7 units will then be used
to evaluate the many possible ways to "float" nurses to the
units and/or "pull" nurses from the units to "float" them
somewhere else.

   a. Will this system require a *nominal, ordinal, interval,* or *ratio*
      scale? Why?
   b. Devise a one-page questionnaire for each head nurse to fill
      out that measures the *seriousness of shortage* for the next
      shift for the 7 possible situations. This instrument must produce
      7 numbers measuring seriousness of shortage which would
      result from the 7 separate situations. Its purpose (exactly what
      it is trying to measure) and how she is to complete it must be
      clearly and easily understood by each head nurse.
   c. Discuss problems of *accuracy, bias, reliability* and *validity*
      (both kinds) with the measures you would obtain with your

questionnaire, and how you might attempt to overcome these problems.

## Additional Reading

Aydelotte, M. K., Tennor, M. E., et al. *An Investigation of the Relation Between Nursing Activity and Patient Welfare.* State University of Iowa, 1960.

Barnes, R. M. *Work Sampling.* New York: John Wiley and Sons, 1957.

Bennett, A. C. *Methods Improvement in Hospitals.* Philadelphia: Lippincott, 1964.

Dalkey, N. D. and Helmer, O. "An Experimental Use of the Delphi Method with a Group of Experts." *Management Science* 9 (1963): 458–67.

Durbin, R. L. and Springall, W. H. Chapter 10, *Organization and Administration of Health Care.* St. Louis, Mo.: Mosby Co., 1969.

Edwards, W. "Conservatism in Human Information Processing." In *Formal Representation of Human Judgment,* edited by B. Kleinmuntz. New York: John Wiley and Sons, 1968.

Guilford, J. P. *Psychometric Methods.* New York: McGraw-Hill, 1954.

Gustafson, D. H., Kestly, J., Greist, J. H. and Jensen, N. "An Initial Evaluation of a Subjective Bayesian Diagnostic System." *Health Services Research Journal.* Fall 1971.

Hayes, W. L. *Quantification in Psychology.* Belmont, Calif.: Brooks/Cole Publishing Company, 1969.

Haussmann, R. K. D., Hegyvary, S. T. and Newman, J. F. *A Methodology for Monitoring Quality of Nursing Care.* DHEW Publication (HRA) 76-25 (January 1974).

Huber, G. and Delbecq, A. "Guidelines for Combining the Judgments of Individual Group Members in Decision Conferences." *Journal of the Academy of Management* 15, (June 1972).

Huber, G. P. "Methods for Quantifying Subjective Probabilities and Multi-Attribute Utilities." *Decision Sciences* 5 (1974).

Ludke, R. *Training Manual for Physician Likelihood Ratio Estimators.* Madison, Wisconsin: Computer-Aided Medical Diagnosis Research Project, University of Wisconsin, 1970.

Nunnally, J. C. *Psychometric Theory.* New York: McGraw-Hill, 1967.

Siegel, S. *Nonparametric Statistics for the Behavioral Sciences.* New York: McGraw-Hill, 1956.

Van de Ven, A. and Delbecq, A. L. "Nominal Versus Interacting Group Processes for Committee Decision-Making Effectiveness." *Academy of Management Journal* 14 (June 1971).

Wolfe, H. *A Multiple Assignment Model for Staffing Nursing Units.* Ph.D. dissertation, John Hopkins University, 1964.

Wolfe, H. and Young, J. P. "Staffing the Nursing Unit, Part I. Controlled Variable Staffing." *Nursing Research* 14 (Summer 1965).

Wolfe, H. and Young, J. P. "Staffing the Nursing Unit, Part II. The Multiple Assignment Technique." *Nursing Research* 14 (Fall 1965).

# Part IV

# Regulation and Control

*In the previous part, we saw measurement, forecasting, and information systems as responses to the need for informed decision making and internal control of the institution. In today's environment, the health care manager must also be familiar with the many controls on the institution and its performance that are externally imposed. Part IV explores regulation by state and federal governments of patient management and financial reimbursement. The value of the cybernetic control framework introduced at the beginning of the text is seen once again in its application to rate, utilization, and quality control.*

# 10

# External Controls through Rate Regulation and Reimbursement

## 10.1 INTRODUCTION

In 1980 the Government Accounting Office published a report entitled "Rising Hospital Costs Can Be Restrained by Regulating Payments and Improving Management." The notion that external regulation was a necessary component in the efficient management of health resources had been substantiated by state-level rate regulation experiments, industry- and consumer-initiated pilot projects, and federally funded research studies. The health care administrator could be assured that regulatory controls on hospital operations would be given increasing consideration.

Institutional survival in an environment of externally imposed decision criteria demands a sensitivity to the possibilities and constraints that accompany rate regulation. This chapter presents a brief account and analysis of the reimbursement system in health care as it impacts decision making and control in hospitals.

## 10.2 BASIC PRINCIPLES OF RATE REGULATION

The principles which underlie reimbursement and payment practices in the external regulation of hospitals include (1) efficiency and effectiveness in the production of hospital output, (2) equity in the payment for that output, and (3) the inability of any one hospital to act in a way which maximizes resource use throughout the "system." These principles have driven regulators to grapple with difficult theoretical and methodological issues in terms of the units and bases of reimbursement summarized in this section.

Efficiency can be viewed as the relation of outputs to inputs: internally, the hospital's goal is to maximize output at minimum cost. But measurement of efficiency has been difficult since there has been little agreement on the definition of output. Treatment given a patient, better health, all services provided to a patient—all have been proposed as possible definitions of outputs. But regardless of definition, the unit of quantification of these proposed outputs has traditionally been the *patient day,* and payment has usually been calculated on this *per diem* basis. Within this mode, reimbursement does not require the "unbundling" and costing of all of the services provided to patients admitted for any number of reasons, but rather requires only the calculation of an average cost for a day of services: a patient in the hospital for four days pays twice as much for hospital services as one who stays two days.

Reimbursing on a per diem basis can be seen as a violation of the equity principle. It has obvious limitations in that it ignores the severity of the patient's illness and thus the range in intensity of services provided to different patients. It also does not accurately capture the varying use of services over time; e.g., that more intense services are often offered in the first few days of the stay, or that services tend to taper off the longer the stay. Thus, patients' payments are not based on the resources they actually consume.

In contrast to a per diem–based payment, reimbursement on a *per discharge* (or admission) basis has been offered as an alternative, although it, too, might be viewed as violating the underlying principles of reimbursement. Under this system, payment is made for a hospital stay irrespective of the length of that stay. This basis demands consideration of the diagnosis of the patient, or the *case mix* of the hospital (the distribution of diagnoses in a hospital), recognizing that an acute myocardial infarction will require a different type and intensity of services than an uncomplicated vaginal delivery, even though both require an admission and similar lengths of stay.

The most recent development in unit of reimbursement is payment on a *per case* basis. This "controls" for diagnosis, in that payment is based on the diagnosis that led to the admission (or the *principal diagnosis*). This measure assumes that resource use (and inherently length of stay) of a patient varies by diagnosis; therefore, payment incorporates costs for all services related to that illness.

Regardless of the unit of payment (per diem, per discharge, or per case), regulators must determine the mechanism for recovering the costs of production. *Charge-based* mechanisms provide reimbursement to the hospital on the basis of the hospital's reported charges. The underlying assumption is that there is a close relationship between charges and actual costs, and little *cross-subsidization* between departments or services occurs. While the payer knows in advance its financial liability per unit of service, there is no incentive for the provider to constrain the availability of services since whatever is ordered and provided will be paid for on the basis of charges.

*Cost-based* mechanisms also have problems. The measurement of outputs and costs is still an issue; determination of which costs are *allowable* by the payer requires rules and regulations as to how costs attributable to a particular patient or group of patients are defined and calculated; and the incentives to the individual organization, provider, and hospital system are viewed as inconsistent with the stated principles of reimbursement. Cost-based reimbursement, and particularly reimbursement based on total incurred costs, transfers to the payer the burden of increasing technological costs, volume of services, and medical treatment experimentation.

Both charge-based and cost-based mechanisms can operate on a retrospective or prospective payment basis. *Retrospective* reimbursement systems pay the provider after the service is delivered; services are provided and an account of charges or costs is then submitted to the payer. Under *prospective* reimbursement, an estimate of the level of resource use or quantity of services is submitted, and payment is made prior to use of services. Under many prospective payment systems, this payment may be adjusted retrospectively for variations in the types of patient served or volume of services provided. Under more "pure" prospective reimbursement, there is no substantial adjustment after the fact: the provider is responsible for the cost of services which exceed the prospectively determined payment.

The principle of external efficiency or "system" efficiency has generated its own requirement for an industry-wide monitor, with an accompanying standard of reward and penalty for hospitals. This monitor can consist of payers, hospital executives, consumers, or other regulators, and functions with or without sanctioning power. As a group, the monitoring bodies function as budget reviewers, rate reviewers, or rate setters, using three common mechanisms for controlling budgets or rates.

The first is to set for each hospital under their purview an *allowable rate of increase* (or target rate) in expenses per admission, in charges, or in revenues. This technique establishes a base year status quo and allows for escalation from that base year. The second mechanism involves setting an average cost per unit of reimbursement (day, case, or discharge) comparable with that of peer hospitals and allowing a *percentage of the mean* as an acceptable limit for increases in costs. For instance, suppose the mean per diem costs for all hospitals in community A are $1,000. Incurred costs more than 10 percent above this mean level would not be allowed by the monitoring body. This limit could apply to each unit of service or to the entire hospital budget. A basic underlying assumption is that the community mean is an appropriate standard of care and costs.

The third common method of rate control is an overall *cap on total expenditures*. In its purest form, this method inherently limits increases in volume of services and relies on the substitutability of less expensive services for more expensive services.

The effectiveness of health services delivery implies consideration of the quality of care. The issue of quality has been difficult to incorporate into reimbursement systems because of its subjective nature and the difficulty of measuring it. But the problems of reimbursing on the basis of quality are not just technical problems; they are policy issues. Who is qualified to judge quality, and what mechanisms can be implemented to systematically monitor quality? Because of the inability to resolve these issues, quality has been included in regulation primarily as a peripheral constraint: the use of professional standards review organizations (PSROs) to monitor cases for appropriateness of care, and now peer review organizations (PROs) for review of various medical services (Section 143, P.L. 97-248). If the "experts" perceive that a hospital is providing services that are medically unnecessary or that do not meet professionally recognized standards of care, then the organizations can recommend that hospital's exclusion from the reimbursement program. It is clear that the objectives of a reimbursement system—high quality and cost containment—may indeed conflict.

The discussion of reimbursement presented here illustrates the emphasis on controlling hospitals and payers, and the relative lack of effort to control physicians and consumers. It has been recognized for some time that a major weakness in all the methods of reimbursement used in the American health system is the separation of decision maker from payer. The physician decides on the timing and extent of resource use and a separate entity pays the bill for that use. A historical view of rate regulation will show the underlying assumptions, the results of that separation, and the most recent attempts to correct this weakness.

## 10.3 HISTORY OF HEALTH CARE REIMBURSEMENT

The reimbursement system for health services has revolved around three major actors: (1) the consumer of health care services, whose responsibility it is to see that payment is made for the services; (2) the provider of services—in this case, the hospital; and (3) those who pay for the services: the consumer without complete insurance coverage and the "third parties," consisting of Medicare, Medicaid, Blue Cross, and commercial insurers. The history of reimbursement policy for the hospital industry has been one of a shift in control among these actors, in terms of both who makes the decisions related to resource use and its compensation, and how these decisions are implemented.

Prior to the recent expansion in the health care industry and the accompanying escalation in costs, administrators set the charges for the services provided to their consumers, unencumbered by massive state and federal intervention. All payers reimbursed the provider on the basis of these charges, which incorporated the cost of labor, equipment, capital expansion, and other service components believed necessary to provide quality care in what was often a captive marketplace. Whatever technology was adopted, whatever patient groups needed service, the costs were transferred to the payer and, eventually, the consumer. As the costs of providing care increased over time, the charges reflected those increases. But as the payers (and consumers) became unable or unwilling to absorb those increases, the hospitals found themselves sharing control with those payers over that portion of the costs of care the hospitals could expect to recover.

The shift in control extended beyond the administrator-payer realm; it occurred within payer groups as well. Medicare, a federal program, and Medicaid, a state-federal program, reimbursed hospitals on the basis of "allowable" costs—those which, according to the regulations, could be directly attributable to the program enrollees. Blue Cross plans, through their contracts with participating hospitals, paid a discounted cost-based rate. Hospitals still had to recover their costs, and so the costs not covered by these programs were subsidized by those who paid on the basis of charges: commercial insurers and consumers without insurance coverage.

Even though some control over revenues had been preempted by the partial shift from charge- to cost-based reimbursement systems, hospitals were still, for the most part, not constrained in the amount of services which could be provided for any given patient, since reimbursement was retrospective: whatever services were provided would be reimbursed after the fact. The incentive to maximize utilization, and thus revenue, was (and in many states remains) intact. However, efforts to slow the spiraling costs of health care and correct the inefficiencies that feed that spiral have resulted in a further shift in control from the individual hospital to a separate body of decision makers.

## Rate Regulation

Hospital rate regulation has varied by state in terms of the control allowed to and exercised by each of the affected parties. The degree of control placed in the hands of the health care provider can be viewed within a continuum of rate regulation options. Maximum hospital autonomy might be represented by a voluntary budget review process, in which participating hospitals allow a hospital-controlled body to screen budgets for excessive or inequitable costs. Some hospital associations and state governments have encouraged such regulatory methods to stave off federal intervention in hospital decisions or to equalize payer contributions (and therefore decrease cross-subsidization by commercial carriers). Less hospital control might be represented by state-mandated budget review programs that use formulas for screening, offer minimal opportunity for appeal or negotiation, and whose budget decisions can be tied to capital expansion approvals (certificate of need) or special program participation. The maximum shift in control from the individual hospital to a separate decision-making body might be represented by a state-mandated prospective rate-setting commission. Here, rates of payment are established in advance for the subsequent year and the hospitals receive these amounts regardless of actual costs (see the study by Dowling listed in Additional Reading). The hospital has various incentives and sanctions to control its services, admissions, or types of patients treated. The prospective nature of the method places the majority of the risk of loss of revenue on the hospital.

State hospital rate regulatory programs have been conceived of and modified on the basis of several motives: a desire to preempt federal involvement in state decisions, an awareness of pending crises in state Medicaid costs, pressure from health care payers to control costs, and a general concern over equity in allocation of resources.

The organizational forms for these programs differ according to the initial motives and how these were transformed into action, whether by legislative mandate or voluntary compliance. The most common models are the commissions, either mandated and administered by the state (usually by the Department of Health) or sponsored and administered by the voluntary hospital association. Which payers participate also varies by the authority: in Maryland, for example, all payers are covered by the rate-setting commission; in Connecticut, only self-payers and commercial insurers are covered; in western Pennsylvania, only Medicare, Medicaid, and Blue Cross participate.

The rate regulatory methods used in the programs, including budget review, rate review, and rate setting, determine which activities are monitored; whether sanctions are imposed, and what they are; and, in some cases, what their future reimbursement must be. Sometimes only selected departments are reviewed, but more often budget review programs examine all cost centers to assess cost shifting within the institution. The process is time-consuming, however, and many budget review programs are moving from reviewing every portion of every budget to reviewing only exceptions—those departments or costs which fall outside predetermined guidelines. Rate-setting programs have also sought to minimize some of the more time-consuming aspects of the process by automatically adjusting a formerly approved base rate by an inflation formula (controlled for volume and some other factors) to arrive at the next period's approved rates. In both budget review and rate setting, the acceptability and extent of negotiations are somewhat dependent on the size of the staff and the formality of the program. In Washington state, informal meetings between hospital personnel and regulators are held to discuss key issues or differences prior to the formal hospital commission hearings during which the approved rates are finalized. In states where reviews rely heavily on formulas, the appeal process is often seen as a substitute for prenegotiations.

One of the major challenges in budget reviews or prospective rate-setting programs has been to establish an equitable means of comparing hospitals and/or their departments.

## 10.4 CASE-MIX MEASUREMENT

The determination of peer groups for interhospital comparisons relies on the assumption that differential costs of delivering care can be explained by some combination of characteristics of the hospital—percentage of each type of payer, bed complement, teaching status, composition of medical staff specialties, profit status, case mix of patients—and its environment—urban/rural location, sociodemographic attributes of the service area population (income, age, sex), number of physicians per capita. Most state commissions use some of these variables in establishing peer groups, but the accuracy of the data and the extent to which these variables reflect service and cost differentials are often questioned. Hospital challenges often result in lengthy negotiations, legal battles, or noncompliance. Many challenges are based on claims that the hospitals are unique in ways that have not been adequately measured, particularly the type and severity of the cases they treat. The desire to accurately reflect the hospitals' complexity of case mix (the proportion of patients or cases in each diagnostic category) led to the use of proxy or correlate measures of case mix, such as teaching status, service mix, or bed size. Efforts to avoid proxies and measure the actual "product" of the hospital— its patients' treatment episodes—have resulted in several diagnosis-based case-mix classification methods, such as (1) the CPHA List A, (2) isocost groupings, (3) disease staging, and (4) diagnosis related groups. The methods differ in their construction, their dependent variables, their use of physician expertise, and the feasibility of their widespread adoption.

## CPHA List A

The Commission on Professional and Hospital Activities (CPHA) in Ann Arbor, Michigan, has produced from their extensive hospital-based Professional Activity Study (PAS) data base a list (List A) of 350 diagnostic groups. These groups were further partitioned by whether or not surgery was performed, the presence of comorbidities, and five age groupings. Although the resulting 3,500 or so categories have been used in some research on hospital costs and length of stay by researchers at the University of Michigan and elsewhere, the number of categories makes their use for peer groupings cumbersome.

## Isocost Groups

The isocost grouping method of classifying patients is one of the newest methods, and seeks to correct what its originators see as defects in some of the other methods, namely, their dependent variables. The isocost method uses total cost per case as the dependent variable and relies heavily on physicians to establish the diagnostic groupings. For each major disease area, board-certified specialists in that area are asked to identify important variables that can be used to classify within the disease type. The variables are evaluated so as to minimize the variance in cost per case within the diagnostic area. At present a research group at Johns Hopkins University is using an expanded data base to further test its model, with the intention of eventually comparing the results with those of other methods being developed.

## Disease Staging

The staging method of case-mix analysis produces a distribution of patients in a particular institution by state of illness. By examining this distribution, a hospital can analyze and compare the severity of its patients, its costs in treating different types of patients, and trends in utilization of specific services.

Medical school faculty in several specialties used over 600,000 hospital discharge records to separate medical and surgical conditions into 426 "staged" conditions, using three stages:

State 1: diseases with no complications or problems of minimal severity

Stage 2: diseases with local complications or problems of moderate severity

Stage 3: diseases with systematic complications or serious problems

Diseases recorded on hospital discharge abstracts are then assigned to one of these three classifications and coded according to the International Classification of Diseases.* If an abstract reveals disease codes that reflect more than one stage, the more serious stage for the patient is recorded.

Research on disease staging has been shown to have a variety of uses since its conception in the early 1960s. Its application as a tool for case-mix analysis shows promise, in that the technique is clinically acceptable and uses data now available in most hospitals.**

## Diagnosis Related Groups

Diagnosis related groups (DRGs) are the result of a classification scheme developed by Yale University researchers to reflect the type and amount of hospital resource use per patient treatment episode. Cases were grouped so as to minimize the variance in resource use, as measured by length of stay (the dependent variable).

Early work in the 1970s grouped codes of the ICDA-8 system into 383 DRGs; in January 1982, regrouping was completed on the new ICD-9-CM coding system using a revised methodology which ad-

---

*The International Classification of Diseases is a system developed by the World Health Organization to classify diseases and operative procedures for the purpose of indexing medical and hospital records. Diseases are grouped by problem area. For example, all malignant neoplasms of the different organ systems are listed together, as are all benign neoplasms, and all infectious and parasitic diseases. Every ten years the system is revised; the most recent is the ninth version or ICD-9-CM (International Classification of Diseases, Ninth Revision, Clinical Modification).

**Gonella, J.S., personal communication, 1982.

dressed most of the criticisms of the early groupings. Decision criteria for grouping included (1) that the groups be "clinically coherent"—that is, that clinicians could agree on patterns of treatment for each disease group; (2) that the groups be defined by resource use, mainly length of stay; (3) that the groups be statistically stable; and (4) that there be a manageable number of groups which would encompass the more than 30,000 diagnoses and procedures which appear in the ICD-9-CM system. Using over one million patient abstracts provided by the Commission on Professional and Hospital Activities (CPHA), as well as cost information from New Jersey hospitals, cases were grouped into 23 major diagnostic categories (MDCs) which were based on the principal diagnosis appearing on the discharge abstract. The MDCs were subsequently partitioned into DRGs by (1) presence or absence of a surgical procedure performed in the operating room, (2) complications/comorbidities which would affect use of resources, and (3) age. There were 467 acceptable DRGs and 3 DRGs which consisted of diagnoses not meeting the partitioning criteria. A "substantial comorbidity" was defined as "a preexisting condition that will, because of its presence with a specific principal diagnosis, cause an increase in length of stay by at least one day in approximately 75 percent of the cases" (Fetter et al. 1982). Examples of a substantial comorbidity include alcohol-induced cirrhosis of the liver, chronic airway obstruction, and angina pectoris.

Each DRG was designed to reflect a unique, homogeneous group of cases with similar disease characteristics, length of stay, and therefore resource use. Disputes as to its clinical meaningfulness have been based on claims that clinically dissimilar diseases were aggregated, or that differing levels of severity of the same diseases were included in a single DRG.

Application of the DRGs as a case-mix measure for peer grouping requires the collection of certain clinical data elements. Efforts instituted in 1969 by the then Department of Health, Education, and Welfare to establish a minimum hospital data set have proven extremely useful for these purposes (see National Center for Health Statistics in Additional Reading). The goal of their efforts was to arrive at a common core of uniformly defined and collected hospital data that would satisfy the needs of many users. The selection of data items which formed the Uniform Hospital Discharge Data Set (UHDDS) was based on several criteria:

1. Data must be on individual inpatients discharged from acute general hospitals.

2. Data must have a demonstrated actual or potential utility to multiple users.

3. Items must be readily available and able to be collected with reasonable accuracy and economy.

4. Items must be continuously available on every patient.

5. Data collection should not be unnecessarily duplicative of other resources.

6. Collected data items should preserve confidentiality but enable public accountability.

7. Cost-benefit factors to both data providers and users must be considered.

The application of the criteria by the technical panels resulted in the recommendation and acceptance of 14 items:

1. Personal identification—a unique number

2. Date of birth

3. Sex

4. Race and ethnicity
   a. Asian or Pacific Islander
   b. American Indian or Alaskan native
   c. Black
   d. Hispanic
   e. White
   f. Other

5. Residence—zip code

6. Hospital identification

7–8. Admission and discharge dates—month, day, and year of both

9–10. Physician identification (attending and operating)

11. Diagnosis
   a. *Principal diagnosis:* "condition established after study to be chiefly responsible for occasioning the admission of the patient to the hospital for care" (National Center for Health Statistics, p. 12)
   b. *Other diagnoses:* "designated and defined as associated with the current hospital stay: All con-

ditions that coexist at the time of admission, that develop subsequently, or that affect the treatment received and/or length of stay. Diagnoses that relate to an earlier episode which have no bearing on current hospital stay are to be excluded." (National Center for Health Statistics, p. 12)

12. Procedures and dates—All significant procedures are to be recorded using Clinical Modification of ICD-9. A significant procedure is one that carries an operative or anesthetic risk, requires highly trained personnel, or requires special facilities or equipment.

13. Disposition of patient
    a. Discharged to home
    b. Left against medical advice
    c. Discharged to another short-term hospital
    d. Discharged to a long-term-care institution
    e. Died

14. Expected principal source of payment
    a. Self-pay
    b. Worker's compensation
    c. Medicare
    d. Medicaid
    e. Maternal and Child Health coverage
    f. Other government payments
    g. Blue Cross
    h. Insurance companies
    i. No charge
    j. Other

SOURCE: National Center for Health Statistics, 1980.


The Department of Health, Education and Welfare adopted the Uniform Hospital Discharge Data Set in 1974 for Medicare and Medicaid programs. While certain definitions or categories of classification have changed since that date, hospitals that participate in the federal programs have the abstract-based data collection in place.

The UHDDS contains the diagnostic and procedural elements necessary to apply the DRG methodology to the records and makes the use of a DRG case-mix variable feasible for rate regulatory activities. More direct links, however, between the case-mix measure and reimbursement require additional data on costs and charges. These data can be gathered from patient bills if they detail charges per service provided, and from cost-charge ratios per department. In order to make interhospital comparisons on case mix and cost effectiveness of treatment, a standard chart of accounts and some uniformity in reporting are necessary.

It is becoming clear that payers of health care, administrators of facilities, and state and federal regulators desire a means for acknowledging and comparing the intensity of services provided in health care facilities. Of the methods presented, the DRG system has received the broadest empirical examination. In the next two sections we will discuss its implementation at the state and national levels.

## 10.5 DEVELOPMENTS AT THE STATE LEVEL

DRGs have been used as the basis for an ongoing experiment in case-based reimbursement in New Jersey and as one option for case-mix measurement in the prospective rate-setting program in Maryland.

### The New Jersey Experiment

In 1976, the New Jersey Department of Health adopted a rate regulatory program known as SHARE—Standard Hospital Accounting and Rate Evaluation—a prospective budget review system which required that hospitals report costs using uniform functional cost center accounting. "Controllable costs" per patient day were aggregated by cost center, adjustments were made for volume variance and inflation, interhospital comparisons were made within peer groups, and rates were set for the two cost-based payers over which the Health Department had jurisdiction, Blue Cross and the state. Medicare remained a retrospective per diem–based program, while other payers operated on the basis of charges.

Despite the commitment to and success of the SHARE program, the Commissioner of Health of New Jersey was intent on implementing a system of reimbursement which would correct what was perceived as the unfairness and inefficiency induced by per diem reimbursement. A DRG-based system was introduced in January 1980; 26 hospitals in the state were used for the first phase of the experiment, which was to include all New Jersey hospitals by 1983. Standards for hospital performance were to be based on the costs of treating a particular type of patient as described by the DRG case types. The supporting legislation alluded to equity among payers and efficiency in the delivery of care; the "pot" of money for health care would merely be redistributed to the efficient hospitals rather than increased to absorb escalating costs.

To implement a case-mix-based system, participating hospitals first had to produce the information necessary to apply the DRG "grouping" method to their discharge abstracts to arrive at a distribution of DRGs for the hospital. In addition, derivation of the total patient care costs per case for each hospital was undertaken, adjusting for direct patient care costs (routine, ancillary, and ambulatory services), indirect patient care costs (general services, i.e., dietary, housekeeping, laundry), institutional costs (research and education, plant maintenance, utilities, etc.), and capital facilities costs (costs of depreciation, leases on buildings, land, and fixed and movable major equipment).

From the hospitals' records, a distribution of costs per DRG was derived, outliers were examined and removed, and the standard for any incentive system was set at the mean total patient care costs per case. The rate for a particular hospital was based on a combination of this standard and the hospital's own reported costs in a particular base year. The proportion of the rate that was based upon the standard rather than the hospital-specific data varied by the degree of confidence in the validity of each DRG (based on the coefficient of variation in costs for that DRG). Costs per DRG that had little variation, and were thus believed to be highly valid, were more heavily weighted toward the standard; those with more variation were more heavily weighted by the hospital's own costs. For instance:

**DRG 373:** Normal delivery without complications
Industry's mean costs per case = $567
Hospital's mean costs per case = $800
This is a "low-confidence" DRG; therefore, the standard is weighted 78 percent (in teaching hospitals):
Standard: .78 x 567   = $442
Hospital: .22 x 800   =   176
Allowed rate per case = $618

**DRG 202:** Cirrhosis and alcoholic hepatitis
Industry's mean costs per case = $1,010
Hospital's mean costs per case = $1,500
This is a high-confidence DRG; therefore the standard is weighted 48 percent (in nonteaching hospitals):

Standard  .48 x $1,010 —    $485
Hospital:  .52 x $1,500 =    $780
Allowed rate per case  =  $1,265

In May 1980, all bills to all payers used a DRG-specific rate per case. The regulations promulgated under the state law that created the system are being modified as new data on the system's progress become available. By the end of 1982, all hospitals in New Jersey were using the DRG-based method, incorporating the new DRGs based on ICD-9-CM. Research on the New Jersey experience continues to assess the impact of case-mix-based prospective reimbursement on hospital costs.

## Maryland Rate-Setting Program

The Health Services Cost Review Commission (HSCRC) in Maryland is responsible for the review of nongovernmental hospital rates. Its uniqueness, however, lies not in the fact that budgets are reviewed annually, with accommodations made for inflation and volume; rather, it is the commission's institution of a voluntary incentive program for hospitals to reduce utilization within case type and slow the escalation of costs that makes a review of Maryland's program of interest.

Since 1974, all hospitals have been subject to the budget review process of the HSCRC; all payers have participated since 1977. In 1976, the commission introduced a voluntary program, the Guaranteed Inpatient Revenue Program (GIR), which utilizes an admission-based (rather than service-based) reimbursement system adjusted for case mix.

Each hospital participating in the GIR program selects a 12-month base period from the past, whose rates were, at that time, approved by the commission. The hospital also selects one of several available case-definition methods and applies it (with some exclusions) to its admissions from the chosen base year. The average charge per case type from the base year is calculated, and then adjusted for inflation to the current or proposed period. That rate becomes the basis for the allowable revenues for the proposed period. At the end of the proposed period, admissions are again aggregated into case type, and actual per-admission revenues are compared with the approved revenues. If the actual are less than the approved, the hospital receives 50 percent of the revenue as discretionary income; if the actual are greater than the approved, the hospital is required to return 50 percent of the related revenue to the commission.

The program is an attempt to encourage hospitals to establish, monitor, and improve controls over the costs of patient care. By allowing hospitals to select not only the base year but the method of case definition (DRGs, the first three or four digits of ICD-9-CM, service department [medicine, surgery, obstetrics, etc.]) and the divisions on which those disease categories can be segmented further (age, payer categories, others), the commission is encouraging hospitals to examine and determine the most accurate and advantageous patient-type description for recovering the maximum revenue while controlling the rate of cost increases.

At present, over half of Maryland's hospitals are participating in the voluntary program. All but a few have collected the discretionary income that results from having provided services at less than the approved GIR rate.

## 10.6 DEVELOPMENTS AT THE NATIONAL LEVEL

Three federal actions have contributed significantly to the trend from cost-based reimbursement to case-based reimbursement: the Omnibus Budget Reconciliation Act of 1982 (P.L. 97-35), the Tax Equity and Fiscal Responsibility Act of 1983 (TEFRA) (P.L. 97-248), and the Social Security Amendments of 1983 (P.L. 98-21).

P.L. 97-35 was signed into law on August 13, 1981. It contained a number of amendments to the federal Medicaid program, particularly increased flexibility for states in the implementation of their plans, as well as several significant amendments to the Medicare program. Increased cost sharing by beneficiaries, assessment of PSRO performances, and adjustments in payments for inappropriate hospital services were specified by the act, and some key provisions relating to hospital reimbursement were changed. In 1972, the Social Security Amendments established the authority of the Secretary of Health and Human Services to establish prospective limits on specific services delivered to Medicare beneficiaries. These limits were called "Section 223 limits," after the section of P.L. 92-603 in which they were outlined. The limits on reimbursements for routine inpatient operating costs were set at 112 percent of the mean labor-related and the mean non-labor-related costs of each peer hospital group. Section 2143 of the 1981 law lowers the limits to 108 percent of the mean and permits use of alternative methodologies if Medicare's costs are no more than they would be under the 108 percent limit.

The Tax Equity and Fiscal Responsibility Act of 1982 (TEFRA), signed into law on September 3, 1982, contained a significant number of amendments intended primarily to reduce spending in the Medicare program. Section 101 of the act modified the reimbursement requirements of P.L. 97-35, including, in addition to routine costs covered under Section 223 limits, all other inpatient hospital operating costs (ancillary costs, such as laboratory, pharmacy, etc., and special care units). Costs that exceed a percentage of the average cost *per case* for comparable hospitals would not be considered "reasonable." This percentage varies from 120 percent of the mean for comparable hospitals for the first year (after October 1982), to 115 percent in year 2, to 110 percent in the third and subsequent years. These limits are adjusted for case mix. There are exemptions and exceptions for sole community hospitals, psychiatric hospitals, rural hospitals (as defined by law), and those hospitals serving a significantly disproportionate number of low-income patients or Medicare Part A beneficiaries.

Section 101 of the bill establishes a target reimbursement system. This target rate is based on the previous year's allowable costs per case adjusted by hospital wage and price indices plus one percentage point to accommodate technological innovation. If a hospital operates below the target rate, it is paid its costs plus 50 percent of the savings (not to exceed 5 percent of the target amount). A hospital with costs above the target would be paid 25 percent of its costs above the target amount for the first two years and none of the excess for the third and subsequent years. The law does allow states whose hospital cost control systems meet certain criteria to use the state methodology rather than the federally mandated system.

The 1983 developments address directly the TEFRA's mandate for the Secretary to develop, in consultation with the Senate Committee on Finance and the House Committee on Ways and Means, a prospective case-based reimbursement system for hospitals by December 31, 1982.

The Social Security Amendments of 1983, unlike the TEFRA cost-per-case limits, set prices for each DRG, as opposed to establishing a case-mix-adjusted cost-per-case limit for the hospitals.

A system of prospective pricing, with discharge as the unit of payment, will be phased in over four years. Rates will be computed on the basis of increasingly weighted regional and national contributions to the average price per DRG. For instance, in the first year (beginning October 1, 1983), 75 percent of the payment per discharge will be the hospital-specific cost-per-case amount, while 25 percent will be the regional average price for the patient's DRG. By year 3, the hospital-specific cost-per-case amount will contribute only 25 percent to the price, while the remaining 75 percent will be based equally on the regional average price and the national average price for the patient's DRG. By year 4, the total price will be based on urban or rural national average prices for each DRG, adjusted for wages.

The transition to prospective case-based payment is not complete even for the Medicare program. The Amendments cover only inpatient services. Outpatient, capital, and medical education expenses are, for the time being, reimbursed on the basis of retrospectively determined costs, as are long-term, children's, psychiatric, and rehabilitation hospitals and distinct units of hospitals.

## 10.7 THE MEDICARE CASE-MIX INDEX

The Health Care Financing Administration (HCFA) has also been investigating the feasibility of a case-mix index based on the DRG classification scheme, which could be used by Medicare to distinguish the relative costliness of Medicare cases in hospitals.

### The Medicare Data

In the past, hospitals have been reimbursed by Medicare on the basis of the incurred costs reported to HCFA or a fiscal intermediary. For every enrollee, an itemized bill with charges for the Medicare patient is also submitted, even though payment is not dependent on these charges. In addition, a narrative description of diagnoses and procedures is submitted for those beneficiaries whose social security numbers end in 0 or 5. Upon receipt at the HCFA office, these narratives are coded using ICD-9-CM. These codes and charge data are maintained in the Medicare statistical data file known as MedPAR. Hospitals that participate in the Medicare program also submit a Medicare Cost Report (and will continue to submit the report for nonpatient services under the 1983 Acts). This report details the Medicare share of patient care costs per day, which is estimated using the formulas provided in the regulations, and the cost-charge ratios for each ancillary department. Complete clinical, charge, and cost information is therefore available on 20 percent of the Medicare inpatient cases.

### The Case-mix Index

The proposed case-mix index is based on these data and the Yale-formulated DRGs. Costs of treating patients in each DRG are normalized to a mean value of 1.0 and applied as weights to the proportion of Medicare patients in that particular DRG. These cost-weighted proportions are then summed to arrive at a measure of relative costliness of the hospital's case mix. The ratio of the hospital's case mix to a nationally derived measure of case mix is considered the hospital's case-mix index. The process is as follows.

**Step 1:** Determine the distribution of case types within a hospital. Using one of the computer software routines, a hospital's discharges (based on UHDDS) are regrouped into DRGs. Assume for this example that the hospital's cases fall into only seven DRGs (Table 10.1).

**Step 2:** The costs of treating each patient are adjusted to reflect the sources of the costs associated with a hospital stay. For each case:
Routine cost per day × number of days in regular room = room costs
Special care unit costs per day × number of days in SCU = SCU costs

## Table 10.1

### Case-Mix Index

| $DRGs_h$ | Mean Adjusted $costs/case_h | $W_i =$ normalized $costs/case_h (Mean = 1.0)$ | $P_i =$ × proportion of $cases_h$ | $= W_i P_{i_h}$ |
|---|---|---|---|---|
| 001 (craniotomy, age ≥ 18, no trauma) | 4,000 | 1.01 | .03 | .030 |
| 036 (retinal procedure) | 1,000 | .33 | .24 | .079 |
| 049 (major head and neck procedure) | 2,000 | .48 | .10 | .048 |
| 165 (appendectomy with complications, age ≤ 70) | 4,500 | 1.20 | .16 | .192 |
| 237 (sprain, dislocated hip) | 6,000 | 1.66 | .31 | .515 |
| 251 (fractured forearm, age 18–69, without complications) | 900 | .26 | .09 | .023 |
| 416 (septicemia, age ≥ 18) | 5,000 | 1.27 | .07 | .089 |
| | | | 1.00 $\Sigma =$ | .976 |

normalized case-mix-weighted costs = .976

case-mix index $_{hospital}$ = .976

$$\frac{CMI_{hospital}}{CMI_{national}} = \frac{.976}{1.345} = .75$$

Ancillary service charges $\times$
cost-charge ratio per
department                          $= \underline{\text{ancillary costs}}$

                                    $=$ adjusted $_1$ costs/case

These adjusted costs per case are further adjusted for:

1. Teaching activity of a hospital (using a HCFA-derived index): adjusted $_1$ costs per case $\times$ $I_{residents/bed} =$ adjusted $_2$ costs per case; and

2. Differences in wage rates among hospitals within different labor market areas: adjusted $_2$ costs per case $\times$ $I_{wage\ levels/bed} =$ adjusted $_3$ costs per case.

**Step 3:** A distribution of costs per case for all cases in a DRG is constructed and outlier cases are removed. The mean of the costs of the remaining cases becomes the unnormalized weight for the DRG:

$$\frac{\Sigma_i \text{ adjusted}_3 \text{ \$costs}}{n \text{ cases}} = \text{mean costs.}$$

The mean is then normalized to 1.0.

**Step 4:** This weight per DRG is then applied to the proportion of a hospital's cases falling into that DRG. This process is executed for every DRG,* and the products are summed to arrive at a case-mix-weighted cost measure for each hospital in the 20 percent Medicare sample.

$$\text{normalized case-mix-weighted costs}_h = \sum_{i=1}^{n} \text{mean costs}_i$$
$$\times \text{ proportion of cases}_{ih}$$
$$\text{for all DRGs}$$

**Step 5:** To arrive at an index which compares the hospital's costs and mix with national performance, the ratio of the hospital figure to the nationally derived figure is computed:

$$\frac{\text{normalized case-mix-weighted costs}_h}{\text{normalized national case-mix-weighted costs}} = \text{Medicare case-mix index}$$

---

*In the Medicare data base, some DRGs are seldom used and the numbers of cases with these DRGs are so small as to make the mean unstable or unreliable. These DRGs are removed from calculation of the index.

Values of the index less than 1.0 would reveal a case mix less complex or less costly than the national average; values greater than 1.0 would indicate a relatively more complex or costly case mix.

A percentage difference between any one hospital and the national index could also be calculated to examine the magnitude and direction of the difference:

$$\frac{1.345 - 0.9764}{0.9764} = +4.4 \text{ percent difference.}$$

The index cannot be applied to the assessment of all hospitals because of limitations in the data base on which the index was based. The data base includes only Medicare bills; therefore, children's hospitals are excluded. In addition, the 20 percent sample is not likely to include 20 percent of every hospital's inpatient cases; small hospitals (50 beds), which by definition submit a relatively small number of bills, would be excluded, since the index would also not be representative of them.

Research on the construction of the Medicare case-mix index and the implications of using it continues. If the objectives of such an index are to include efficiency in the provision of services to the Medicare population and cost containment, then the index must not merely reinforce the status quo. A scaler measure such as the index is simple, in that it condenses information for ease of handling—but at what cost? The critics claim that its difficulties lie in the homogeneity in cost structure across hospitals that is imposed by using an overall index. Interhospital differences that might be detected are buried when the detailed case-mix information is aggregated. Other complaints center on the accuracy of the Medicare data base, and the use of DRGs as the clinical descriptor. The index is, however, a good example of the application of the measurement concepts discussed in Part III to broad-scale reimbursement policy.

## 10.8 SUMMARY

The reimbursement and payment systems described in this chapter illustrate the extent to which hospital operations have been and will increasingly be subjected to outside review and control. Regulators and payers are assessing not only the volume of services provided, but the appropriateness and costs of those services for particular patients. Administrators must insure that relevant, timely data about their "product" and how it is changing are available, so that decisions related to services, revenues, and costs will be properly informed. While external controls on reimbursement are strengthening, hospitals must exhibit their own controls over utilization, quality of care, and cost escalation.

## Additional Reading

Bauer, K. G. "Hospital Rate Setting—This Way to Salvation?" *Milbank Memorial Fund Quarterly/Health and Society,* Winter 1977, pp. 117–158.

Bentley, J. D. and Butler, P. W. "Describing and Paying Hospitals: Developments in Patient Case Mix." Washington, D.C.: Association of American Medical Colleges, May 1980.

Coelen, C. and Sullivan, D. "An Analysis of the Effects of Prospective Reimbursement Programs on Hospital Expenditures." *Health Care Financing Review* 2, no. 3 (Winter 1981): 1–40.

Department of Health and Human Services. *Report to Congress: Hospital Prospective Payment for Medicare.* Washington, D.C.: December 1982.

Dowling, W. L. "Prospective Reimbursement of Hospitals." *Inquiry* 11, no. 3 (September 1974): 163–180.

Fetter, R. B., Shin, Y., Freeman, J. L., Averill, R. F. and Thompson, J. D. "Case Mix Definition by Diagnosis-Related Groups." *Medical Care Supplement,* February 1980, pp. 1–53.

Fetter, R. B., Thompson, J. D., Averill, R. F. and Freedman, A. T. "The New ICD-9-CM Diagnosis Related Groups Classification Scheme." Final Report. New Haven, Ct.: Yale University, Health Systems Management Group, School of Organization and Management, May 1982.

Garg, M. L., Louis, D. Z., Gliebe, W. A., Spirka, C. S., Skipper, J. K. and Parekh, R. R. "Evaluating Inpatient Costs: The Staging Mechanism." *Medical Care* 16, no. 3 (March 1978): 191–201.

Government Accounting Office. "Rising Hospital Costs Can Be Restrained by Regulating Payments and Improving Management." Washington, D.C.: September 1980.

Grimaldi, P. L. "Adjusting to Medicare DRG Indexes and Target Ceilings." *Hospital Progress,* January 1983, pp. 42–47.

Haley, M. J. "What is a DRG?" *Topics in Health Care Financing* 6, no. 4 (Summer 1980): 55–61.

Horn, S. D. and Schumacher, D. N. "An Analysis of Case Mix Complexity Using Information Theory and Diagnostic Related Groupings." *Medical Care* 17, no. 4 (April 1979): 382–389.

Institute of Medicine. "Reliability of Medicare Hospital Discharge Records." National Academy of Sciences, NTIS No. PB281680. Washington, D.C.: November 1977.

Klastorin, T. D. and Watts, C. A. "On the Measurement of Hospital Case Mix." *Medical Care* 18, no. 6 (June 1980): 675–685.

Lave, J., Pettengill, J. and Vertrees, J. "Regional Issues in the Construction of the Medicare Case Mix-Index." *Health Care Financial Management,* April 1983.

National Center for Health Statistics. "Uniform Hospital Discharge Data: Minimum Data Set." Report of the National Committee on Vital and Health Statistics, DHEW Publication No. (PHS) 80-1157, April 1980.

Pettengill, J. and Vertrees, J. "Reliability and Validity in Hospital Case-Mix Measurement." *Health Care Financing Review* 4, no. 2 (December 1982): 101–128.

Ruchlin, H. S. and Rosen, H. M. "Short Run Hospital Responses to Reimbursement Rate Changes." *Inquiry* 17, no. 1 (Spring 1980): 42–53.

Warner, D. M. and Kinzer, D. "Factors Affecting Reimbursement under Admission-Based Rate Setting." *Health Services Research,* Summer 1983.

# 11

# Cybernetic Control
# Applied to Facility Management

## 11.1 INTRODUCTION

**Problem:** How would you answer the following job announcement?

Wanted: Health Facility Administrator

Position requires a person with the ability to maintain an average occupancy rate of at least 96 percent on medical/surgical nursing units, 63 percent on ICU/CCU units, and 63 percent on obstetrics units, while scheduling all non-emergency surgical patients and, on the average, 21 out of the 100 medical patients each week. No more than 5 scheduled patients out of every 1,000 can be cancelled and no more than 15 out of 1,000 ICU/CCU patients, 5 out of 1,000 OB patients, or 10 out of 1,000 emergency patients can be turned away.

In addition, the person in this position is responsible for allocating nurses to each of these nursing units (1) so that an average of 5.0 hours of nursing care is maintained for each patient each day, (2) so that registered nurses, licensed practical nurses, and aides are assigned to each unit to utilize their skills fully, (3) so that the nurses' individual work schedules minimize their aversions to working 6, 7, or 8-day stretches with or without 3-day weekends, and (4) so that quality nursing care is provided.

Applicants must have knowledge or skill in setting up systems for physicians to control patient placement in appropriate levels of care, and to control medical necessity of patient services.

This announcement summarizes some of the important measures of performance that previous chapters have introduced. Although the decision framework and appropriate quantitative techniques have been applied to arrive at these desired levels of performance, an important responsibility of the administrator has just begun: to control the facility so that it continues to meet these performance levels. To illustrate the application of the cybernetic control framework for achieving desired performance, we have selected three hospital systems—the admitting system, the nursing care system, and the physician care system. This chapter concentrates on the admitting and nursing care systems, and Chapter 12 will concentrate on the physician care systems. The discussion that follows assumes the reader is familiar with Section 2.3.

The study of how systems should be controlled, or how they should control themselves, and the flow of information necessary to do this is called *cybernetics*—the *science* of control. The *profession* of control is management; it is necessary, therefore, for managers to understand cybernetics.

Students of cybernetics have come to realize that common principles govern systems under control. Control is not an arbitrary exercise of power that requires managers to bully people into operating in a desired way. Rather, control is a process of coaxing a system toward desired performance. Furthermore, because systems are naturally complex and uncertain, as illustrated by the examples and exercises already discussed, they cannot be controlled entirely from the outside.

The satellite outpatient clinic provides a good illustration of the difficulty administrators have in controlling a system's multiple and conflicting objectives. The clinic problem requires that a fine line be maintained between meeting patients' needs, meeting the clinic's needs, and meeting the parent systems' needs, including the hospital, third-party payers, and the community. To demonstrate the trade-offs between the clinic's conflicting measures of performance, consider establishing the budget objective for the clinic, including the desired amount of staff time, equipment, supplies, and facility. (The reader might want to review Section 1.2: the appropriate objectives mega-problem.)

If the budget objective for hours of staff is set too low, patient requests for medical services throughout the day will not be met without undue delay. If set too high, the clinic payroll may not meet third-party reimbursement regulations. There is a reasonable limit to how much the clinic can charge patients and their insurance programs for services. If the budget objective is set too high, the reasonable charge will be insufficient to cover the clinic expenses.

Furthermore, Medicare and Medicaid reimbursements are made only for medically necessary services provided in the most economical level of care—acute hospital, skilled nursing facility (SNF), home health care, or outpatient care. If the budget objective is set too high, there is a chance that medically unnecessary services (or in acute hospitals and SNFs, too high a level of care) will be provided in order to fully utilize the staff and facility. Receiving medically unnecessary services (or too high a level of care) is potentially dangerous for patients. In addition, Medicare and Medicaid may deny payment when review procedures (Section 12.2) determine that services are medically unnecessary or days in acute hospitals and SNFs are unnecessary.

When these trade-offs for budgeting hours of staff are repeated for budgeting equipment, supplies, and examining rooms, the conflict between measures of performance increases. Equipment, supplies, and examining rooms must be matched to staff; equipment must be matched to supplies and examining rooms; and supplies must be matched to examining rooms.

The control problem is further complicated by the large number of choices facing the clinic administrator for achieving desired budget performance. She can change the total number of staff hours available, the staff schedule, or the tasks performed by the staff to match their skill levels more closely. She can change the equipment's capacity, the equipment's scheduled use, or the type of equipment (to make it less specialized). The administrator can change the amount of supplies in inventory, the supply-ordering schedule, or the type of supplies (to disposable, for example). She can change the number of examining rooms, the examining room schedule, or the room sizes and the flow of patients through the rooms. Finally, to a limited extent, she can change the number of patients seen by the clinic, the patient-arrival schedule, and the types of patients seen by the clinic. Limiting the clinic's size and modifying the range of services it provides will change the number and types of patients. Changing the patient-arrival schedule is possible only for nonemergency patients.

As if this complexity were not enough, the clinic's environment adds an additional dimension. The environment includes the systems affecting the clinic's measures of performance but not controlled by the administrator—the availability of physicians and nurses in the community, changes in insurance coverage, changes in the incidence of medical problems (drug abuse, venereal disease, and abortions, for example), and changes in services provided by other clinics that may duplicate the clinic's services.

To make explicit an important role of the administrator in controlling systems, reconsider the megaproblem of appropriate objectives. Since a system is controlled to achieve its objectives, the administrator must see that systems objectives are defined in terms of how the system plays a part in meeting its parent's and siblings' objectives. Its parent's and siblings' objectives must in turn be defined in terms of *their* parent's and siblings' objectives, etc. The important link between systems, therefore, lies in the establishment of their objectives.

The administrator of the satellite outpatient clinic must steer the clinic so that it achieves its objectives for patient waiting time, patient turnaways, budget, range of services, etc. The clinic administrator must do the following:

1. develop or be given explicit measures of performance for these objectives, and establish or be given desired levels of performance;

2. receive feedback about actual performance;

3. be able to solve problems within the clinic so the clinic achieves its objectives;

4. forecast problems that may be encountered in the process of achieving desired performance;

5. learn about the clinic's environment so she can anticipate changes in the availability of physicians and nurses in the community, changes in insurance coverage, changes in incidence of medical problems, changes in demographic characteristics of the surrounding communities, and changes in services provided by other clinics or its own parent system (the hospital); and

6. know when back-up support from the administrator of the clinic's parent system is required.

Why should the administrator of the clinic be able to do all of this? So that she can control the satellite outpatient clinic's performance. Although this may seem obvious, a common alternative is to give the clinic administrator a list of rules to follow under different circumstances, and for the clinic administrator to obtain "permission" from the hospital administrator whenever a deviation from the rules seems necessary.

To see why the clinic administrator must be able to control the clinic herself, consider the administrator of the clinic's parent system, the hospital administrator. Can the hospital administrator control the clinic with rules? Or, in general, can the administrator of a system control its subsystems by prescribing rules to follow under various circumstances? At a practical level, it is unlikely that the hospital administrator could approve exceptions for the clinic to achieve its objectives *and*, at the same time, steer the nursing department, admitting department, laboratory department, physical therapy department, emergency room, operating room, etc., so that they achieved their objectives. There would simply not be enough time, and the hospital administrator would be forced to ignore some of these subsystems—perhaps at the time an unpredicted event occurred that required attention.

At a theoretical level, the hospital administrator cannot control the clinic with rules because of the complexity (the large number of different subsystems and sub-subsystems) and the uncertainty inherent in the clinic. The rules will naturally be too simple. They cannot take into account the large number of factors, and interaction of factors, influencing performance and constantly creating special cases. And they will be too deterministic. Rules by their nature are deterministic and will not account for uncertain events. Therefore, the best way for the hospital administrator to make sure the clinic achieves its objectives is to make sure the clinic administrator can control the clinic's performance.

So what is the hospital administrator's role? His role is to control the hospital system, *including* the satellite outpatient clinic subsystem. Therefore, the administrator must have explicit measures of performance, feedback, problem-solving capacity, etc., for the hospital system. The hospital, even though it is imbedded in the community system, cannot be entirely controlled by rules and regulations specified by outside agencies because of its complexity and uncertainty. Therefore, the best way for outside agencies to control hospitals is by assuring the control structural requirements and process are available to hospitals so that they can control themselves. Self-regulation is the fundamental concept of cybernetic control.

With the above discussion in mind, return to the job announcement and the use of the cybernetic control framework to guide an interview for this position.

## 11.2 Overbedded versus Non-overbedded Facilities

We must determine a primary characteristic of the facility that is offering the job—whether it is overbedded (let's say an average occupancy rate below .80 on the medical/surgical unit) or not overbedded (average occupancy rate above .80). In non-overbedded facilities, attention is usually placed on controlling the flow of admissions, while in overbedded facilities, attention is usually placed on controlling staffing levels.

To raise the occupancy rate from below .80 to the required .96 on overbedded medical/surgical (MED/SURG) units, either additional patients have to be found to fill the beds (e.g. closing down other hospitals, increasing the community's population, increasing people's use of hospital beds, or aggressively "stealing" patients from other hospitals); or the number of MED/SURG beds must be reduced (e.g. closing wards or converting to skilled nursing facility beds). However, if closing wards or converting beds means that patients will be delayed admission, physicians may threaten to take their non-emergency medical, surgical, or gynecological patients to another facility that has empty beds and can immediately admit their patients. Thus, it may not be possible for *one* facility to raise its occupancy rate to .96 in an overbedded region; its survival will be threatened if patients are lost to other facilities with immediately available beds. All facilities in the community may have to raise their MED/SURG occupancy to .96, becoming "correctly" bedded.

The MED/SURG unit census for *overbedded* hospitals is normally subject to large fluctuations reflecting random requests for admission and uncertain lengths of stay. If admissions cannot easily be controlled to damp these fluctuations, attention must be given to controlling personnel staffing levels so that they "track" this census fluctuation. Controlled variable staffing, discussed below, becomes an important control system for overbedded facilities. However, to achieve the .96 occupancy rate in the job announcement, the administrator would have to close beds if the facility was overbedded, in which case controlled variable staffing may not be needed.

For non-overbedded facilities, or facilities that have closed down beds, the census fluctuations are naturally damped because admissions are controlled to keep the census close to capacity. If the average occupancy rate is .96 on MED/SURG units, and if the mix of self-care, intermediate-care, and intensive-care patients remains relatively constant on each unit, personnel staffing levels will remain relatively constant from day to day. Only personnel absenteeism will have to be accounted for to control nursing hours per patient-day.

In any facility, controlling the patient mix between self care, intermediate care, or intensive care on a unit may be accomplished in part by admitting and transferring patients to nursing units specializing only in self-care patients, intermediate-care patients, or intensive-care patients; or by assigning patients to units to maintain a specified mix between these classes. This will help maintain the mix of different skill levels between RNs, LPNs, and AIDEs relatively constant from day to day. However, it is the daily fluctuation in census that most affects the changing need for staff from day to day.

Reconsider the admission control system from Section 5.5 as implemented in an non-overbedded facility. We will describe in Section 11.4 the relatively straightforward nurse staffing system that goes with it. Section 11.5 contains a discussion of controlled variable nurse staffing in an overbedded facility, where admissions cannot be controlled without physicians' threatening to take their patients to another facility. The attendant problems that make it more complicated will be discussed. It may be that the .96 occupancy rate is impossible to achieve in the facility advertising for an administrator, and instead, attention will have to be placed on achieving an average of 5.0 nursing hours per patient.

## 11.3 CONTROLLED ADMISSIONS IN NON-OVERBEDDED FACILITIES

The control process applied to inpatient admissions is diagrammed in Figure 11.1.

Requirement 1: Explicit Measures of Performance

Notice that the job announcement has summarized the desired performance of the admission control system (Figure 5.27) that was discussed in Chapter 5.

$A_1 = .2$ ICU/CCU turnaways/week (TUI)
or, since on the average there are 13.78 ICU/CCU admissions + turnaways/week (Figure 5.35), $(.2/13.78) = 15$ ICU/CCU turnaways/1,000 arrivals;

$A_2 = .5$ ER turnaways/week (TUE)
or, since on the average there are 49 ER arrivals/week, $(.5/49) = 10$ ER turnaways/1,000 arrivals;

# Figure 11.1
## Control Framework Applied to Inpatient Admissions

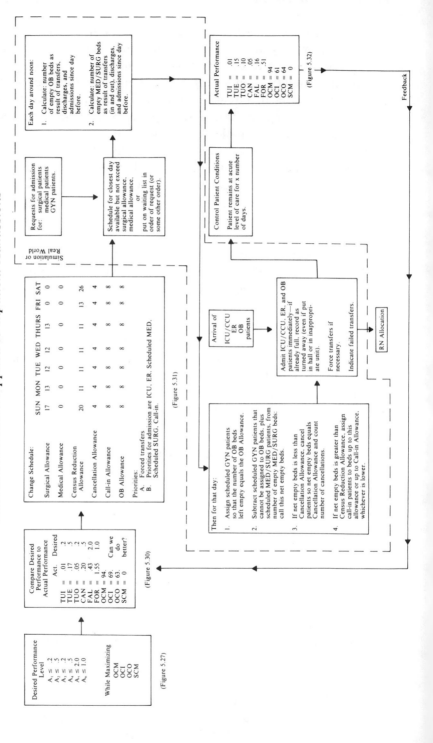

$A_3$ = .2 OB turnaways/week (TUO)
or, since on the average there are 42.20 OB admissions + turnaways/week (Figure 5.35), (.2/42.20) = 5 OB turnaways/1,000 arrivals;

$A_4$ = .5 cancellations/week (CAN)
or, since on the average 21 medical patients and 67 surgical patients are scheduled/week, (.5/88) = 5 cancellations / 1,000 scheduled patients;

$A_5$ = 2 Failed transfers/week (FAL); and

$A_6$ = 1.5 Forced transfers/week (FOR);

while maximizing:

MED/SURG occupancy rate (OCM),

ICU/CCU occupancy rate (OCI),

OB occupancy rate (OCO), and

Number of scheduled urgent medical patients/week (SCM). The highest occupancy rates and scheduled number of patients that were achieved (Figure 5.36) while not exceeding the $A_i$ above was

OCM = 96,

OCI = 63,

OCO = 63, and

SCM = 21.

These then become the desired performance levels for this facility.

Requirement 2: Feedback

A critical requirement of the control process is the feeding back of these performance measures to the admitting system manager. The measurements should describe actual performances: ICU/CCU, ER, and OB turnaways/week; cancellations/week; failed and forced transfers/week; MED/SURG, ICU/CCU, and OB occupancy rates; and number of scheduled medical patients. These measurements should then be compared to desired performance by the admitting system manager and necessary schedule adjustments made.

It should be emphasized that this feedback is about a *real* system. The description in Section 5.5 was of a simulated system; the analyst changed the schedule until the simulated performance met the desired levels. The analyst received feedback about the simulated system; the resulting measures of performance were only *predictions* of how the real system would behave. Each simulation run was for 200 weeks (200 × 7 days = 1,400 times through the section of the diagram enclosed in dashed lines in Figure 11.1) before the schedule was changed, and 12 different schedules were tried before a schedule that met desired performance was found. Certainly this amount of experimentation would have been difficult and expensive to do on the real system.

However, the simulation was only a simplified version of the real system, and the real system may not behave like the simulated system when unanticipated events occur. Controlling the real system requires the cybernetic control framework. Once the admitting department is given the schedule determined best for the simulated system, weekly measurements must be made on the real system and compared to desired performance.

Requirement 3: Problem Solving Capability

Admitting personnel must be trained to use the admitting system, and the schedule may have to be adjusted periodically. The admitting system manager must be able to solve the system's problems, or obtain back-up support, in order to achieve desired occupancy rates, cancellation rates, turnaway rates, etc.

Requirement 4: Forecasting

The question now becomes, How many weeks of actual performance should be observed before a decision to change the schedule can be made? This is a case of forecasting *performance*. As with forecasting demand, there is no simple answer. Recall that Chapter 7 presented three ways to make forecasts:

1. Base the prediction of future performance on measured past performance;

2. Base the prediction of future performance on subjective (expert) opinion; and

3. Base the prediction of future performance on a combination of 1 and 2.

The first method was implicitly used to determine an admitting schedule from the simulation in Section 5.5; the analyst used past simulated performance averaged over 200 simulated weeks. However, waiting more than several weeks before changing a schedule could be disastrous when controlling the real system.

Past performance can be plotted on a weekly basis and performance trends watched to decide whether the schedule should be changed. Testing whether a trend really exists or is simply a variation around desired performance can be done as shown in Chapter 7. As an alternative, the standard deviation based on past performance measurements can be calculated. If performance is outside ± two standard deviations (as an approximation to the 95 percent confidence interval of the normal distribution), the admitting manager might decide a trend exists and an adjustment in the schedule should be made (requiring new simulation runs).

However, just as past data should not be totally relied upon when forecasting demand, past data should not be totally relied upon when forecasting performance. If a trend of deteriorating performance can be explained by a change in admitting department personnel, and if efforts are underway to train these new personnel to use the scheduling system, performance may return to desired levels. As always, subjective opinion would modify the past trend.

Likewise, though performance may be at desired levels today, seasonal variation in demand will affect performance in the future. Plans should be made now to change the schedule in anticipation of seasonal variation. A more dramatic illustration of changing a schedule in anticipation of a performance change is the schedule change made before a nurses' strike. Such performance variation was not included in the simulation used to arrive at the best schedule, and it would not be observed in past performance trends. Yet it would have to be anticipated for the admission scheduling system to come close to desired performance.

Requirement 5: Learn about Environment

Requirement 4 illustrates why the admitting system must be able to learn about its environment. Nurse strikes are just one of the many events outside the admitting system that can affect performance. Other examples include an expanded number of beds in a nearby hospital, a closed-down SNF which forces patients to remain in the acute facility longer, or a new industry moving into the community. When known, these should certainly be incorporated into demand forecasts for inpatient beds and into the simulation. But not all events can be anticipated each time a demand forecast is made.

Requirement 6: Back-up Support

If the admitting system itself cannot achieve desired performance, provisions must be made for back-up assistance. This would be the role of the assistant administrator or administrator; he in turn may wish to consult staff specialists. Previous chapters have presented concepts and techniques for the administrator to use in providing back-up support.

## 11.4 CONTROLLED VARIABLE STAFFING WITH CONTROLLED ADMISSIONS

Nursing hours per patient day are simpler to control when admissions are controlled, because the variance in daily census is small. The average census resulting from controlled admissions using the simulation of Section 5.5 is shown in Table 11.1. These figures incorporate the combined results of forecasting demand and applying the admission scheduling rules. Let us now look at the problem of controlling the daily allocation of nurses (RNs, LPNs, and AIDEs) to these patients.

Recall from Section 6.6 the definition of three nursing manpower decisions.

1. *Staffing Decision:* an annual decision specifying the number of full-time equivalent *positions* of each skill level (RN, LPN, and AIDE) to be funded for each unit.

2. *Scheduling Decision:* a four-week decision specifying when each nurse in each unit will be on duty and off duty for the next four weeks, taking into account weekend policy, requests for days off, and the minimum number of nurses of each skill class that must be on duty in each unit during each day and shift.

3. *Reallocation Decision:* a shift-by-shift decision specifying how a float pool of nurses is to be allocated among various units, to account for unforecastable changes in nursing care needs and in absenteeism. Recall that float nurses do not report directly to a unit when arriving for work, but report instead to the nursing office which allocates them to where need is greatest that day and shift.

The output of the staffing decision provides the desired performance for the nurse staffing system. The staffing decision would determine the number of RNs, LPNs, and AIDEs to fund for a unit, based on the average number of self-care, intermediate-care,

## Table 11.1

### Average Census from Controlled Admissions

| | TOTAL | SUN | MON | TUES | WED | THURS | FRI | SAT |
|---|---|---|---|---|---|---|---|---|
| Average number of MED/SURG beds occupied | 204.7 | 202.7 | 208.6 | 208.4 | 208.6 | 208.6 | 203.1 | 192.7 |
| Average number of OB beds occupied | 22.6 | 22.1 | 22.5 | 23.0 | 23.2 | 23.7 | 22.5 | 21.2 |
| Average number of ICU/CCU beds occupied | 11.5 | 11.6 | 11.5 | 11.6 | 11.5 | 11.8 | 11.5 | 11.5 |

and intensive-care patients in that unit each day, and on the cost of quality lost by tasks being performed by persons in inappropriate skill classes. (The mathematical programming formulation of Section 6.6 addressed this decision.) Section 9.2 presented a work sampling method for measuring the hours required on a unit to perform 16 task categories. Section 9.3 presented a scaling method for measuring the cost of lost quality.

Since we are discussing a non-overbedded facility with controlled admissions, the variation in total patients on the medical and surgical units is small. If, in addition, the mix of self-, intermediate-, and intensive-care patients is kept relatively constant by the admission process, using work sampling to measure required nursing hours provides fairly accurate input to the staffing decision. By not controlling admissions or patient mix, the variation in patient numbers and dependency may be so great that the staffing decision would have to be made daily (or made for many different situations, generating a table to be used daily for allocating a skill-level mix that corresponds to patient mix and number).

For a non-overbedded facility, then, we would end up with a table like Table 11.2. This table, especially if it incorporates the cost of lost quality due to inappropriate skill levels performing tasks, would become one measure of performance. It would also provide a basis for establishing another measure of performance, nursing hours per patient day. For the day shift, since on the average there are 204.7 MED/SURG patients/day (Table 11.1) and 95 Full-Time Equivalents (FTEs), the standard for nursing hours per patient day is

### Table 11.2

*Coverage Requirement on Day Shift:*
*Full Time Equivalents*

| MED/SURG | RN | LPN | AIDE | TOTAL | AVERAGE CENSUS |
|---|---|---|---|---|---|
| Unit 1 | 3 | 8 | 10 | 21 | 46 |
| 2 | 2 | 6 | 8 | 16 | 35 |
| 3 | 1 | 3 | 4 | 8 | 17 |
| 4 | 4 | 5 | 6 | 15 | 32 |
| 5 | 2 | 3 | 3 | 8 | 17 |
| 6 | 2 | 3 | 3 | 8 | 17 |
| 7 | 1 | 4 | 3 | 8 | 17 |
| 8 | 2 | 5 | 4 | 11 | 24 |
| | | | | 95 | 205 |

$$\frac{95 \text{ FTE} \times 8 \text{ hours}}{204.7 \text{ patients/day}} = 3.71 \text{ hours/patient day}$$

for the entire hospital. Each unit would have a different standard based on its average mix of self-, intermediate-, and intensive-care patients and on the time required to perform the 16 task categories. After adding in student nurses and ward clerks and taking into account the second and third shifts, the average number of hours per patient day was 5.0 hours in the job announcement.

Once the coverage requirement is determined for each unit and each shift (Table 11.2), the scheduling decision is made every four weeks, so that each RN, LPN, and AIDE is assigned to meet the coverage requirement, while taking into account weekend policy, requests for days off, and aversion to particular work stretches. Section 6.6 discussed this decision in detail.

In the non-overbedded facility with controlled admissions, as long as the patient mix does not vary greatly from day to day, there is likely to be no need to reallocate nurses each day. The RNs, LPNs, and AIDEs go to the unit where they were scheduled. However, absent nurses will have to be replaced. Depending on the hospital's policy and the availability of nurses in the community, a nurse could be obtained from a float pool, from a nursing registry (an organization within some communities that has a list of nurses who will work whenever they are called for as long as they are needed), or by overtime. Pulling a nurse from one unit and reallocating her to replace the absent nurse is unlikely when there is a 96 percent occupancy rate and a constant patient mix on each unit. A rule could be established that changes would not be made if the difference between hours required on a unit and hours allocated to the unit is ± 4 hours (for a 30-bed unit). For a larger unit it could be greater. If the difference is greater than ± 4 hours only a few times a month, a daily reallocation system is obviously not warranted.

The control process is diagrammed in Figure 11.2. A nursing unit with admissions controlled is better able to control its performance; controlling admissions reduces much of the uncertainty about the number of patients assigned to the unit.

## 11.5 CONTROLLED VARIABLE STAFFING
### WITHOUT CONTROLLED ADMISSIONS

When admissions are not controlled, the burden of controlling nursing hours per patient day lies with the nursing unit and its back-up support from nursing administration. A re-examination of Figure 11.2

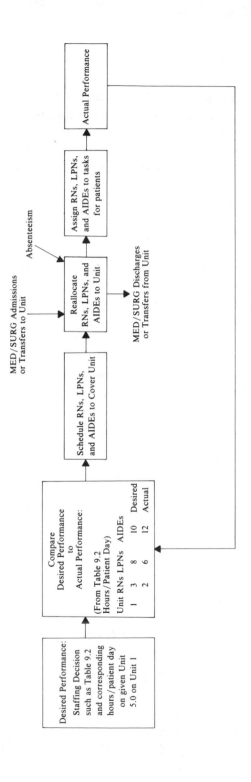

*Figure 11.2*

*Control Framework Applied to Variable Staffing*

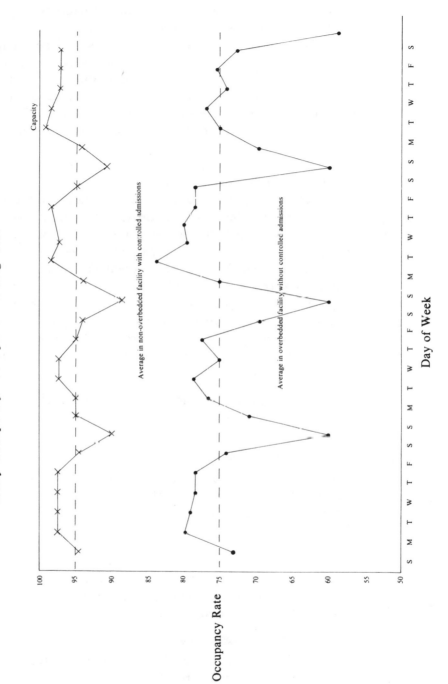

*Figure 11.3*

## Daily Occupancy Rates for a Nursing Unit

highlights the problem. An uncertain number of patients on the unit from day to day makes it difficult to adjust the nursing hours and the skill-level mix. Figure 11.3 illustrates how, as average occupancy nears 100 percent, the variation from day to day is naturally damped. As average occupancy drops, there is more opportunity for fluctuation. This would be less serious if each day of the week always had about the same occupancy rate—i.e., if Sundays averaged 75 percent with a small variation. We could then plan for this situation by scheduling nurses every four weeks to account for the differing occupancy rates on Sunday, Monday, Tuesday, etc. But even this is unlikely to happen if admissions are not controlled.

To control staffing when admissions are not controlled, the staffing and scheduling decision must provide enough nursing hours to care for a prespecified number of patients on each unit, with nurses added each day if the actual patient census is greater than the prespecified number. Nurses can be obtained from a float pool, by pulling nurses from a unit with low staffing needs, by hiring nurses from a nursing registry, or by having nurses work overtime. The measure of performance is how well the nursing hours *track* the census (or census weighted by patient dependency class). However, not only must hours of nursing track census, but the skill level mix must track the patient mix.

**Problem:** How should the head nurse be supported to control her unit's performance?

Requirement 1: Explicit Measures of Performance

The head nurse must establish or be given explicit measures of performance and desired levels of performance. These will be discussed in more detail below.

Requirement 2: Feedback

The head nurse and nursing unit must know how they are doing on the measures of performance. Plotting the information each week or every two weeks is probably sufficient, depending upon how close the unit is to achieving desired performance.

Requirement 3: Problem-solving Ability

Naturally, the head nurse must be given time to solve problems. She must know how to assign nurses to each patient or task category. She must know how to improve quality, how to make use of the nurses allocated to her unit, and how to acquire additional nurses, if needed, or where to send extra nurses, if not needed. She must know how to use the dependency categories to establish needed hours for her unit.

Requirement 4: Forecast

The head nurse must be able to anticipate changes in patients' dependency categories, changes in nursing personnel, and changes in admissions or discharges to her unit. She should forecast future performance problems and be able to begin solving them.

Requirement 5: Learn About Environment

The head nurse must know how the admitting department can affect her unit's performance; how the ancillary departments depend on her unit and how she depends on them; and how the availability of SNFs, home health agencies, and other community health resources affect her unit's performance.

Requirement 6: Back-up Support

Finally, when desired performance cannot be achieved, the head nurse must know where to obtain back-up support. Additional training may be required. Help from other nursing units, ancillary departments, the business office, or social services department may be required.

It would be inappropriate to develop a set of rules for head nurses to follow and then require them to justify exceptions to those rules. Such rules cannot capture the complexity and uncertainty of nursing units.

**Reallocation Decision**

**Problem:** How can nursing hours and skill-level mix for a unit be adjusted to track patient census and patient mix?

Figure 11.4 illustrates the control process applied to reallocating nurses to units each day. Each day about noon, the head nurse categorizes patients as self care, intermediate care, and intensive care, using the guidelines in Table 11.3. Since most patients will be in the same category as the day before, it is a matter of changing the category for the few patients with worsened or improved conditions, and making assignments for recently-admitted patients.

One study found that when 96 adult patients on typical MED/SURG units were observed continuously for four days, self-care patients averaged .50 hours of direct care (range was 0 to 1 hours), intermediate-care patients averaged 1.00 hour of direct care (range was .16 to 1.75 hours), and intensive-care patients averaged

*Figure 11.4*

## Control Framework Applied to Reallocating Nurses

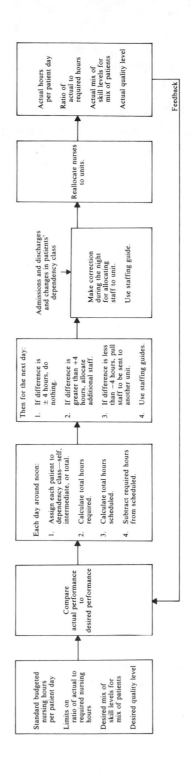

Standard budgeted nursing hours per patient day

Limits on ratio of actual to required nursing hours

Desired mix of skill levels for mix of patients

Desired quality level

→

Compare actual performance to desired performance

→

Each day around noon:

1. Assign each patient to dependency class—self, intermediate, or total.
2. Calculate total hours required.
3. Calculate total hours scheduled.
4. Subtract required hours from scheduled.

→

Then for the next day:

1. If difference is ± 4 hours, do nothing.
2. If difference is greater than +4 hours, allocate additional staff.
3. If difference is less than −4 hours, pull staff to be sent to another unit.
4. Use staffing guides.

Admissions and discharges and changes in patients' dependency class
↓

Make correction during the night for allocating staff to unit.

Use staffing guide.

→

Reallocate nurses to units.

→

Actual hours per patient day

Ratio of actual to required hours

Actual mix of skill levels for mix of patients

Actual quality level

Feedback

## Table 11.3

## Characteristics of Patients in Dependency Categories

Category I Self-care

Any of the following combinations checked
a. Ambulatory, or up in chair—self (without assistance)
   Feeding self, or requires food cut
   Bathing in bathroom, or at bedside—partial self
   (can bathe self except for back and perhaps extremities)
b. Ambulatory—with assistance
   Up in chair—self
   Bathing in bathroom, or at bedside—partial self
c. As in (a and b) with
   Vision inadequate
   Oxygen therapy
   I.V. feeding
   but no two of these factors simultaneously

Category II Partial or intermediate care

Any of the following combinations checked
a. Ambulatory—with assistance
   Bathing in bathroom, or at bedside— partial self
   Feeding—complete assistance (except I.V. feeding)
   Vision inadequate ⎫
   Oxygen therapy   ⎬ optional (does not affect classification under these conditions)
b. Up in chair—self
   Bathing at bedside—complete assistance
   Feeding self, or requires food cut or I.V. feeding
   Oxygen therapy   ⎫ optional
   Vision inadequate ⎭
c. As in (b) with the following changes
   Up in chair—with assistance
   Bath at bedside
d. Up in chair—with assistance
   Bath at bedside—partial self
   Feeding—complete assistance
   Vision inadequate ⎫ optional
   Oxygen therapy   ⎭
e. Bath at beside
   Feeding—self, or requires food cut, or I.V. feeding
   Vision inadequate ⎫ optional
   Oxygen therapy   ⎭
f. Requiring special care by necessity (patient has continuous nursing assistance to the
   extent that meal relief must be provided for special duty nurse)

NOTE: Any patient who otherwise falls into Category I or II, but who is under suction
therapy or is in isolation, incontinent (including wound drainage necessitating change
of bed linen), or markedly emotionally disturbed (needs almost constant observation,
in single room, creates disturbance) will be dropped to the next category.

Category III. Intensive, or total, care

All combinations not previously mentioned.

SOURCE: Wolfe, H. and Young, J. P., "Staffing the Nursing Unit, Part I. Controlled
Variable Staffing," *Nursing Research,* vol. 14, no. 3, Summer 1965.

2.5 hours of direct care (range was .83 to 3.66 hours; see Wolfe and Young). This study also found through work sampling that, for a typical 30-bed nursing unit, the time required to perform all activities other than direct care remained fairly constant at 20 hours for the day shift regardless of the number of patients or their degree of dependency. This example provides an illustration for calculating the average nursing hours per day required by one hospital unit. We multiply the number of self-, intermediate-, and intensive-care patients on a unit by .50 hour, 1.0 hour, and 2.5 hours respectively, and add the results to 20 hours of indirect care. This provides the required hours of nursing for the unit for the next *day* shift.

The required hours are compared to the actual hours scheduled for that unit on the next day. If more than, say, 4 additional hours are required, nurses are reallocated to that unit. If more than 4 hours are scheduled but not required, nurses are pulled from that unit and reallocated to another. If there is a nursing registry in a community, it is often less expensive to call the registry to obtain additional nurses from outside the hospital for a few days at a time. When no longer needed, these nurses return to the registry, and the hospital no longer pays them.

Although the above calculation gives us the number of additional nursing hours needed (or not needed), it does not tell us what type of nurses are needed (RNs, LPNs, or AIDEs). In this situation, the staffing decision needs to be made each day to establish the skill-level mix for differing combinations of patient dependency. A range of required nursing hours and patient mixes must be considered in producing a table of the corresponding skill-class mix. The table can then be used as a guide for selecting the skill class to allocate to a unit, or to pull from a unit.

Since this initial patient assessment and reallocation is done on the preceding day, all admissions and discharges from the unit, as well as changes in patients' conditions, will occur before the next morning. These adjustments are made during the night. The following morning, nurses are reallocated to the units that need them the most or are sent back to the registry if no longer needed.

Measures of performance are more complex than when admissions are controlled. A measure of the quality of nursing care should be employed (Section 9.6) since the daily changes in nursing staff (whether they come from a float pool, another floor, registry, or overtime) make it more difficult to manage quality care. There is constant turnover of personnel with new faces, new procedures, and new (to the personnel) patients. The trade-off, of course, is the cost of not reallocating nurses each day. To obtain adequate nursing coverage without reallocating nurses each day requires that each unit be staffed in relation to the peak nursing loads. This increases the required nursing hours per patient day and, therefore, the cost.

Not only should a standard be set for the number of nursing hours to budget per patient day (as with controlled admissions), but the number of nursing hours should match the number of required hours *each day*. It is possible for the *average* hours per patient day to meet the standard exactly, yet, every time required nursing hours increase, available nursing hours decrease, and vice versa. Figure 11.5 illustrates two points where this happens. The first two peaks are fairly close. The third indicates insufficient nursing hours and the next valley indicates excess. If the ratio of actual to desired nursing hours is calculated each day, the above fluctuations will be seen in Figure 11.6. A ratio dropping below 1.0 indicates too *few* hours, and quality is likely to suffer. A ratio exceeding 1.0, indicates too *many* hours, so the budget is likely to suffer. A standard for the upper limit and lower limit of this ratio should also be set and used as a measure of performance.

The difficulty of achieving desired performance on hours per patient day, ratio of desired to actual hours, and quality on each unit when admissions are not controlled is exacerbated by several practical problems.

1) Generally, nurses do not like to float from one unit to another, or be pulled from their home unit and sent to another. It is also difficult for some to work overtime. In addition, it is difficult to control the competence of nurses called in for short periods of time from a nursing registry. They usually do not participate in the facility's inservice education programs and may not be properly oriented to the facility.

2) Because of the first problem, it is difficult to control the quality of nursing care on a unit, making the measurement of quality and its control that much more important.

3) Since nurses on a unit assign patients to self-, intermediate-, or intensive-care categories resulting in, for example, .5, 1.0, or 2.5 hours of nursing respectively, patients are commonly assigned to categories that will result in more nursing hours. This may mean that the numbers .5, 1.0, and 2.5 are not high enough and nurses on a unit must assign patients to higher dependency categories in order to obtain sufficient nursing. It may also mean that the nurses on a unit are trying to obtain as many hours as possible, just in case they are needed. Whatever the reason, the usual attempted

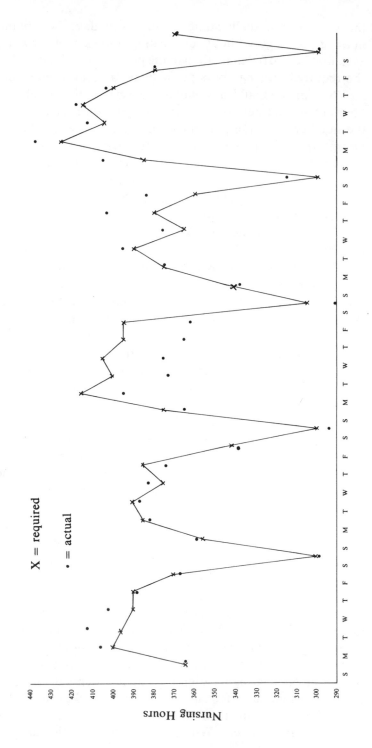

*Figure 11.5*

*Comparison of Actual Hours to Required Hours*

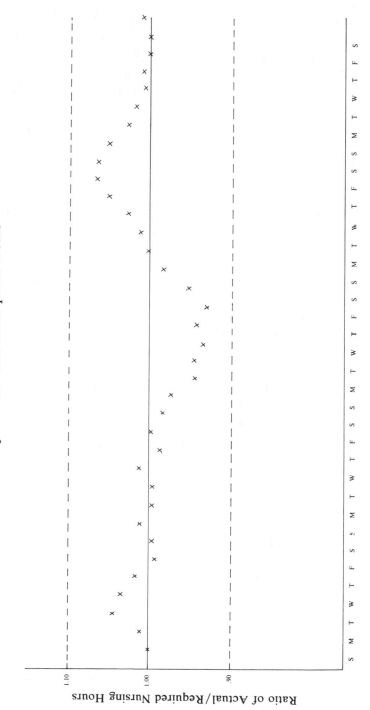

Figure 11.6

*Ratio of Actual Hours to Required Hours*

remedy is for the central nursing administration office to audit the assignments to insure they are not being inflated. The nurses usually have good justification for assigning a patient as they do, so an audit is less satisfactory than making the unit responsible for its budget, thereby decreasing the chance that assignments will be inflated without good reason.

4) Because of 3), achieving the standard budgeted number of nursing hours per patient day is difficult. As patient assignments are inflated, more hours are allocated to a unit than originally budgeted. If the nursing hours per patient day budget is adjusted to account for the average increased dependency of patients, eventually most patients may be assigned to the intensive-care category, and there is no longer a need to go through the process of assigning patients to dependency categories.

5) A unit's ability to achieve its performance is heavily dependent on the admitting department (usually not controlled by the nursing units themselves). Admitting can inadvertently help some units and hurt others by the way patients are assigned. Units maintaining occupancy rates of 96 percent have the same advantages as if admissions were controlled. Few float nurses will be required. Actual nursing hours will track desired nursing hours. Quality will most likely be consistent and easier to manage since the same nurses can be sent to the unit each day. Because the MED/SURG occupancy rate for overbedded hospitals is below 80 percent, if some MED/SURG units have an average occupancy rate of 96 percent, others will have an average occupancy rate of 70 percent or lower, with large fluctuations. (They will have to absorb all the fluctuation for the hospital since the high-occupancy units will not fluctuate much at all.) This compounds problems 1) through 4) for the low-occupancy units.

Thus, admitting and nursing cannot be viewed as separate, independent systems. A nursing unit's performance is dependent on the admitting department's patient assignments: at one extreme, assignments may be made so that occupancy rates stay at 96 percent; at the other extreme, occupancy rates may be allowed to fluctuate around 70 percent or lower. The consequences have already been discussed.

6) In an overbedded facility, with a nursing registry in the community, a unit's ability to achieve desired performance is heavily dependent on the head nurse's managerial competence. Problem 5 is compounded if the managerially less competent head nurses are on the low occupancy units.

A nursing unit in an overbedded facility, and especially one with a nursing registry in the community, must be able to control its own performance because of the complexity and uncertainty in the assignment of individual nurses to take care of individual patients. Control from the central nursing administration office cannot take this complexity and uncertainty into account. Head nurses in these units can manipulate the assignment of patients into dependency categories in order to obtain whatever number of nursing hours they feel they need. There is essentially no control of this measure of performance unless head nurses are also responsible for achieving a budgeted number of hours per patient day, a desired level of quality, and a ratio of actual to required nursing hours within desired limits. No matter what the central office does to control a unit's performance, the nurses on the unit—and the head nurse in particular—are ultimately responsible for assigning individual nurses to individual patients and justifying the assignment.

## 11.6 OTHER EXAMPLES OF MANPOWER CONTROL SYSTEMS

Each department or cost center needs to control its productivity, just as the nursing units need to control nursing hours per patient day. The measure of productivity is a ratio of resources used per unit of service delivered, or vice versa. The second column of Table 11.4 lists some of the measures reported by the Hospital Administration Services (HAS) (see Wilkins in Additional Reading). We have already provided the background needed to design a system to control man hours used per unit of service delivered in these departments.

The *standard* man hours per unit of service is established using work sampling, continuous observation, subjective estimation, or a combination of the methods. To arrive at the *standard workload,* the standard man hours per unit of service is multiplied by the volume of service. This is compared to actual man hours worked. The difference is sometimes called the *variance,* although the term should not be confused with statistical variance. Table 11.4 illustrates *actual* man hours per unit of services for typical hospital departments reported by Baptist Hospital, Pensacola, Florida; Florida Hospitals; and U.S. Hospitals (see Wilkins). Baptist Hospital has had a productivity incentive program that results in monthly bonus pay to those employees who work in a department where the standard man hours budget is higher than the actual man hours worked. The difference, or hours saved, is multiplied by the entry-level pay rate for the department, divided in half as a way to share the savings with the patients or institution, and divided among the number of full-time-

## Table 11.4

### August 1973 Hospital Administration Services Data

| Department | Productivity Measure | Baptist Hospital | Actual Productivity | |
|---|---|---|---|---|
| | | | Florida Hospitals | U.S. Hospitals |
| Nursing Service | MED/SURG nursing hours per patient day | 4.77 | 5.30 | — |
| Operating Room | Manhours per O.R. visit | 8.05 | 11.44 | 10.44 |
| Laboratory | Tests per manhour | 14.11 | 6.79 | 5.20 |
| Radiology | Manhours per procedure | 1.02 | 1.40 | 1.30 |
| Physical Therapy | Treatments per manhour | 1.73 | 1.23 | 1.24 |
| Medical Records | Manhours per discharge | 1.19 | 2.10 | 2.05 |
| Housekeeping | Manhours per 1000 feet | 33.47 | 44.54 | 42.18 |
| Dietary | Meals served per manhour | 3.35 | 3.35 | 3.40 |

equivalent employees in the department. The use of supplies that the department can control was also included in the bonus pay formula. Further discussion of productivity incentive programs is beyond the scope of this book and the interested reader is referred to Gustafson, Doyle, and May.

The application of the cybernetic control framework to controlling the productivity in these departments is left as an exercise, since the background material has already been presented in this and previous chapters.

We have now considered the knowledge and skill required of an administrator to control the performance of the admitting system, nursing care system, and other hospital departments. We wish to re-emphasize that the administrator must be aware of what this chapter has described about the interrelationships between these systems. One cannot be controlled without considering the others.

In addition, however, the administrator must be aware of how physician control systems, both utilization control and quality control, affect the admitting system, the nursing care system, and ancillary services, and vice versa. The job announcement stated that applicants must have knowledge and skill in setting up systems for physicians to control patient placement in appropriate levels of care, and for physicians to assure the medical necessity of patient services. We will apply the cybernetic control framework to utilization control in the next chapter.

## Exercises

In each of the following questions, two alternatives are presented for the design of a control system. Select the alternative that you believe should be implemented. Justify your selection, applying the six structural requirements and/or the process of cybernetic control.

When deciding the number of nurses to assign to a unit, an assessment is made of the level of need for nursing required by each of the patients on the unit. The patients are categorized into three levels: self care, intermediate care, and intensive care. Each category of patient requires a different number of nursing hours to be assigned to the floor.

11.1 a. The assignment of a patient to one of the three levels of need would be made by the team leader of the nursing team caring for the patient, based on his/her best judgment.

    b.  Using criteria established for assigning patients to one category versus another, the nursing specialist in the staffing department would review the nursing notes and nursing care plans and assign the patient to one of the categories.

11.2  a.  The basis for assigning a patient to one need category versus another would be made using a nursing care plan.

    b.  The basis for assigning a patient to one need category versus another would be made using the medical record and the nurses' notes left at the nursing station.

11.3  a.  In an ancillary department, the comparison of actual expenditures to budgeted expenditures would be made at the end of each month.

    b.  In an ancillary department, the actual expenditures would be compared to the budgeted expenditures on a daily basis.

11.4  a.  The head nurse of a unit would be solely responsible for meeting the budget and would meet with her/his supervisor only once a month to go over the actual expenditures.

    b.  The head nurse of a unit would be solely responsible for meeting the budget and, as actual expenditures were fed back to the head nurse, the head nurse would go to her/his supervisor when a problem occurred in meeting the budget that the head nurse could not solve alone.

11.5  a.  In establishing the standard number of hours per patient day to budget for nurses, a work sampling study was performed.

    b.  In establishing the standard number of hours per patient day to budget for nurses, the head nurse was asked to estimate the time required for the activities of the unit.

11.6  a.  The head nurse would be familiar with his/her unit only and be completely knowledgeable about how nursing time was being spent on the unit.

    b.  The head nurse would spend time in each of the major ancillary departments (X-ray, laboratory, physical therapy, etc.) on a weekly or monthly basis, learning about how these departments are providing service.

11.7  a.  The head nurse would participate in an inservice training program for learning methods of meeting the budget.

    b.  The head nurse would attempt to meet the budget by using her previous experience in managing the unit.

11.8    Design a system to control the productivity of one of the departments (not nursing) listed in Table 11.4 using the cybernetic control framework (structural requirements and process). How would you handle the problem of also controlling the quality of the service?

## Additional Reading

Anthony, R. N. *Planning and Control Systems: A Framework for Analysis.* Boston: Harvard University Press, 1965.

"Examination of Case Studies in Manpower Control Systems." In *Proceedings* of a forum held in Boston, Massachusetts, April 21–22, 1975; Richmond, Va.: National Cooperative Services Center for Hospital Management Engineering.

Griffith, J. R., Hancock, W. M. and Munson, F. C., editors. *Cost Control in Hospitals.* Ann Arbor, Michigan: Health Administration Press, 1976.

Gustafson, D. H., Doyle, J. and May, J. *Incentives for Hospital Employees.* American Hospital Association monograph, U.S. Printing Office, 1972.

Wilkins, M. C. "Productivity in Health Care—A Hospital's Approach." *Collection of Case Studies in Improvements in Productivity.* National Cooperative Services Center for Hospital Management Engineering, 1975.

Wolfe H. and Young, J. P. "Staffing the Nursing Unit, Part I. Controlled Variable Staffing." *Nursing Research* 14 (Summer 1965).

# 12

# Cybernetic Control
# Applied to Patient Management

## 12.1 INTRODUCTION

Administrators and governing boards must ensure that attending physicians within their hospitals are achieving desired performance in patient care systems. It is one of the most complex and uncertain systems they will have to deal with. In prior chapters, we discussed the decision and control frameworks applied to facility management. We ignored *patient* management and assumed that physicians admit patients and continue patient stay in a facility because it is the most economical level of care. We also assumed that physicians order services from the facility that are medically necessary and consistent with professionally recognized standards of care. In this chapter, we will examine the first assumption by applying the cybernetic control framework to the concurrent (before discharge) utilization review (UR) systems that are designed to ensure that patients are in the most economical level of care. We will not deal with the question of whether the services ordered by physicians are medically necessary. Retrospective (after discharge) medical care evaluation studies can be designed and performed to determine whether the services were needed. The cybernetic control framework provides an excellent basis for designing and evaluating these retrospective studies, which are important control processes themselves; but this application of the framework will be left as an exercise.

Possible levels of care, each with its own combination of physician, skilled nursing, and ancillary services, include: acute hospital, surgicenter, hospital-based skilled nursing facility (SNF), freestanding SNF, intermediate-care facility, home health agency, ambulatory care, and home with no care. The level-of-care decision requires the selection of one of these facilities in which to admit or continue the stay of a patient. Since, on any given day, each person receiving medical care may be thought of as receiving a certain level of care, as defined by the combination of physician, skilled nursing, and ancillary services being provided, the level-of-care decision is a matter of matching patients to the facilities that provide their required levels of care. For example, while in an acute facility, one patient might require a level of care available only in that setting, while another might only need a free-standing SNF level of care; a third patient might need a home health agency level of care. The level-of-care decision answers the questions, Are the services that are needed or being received available only in the facility where the patient will be admitted or is now? Are these services available in a less expensive setting?

Our assumption that medical necessity and professionally recognized standards of care will be controlled separately from the level-of-care decision fits well with the organizational structure in most hospitals. Two different medical staff committees are usually established to handle these two functions—the medical audit committees perform retrospective chart review to assess medical necessity while the UR committees perform concurrent reviews to assess appropriate level of care.

## 12.2 CONCURRENT FEEDBACK TO PHYSICIANS ABOUT THEIR LEVEL-OF-CARE DECISIONS

If the concurrent UR system were designed using the cybernetic control framework, it would work as follows (the reader might want to reread Section 2.3). UR coordinators (usually registered nurses or record administrators) would focus on gathering information and providing it to the attending physician—or UR physician if back-up support is required. The control process is diagrammed in Figure 12.1. To determine whether a specific patient is in the desired level of care, UR coordinators would compare explicit levels-of-care criteria to the actual level of care (Box 1). If no problem is found, UR coordinators would acquire information enabling them to forecast if and when problems can be expected to occur (Box 2). The process of comparing the actual to the desired level of care, identifying problems, acquiring information, and anticipating problems would occur within the first two or three days following a patient's admission and whenever follow-up reviews (commonly called continued stay reviews) were made.

UR coordinators would not depend solely on a length-of-stay rule for telling them when to make continued stay reviews; other

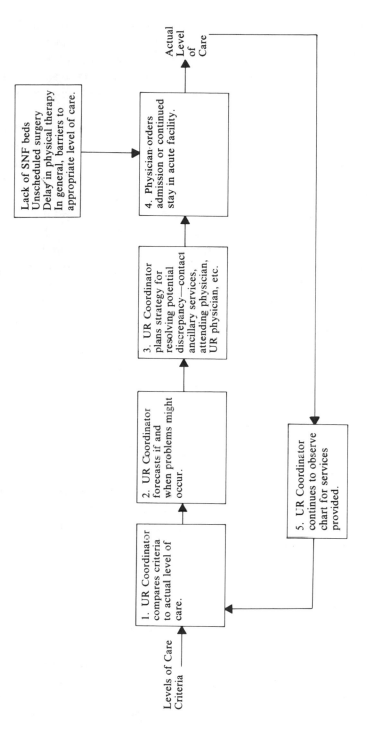

*Figure 12.1*

Concurrent Utilization Review System

Levels of Care Criteria →

1. UR Coordinator compares criteria to actual level of care.

2. UR Coordinator forecasts if and when problems might occur.

3. UR Coordinator plans strategy for resolving potential discrepancy—contact ancillary services, attending physician, UR physician, etc.

Lack of SNF beds
Unscheduled surgery
Delay in physical therapy
In general, barriers to appropriate level of care.

4. Physician orders admission or continued stay in acute facility.

Actual Level of Care

5. UR Coordinator continues to observe chart for services provided.

factors would also trigger their concern—an unscheduled patient admitted for surgery; a patient for whom physical therapy had been ordered but had not been provided; a patient admitted with an unpredictable (from the UR coordinator's standpoint) diagnosis; a patient admitted by a physician who generally admits patients that could be in an SNF, etc.

Whenever a problem arises, UR coordinators would plan a strategy for resolving it (Box 3). They would determine what is responsible for the problem by contacting the attending physician, the floor nurse, the patient, physical therapy, laboratory, radiology, etc. As they obtain this information, coordinators would communicate the effect of the problem to the responsible hospital department.

UR coordinators might also find that the problem is outside the physician's control. For example, this would be true in cases of nonpayment by third parties, lack of SNF beds, or insufficient nursing staff in available SNFs. This information would be fed back to the physician, along with suggestions for solving the problem. UR coordinators could assist physicians in dealing with environmental problems, for example, by documenting the problem's cause in the physician's progress notes. This documentation would then be available in the record so that outside reviewers could see the justification of physicians' decisions (Box 4).

In the process of problem solving, UR coordinators would allow time for the physician or hospital departments to correct the problem. Therefore, they would forecast how long it will take for the problem to be resolved, establish a re-review date, and continue observing the patient's situation to determine whether the desired level-of-care criteria are met (Box 5). If, on the follow-up review, progress has not been made, for whatever reason, and coordinators feel they cannot resolve the problem, they would contact a physician member of the UR Committee. The review physician would act as the UR coordinator's back-up support, assisting the attending physician to meet desired levels-of-care criteria.

The review physician would consult the attending physician and obtain another review physician's advice to determine whether the patient's care should continue to be paid for by the Medicare, Medicaid, or Maternal and Child Health Programs. If review physicians determine that services are not covered, they notify the attending physician. The attending physician might determine that the payment's being covered is not a factor, and that the patient may remain in the hospital and pay his own expenses. (What would you do if you were the hospital administrator?)

By providing feedback (Control Requirement 2) using explicit levels-of-care criteria (Requirement 1), UR coordinators would actually expand the physician care system. Physicians would have the capacity to obtain information in a timely manner about the environment, including factors related to the hospital, the community, and reimbursement for services (Requirement 5). They would also have the capacity to forecast future problems in these areas (Requirement 4). In addition, the coordinators' problem-solving role would help ensure that physicians and patients will find solutions to identified problems (Requirement 3). In this role, coordinators would provide administrator-arranged back-up support rather than strictly external control (Requirement 6).

Like admission scheduling and nurse staffing systems, UR systems also operate differently in overbedded and non-overbedded facilities. In non-overbedded facilities with controlled admissions, UR coordinators would work closely with the admitting department. In order to open beds as soon as possible, thereby reducing cancellations of scheduled patients and waiting time for called-in patients, UR coordinators would review patients more often during their stay and would contact attending physicians if they anticipated a patient could be transferred to a lower level of care. In overbedded facilities, UR coordinators would apply the levels-of-care criteria and obtain a count of the percent of patient days that could have occurred in SNFs. This would provide part of the information necessary for deciding whether to convert acute beds to SNF beds. In addition, UR coordinators would keep track of where patients are transferred and whether any could remain in an acute-based SNF. Because overbedded facilities present no urgent need to obtain beds, coordinators have more time to work on the systemic problems that prevent appropriate patient placement.

Whether the facility is overbedded or not, when an acute-based SNF, a self-care unit, an intermediate-care unit, or an intensive-care unit already exists within the acute facility, UR coordinators would also provide feedback to attending physicians about the appropriate placement of patients in these units.

## 12.3 ADMINISTRATOR'S ROLE IN CONTROLLING PHYSICIANS' DECISIONS

Recall the administrator's role in controlling any system. The hospital administrator designed the satellite outpatient clinic to regulate itself. To achieve self-regulation, the *clinic* administrator needed (1) explicit measures and desired levels of performance, (2) feedback on actual performance, (3) the ability to solve problems, (4) the ability to forecast future events, (5) the ability to learn about the clinic's environment, and (6) back-up support when the clinic could not achieve desired performance.

The clinic had to regulate itself because the hospital administrator could not control the clinic without becoming a part of it—in which case, the administrator could not attend to other hospital subsystems. The clinic is too complex and uncertain to control entirely from outside the clinic. Rules provided by the hospital administrator for the clinic administrator to follow would, in general, be too simplistic and deterministic to cover the clinic's complexity and uncertainty.

Likewise, attending physicians have to regulate their own performance because UR physicians could not treat the patient without becoming a consultant (without becoming part of the system)—in which case, the UR physicians could not attend to their own patients. Furthermore, any diagnostic or therapeutic rules written by the UR committee for the attending physician to follow would naturally be too simplistic and deterministic to cope with the complexity and uncertainty of the patient's physical, psychological, social, and economic condition. Certainly rules could be written, but the physician would soon have to abandon them when an unanticipated change in the patient's condition occurred.

The administrator's role is to provide support so that attending physicians can regulate their own performance. Provisions need to be made so that each of the six structural requirements for control exist and the control process can operate. Regardless of whether the administrator is a physician or not, he should make arrangements for medical back-up support, and should provide administrative or facility management back-up support when needed. Not all problems that keep physicians from transferring their patients to the most economical level of care are medical.

What type of assistance should administrators provide to physicians within hospitals? The answer should be based on the application of the cybernetic control framework. As seen above, the framework for controlling physicians' decisions is no different than for controlling satellite outpatient clinics, nursing units, patient admissions, or any of the other subsystems within a facility. Arrangements should be made so that attending physicians can control their own performance, with back-up support when they need it.

Application of the cybernetic control framework leads to the following crucial areas in which physicians require support from the administrator:

1. The cybernetic control framework and the concept of self-regulating systems are not explicitly understood by physicians, although many understand them implicitly. Medical staffs need support to design concurrent review systems that will support attending physicians as described in Section 12.2.

2. Physicians need support to construct explicit measures of performance, i.e., to make their decision criteria explicit (Control Requirement 1).

3. Administrators must make arrangements for feedback to attending physicians about actual performance (Requirement 2). For retrospective medical care evaluation studies, this support usually comes from personnel in the medical records department and computerized medical record abstracting services such as the Professional Activity Study—Medical Audit Program (PAS-MAP) or the California Health Data Corporation (CHDC). For concurrent feedback to individual physicians, this support comes from UR coordinators. The UR coordinator's role, designed by application of the cybernetic control framework, needs to be made explicit for the UR committee.

4. Because physicians are part of the medical care system, they tend to start (remember the where-to-start megaproblem) solving problems from their limited view of the system. Physicians therefore need support in order to see how other systems affect their system's performance (Requirement 5). In addition, when the problem lies within their system, physicians need support to analyze decisions (Requirement 3). Physicians are experts in making decisions about controlling patients' conditions, not in making decisions about controlling medical care delivery systems.

5. Physicians need support to forecast the medical care system's performance (Requirement 4). Again, they are experienced in anticipating changes in patient conditions or their own personal physician care system, not in anticipating changes in medical care delivery systems.

6. Physicians need support to keep track of the medical care system's environment (Requirement 5), such as other health resources available in the community, insurance coverage under Medicare and Medicaid, PROs, Health Systems Agencies, etc.

What may be surprising is that practicing physicians in hospitals will often seek back-up support if such support is available. It is crucial, therefore, for administrators to be able to provide it.

We will now discuss two specific examples of back-up support: the application of the decision framework to develop levels-of-care criteria (Control Requirement 1), and the identification of barriers to achieving desired performance (Control Requirement 5). We have already presented (in Section 12.2) the feedback strategy used by the UR coordinator in a cybernetic UR system, and we will describe its evaluation in Section 12.7.

Before going into more detail, a brief description of current legislation and the resulting regulations in this area is necessary. However, our purpose is to illustrate the application of the control framework, to report the results of its application, and to provide an approach to dealing with the complexity and uncertainty inherent in controlling patient management. Legislation and regulations will undoubtedly be altered; so their description should not be viewed as a statement of the problem, but as a response to a general problem— how to control physicians' management of patients' conditions when they use services provided by a medical facility.

## 12.4 FEDERAL REQUIREMENTS FOR CONTROLLING PHYSICIANS' DECISIONS

Public Law 92–603, the Social Security Amendments of 1972, provided for the establishment of a national system of medical peer review conducted through regionally based Professional Standards Review Organizations (PSROs). Overall, the PSRO objective was to assure that health services paid for under Medicare, Medicaid, or Maternal and Child Health Programs were appropriate (medically necessary and consistent with professionally recognized standards of care) and were provided at the most economical level of care.

Sections 141 through 150 of P.L. 97-248 (TEFRA) repealed the existing PSRO provisions and established a utilization and quality control peer review program under Sections 1151–1163. The new program defines a peer review organization (PRO) as an entity which is either composed of a substantial number of licensed doctors of medicine and osteopathy, or has access to these persons so that adequate peer review of the professional activities of physicians, other practitioners, and institutional and noninstitutional providers takes place. The review is to focus on the necessity and reasonableness of care, quality of care, and appropriateness of the setting. The determinations as to whether benefits for services are paid will be binding.

As of this printing, the final program regulations have not yet been promulgated, nor has the program been implemented. The PSROs as they existed prior to TEFRA still exist—for the time being—and are therefore discussed in detail in this chapter. The reader should stay abreast of the new regulations as they become available.

In March 1974, the country was divided into 203 PSRO areas, each consisting of at least 300 physicians. These regional PSROs concentrate on controlling medical services in the acute hospitals within their areas. As established by the 1965 Medicare legislation, each acute hospital in the country has a medical staff committee referred to as the UR committee. These committees usually consist of eight to twelve physicians and other, nonvoting members, such as hospital administrators, medical record administrators, discharge planners and nursing personnel. Each PSRO is to delegate its control function to these UR committees whenever the committees meet certain measures of performance. Each committee or, when a committee has not been so delegated, the regional PSRO itself, must perform review activities to assure that physicians within their area are providing services appropriate to each patient's problem or diagnosis, and that each patient is located in the appropriate level of care.

According to the *PSRO Manual,* there are several review activities that must be performed for each facility; these include certification upon admission, continued stay review, and medical care evaluation studies.

On-admission certification is performed to assure that patients requiring acute care are admitted to an acute facility; that care being provided at the acute care level cannot be provided at a lower level of care (SNF, home health care, or outpatient clinic); that admissions are not inappropriately delayed; that a diagnosis-specific or problem-specific length of stay review date is assigned to perform the continued stay review; and that discharge planning is begun as soon as possible after admission. Medically necessary admissions are assigned a length of stay, and Medicare, Medicaid, or Maternal and Child Health payments stop on that day unless the admission is recertified. When an admission is determined to be medically unnecessary, the physician in charge is to be so notified by the UR physician shortly after admission.

Continued stay reviews are performed during a patient's hospital stay to assure that the services the patient is receiving can still only be provided by the acute hospital; that the patient is receiving care necessary for his/her condition; that services are delivered at the appropriate times; that discharge planning is being carried out; and that data are collected for medical care evaluation studies. These reviews are to be performed for patients on or before the review date assigned on admission.

Medical care evaluation studies are retrospective reviews of patients' charts performed to assure that services provided by the medical staff are necessary and meet quality standards, and that the facility is providing the services on a timely basis. According to the *Manual*, at least one such study must be in progress in each hospital at all times, although the number is likely to increase.

Regarding reimbursement to hospitals for Medicare, Medicaid, or Maternal and Child Health patients, any determination made by the PSRO is binding on the institution, the attending physician, and the Medicare or Medicaid intermediary (the fiscal agent contracted by the Federal Government to process claims). Therefore, PSROs or their delegated hospital committees also control what will and will not be paid for under these programs.

The concept of "level of care" is not new. Medicaid programs which provide coverage for various types of nursing facilities (including home health agencies) have understood that these facilities may be defined by the services they provide, and that the "appropriate location" for an individual patient is the most economical facility that can still provide the sufficient types and amounts of services (level of care) needed by that patient. In the Medicare program, the legal determinant for reimbursement for continued hospital stay has always been the level of care that is medically needed by the patient.

PSROs are responsible for ensuring that hospital UR systems perform effectively, and they are expected to extend their responsibility gradually to SNF and ambulatory care review systems. In order to fulfill this mandate, PSROs have to measure the performance of UR systems, identify facilities that are having problems, and recommend changes for improving their effectiveness. One measure of performance is the appropriateness of the UR committee's decisions to grant or deny admissions and continued stays.

Medicare intermediaries have been required by the Social Security Administration to use a measure of performance that is typically calculated as the percent of Medicare patient days submitted for payment by the facility but deemed inappropriate by the intermediary. Note that this is only a partial measure of inappropriate days, since patient days that have been denied by the UR committee but would have been approved by the Medicare intermediary would also be considered inappropriate. Nevertheless, the level-of-care decision is a basis for measuring the performance of the UR systems, and, therefore, the performance of individual physicians.

## 12.5 LEVELS-OF-CARE DECISION

According to federal regulations, concurrent utilization review in acute hospitals must be performed with reference to explicit, written review criteria. UR physicians as well as UR coordinators must refer to these review criteria before making a recommendation (in the case of a coordinator) or decision (in the case of a UR physician) as to whether further stay in the hospital is medically justified. Example sets of diagnosis-specific or problem-specific criteria for review of admission and continued hospital stay have been developed. However, a serious drawback to these criteria is that they are not formulated so that a decision between an acute facility, SNF, or home health care can be made. Recall Step 1 of the decision framework. After identifying the objectives to be served, the available alternatives need to be identified. The decision to admit or continue the stay of a patient in an acute facility depends on whether the needed services can be obtained at an *alternative* level of care. Therefore, criteria for acute hospitals must include levels-of-care criteria for admission to, or continued stay in, SNFs and home health care as well.

There are two major kinds of written review criteria—*diagnosis-specific* criteria, sometimes called problem-specific, and *facility-specific* criteria. In general, most efforts at criteria development have been directed toward the construction of sets of criteria on a diagnosis/problem-specific basis. For example, the major national medical specialty societies have worked on such model sets through a government contract with the American Medical Association (AMA). On the AMA list, physician orders thought necessary to achieve desired outcomes are often referred to as *process* criteria. Process criteria are broken down further into physician orders and patient conditions required to justify a *diagnosis*, physician orders appropriate to *treatment*, physician orders and patient conditions required to justify *admission* to acute facilities, and physician orders and patient conditions required to extend *length of stay* in acute facilities beyond the 50th percentile for this diagnosis.

These sets, in addition to containing diagnosis/problem-specific model criteria for use in performing medical care evaluation studies, are also intended for use in concurrent review. Figure 12.2 provides an example of diagnosis-specific criteria for justifying admission and continued stay for patients with asthma.

It is assumed by some that review criteria specific to the diagnosis or problem under review will, when available, always take precedence over the facility-specific criteria. What the AMA criteria overlook, however, is that the diagnosis-specific criteria are not yet formulated so that a decision between a hospital, SNF, or home health agency *can* be made. These criteria provide indicators for admission and continued stay in an *acute* hospital, but compared to where else? What are the indicators for admission and continued stay in SNFs or the indicators for home health visits for these same diagnoses?

Figures 12.3 and 12.4 contain the facility-specific levels-of-care criteria for coverage in the Medicare program. These criteria have been extracted and, for the most part, directly quoted from the UR regulations of September 24, 1975. These will no doubt be modified and should be viewed as illustrative only. In Figure 12.3, the criteria are displayed in a flow sheet to facilitate deciding in which of the three levels of care recognized by the Medicare program—acute hospital, SNF, or home health—a patient is appropriately located. Figure 12.4 contains questions that, when applied to corresponding footnoted items in Figure 12.3, clarify the meaning of these items.

Although the Medicare criteria provide the basis for deciding between alternative levels of care, they are currently deficient in several respects. First, they fail to consider the difference in skilled nursing and rehabilitative services available in a hospital and in an SNF. Although the constant availability of a nurse can be provided in an SNF as well as in a hospital, there is often inadequate staffing in an SNF to provide the level of care needed by patients. Thus, the patient's nursing needs, measured by the number of required nursing hours per day, must be assessed before transferring the patient to an SNF. The Medicare program does not formally take this distinction into account, and implies that the same skilled nursing services that are provided in a hospital can also be provided in an SNF.

The second, and more serious, deficiency of these Medicare criteria is the lack of any listing of the medical services provided by a hospital and not provided by an SNF. A program officer of the Bureau of Health Insurance in the Social Security Administration said in a letter:

> The Social Security Administration does not use listings which itemize those medical services peculiar to hospitals and those indigenous to skilled nursing facilities . . . In considering any given medical-service

## Figure 12.2

### AMA Diagnosis Specific Criteria for Asthma

The information under the following criteria elements will be used for *concurrent screening for admission certification and continued stay review* for individual patient charts:

I. JUSTIFICATION FOR ADMISSION
   A. Failure of patient to obtain sustained relief by outpatient therapy with bronchodilator drugs
   B. Status asthmaticus
   C. Pulmonary complications
   D. Suspicion of or diagnosis of associated medical problems complicating management of Asthma
   E. Preparation of asthmatic patient for elective surgery

II. LENGTH OF STAY
   A. *Initial Length of Stay Assignment for Primary Diagnosis or Problem* (numerical determinations to be established locally based on statistical norms)
   B. *Extended Length of Stay Assignment* (numerical determinations to be established based on the individual patient's condition at the end of the initial length of stay period)
      1. Reasons for Extending the Initial Length of Stay
         a. Failure to respond to initial therapy
         b. Pulmonary complications (e.g., respiratory insufficiency as defined by significant hypoxia or hypercapnea, atelectasis, pneumothorax)
         c. Persistent fever or infection
         d. Tracheostomy
         e. Adverse reactions to therapy

The information under the following criteria elements *could be used in concurrent review* if desired by a local PSRO and within its capability; however, their primary use is for screening in the *retrospective evaluation of medical care:*

III. VALIDATION OF:
   A. Diagnosis
      1. Documentation of characteristic historical features (e.g., persistent or recurrent tight chest, dyspnea, wheezing), or
      2. Characteristic physical findings (e.g., wheezing and labored breathing or tachypnea with prolonged expiratory phase with or without distant breath sounds
   B. Reasons for Admission
      1. Wheezing and dyspnea, unimproved or recurrent despite therapy (IA, B)
      2. Chest x-ray characteristic of pulmonary infection, pneumothorax, or atelectasis (IC)
      3. Arterial blood gases characteristic of hypoxia and hypercapnea (IC)
      4. Wheezing and dyspnea plus evidence of associated medical or surgical disease (e.g., cardiac or unfavorable reactions to medication, preparation for elective surgery) (I.D and I.E)

IV. CRITICAL DIAGNOSTIC AND THERAPEUTIC SERVICES

|  | Screening Benchmark |
| --- | --- |
| A. Administration of bronchodilators | 100% |
| B. Chest x-ray during this acute illness | 100% |
| C. Administration of narcotics (except for the purpose of preoperative medication or in patients who are undergoing controlled ventilation) | 0% |

SOURCE: American Medical Association, *Model Screening Criteria to Assist Professional Standards Review Organizations,* AMA, 535 North Dearborn Street, Chicago, Illinois 60610.

## Figure 12.3

### Medicare Levels of Care Criteria

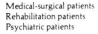

Medical-surgical patients
Rehabilitation patients
Psychiatric patients

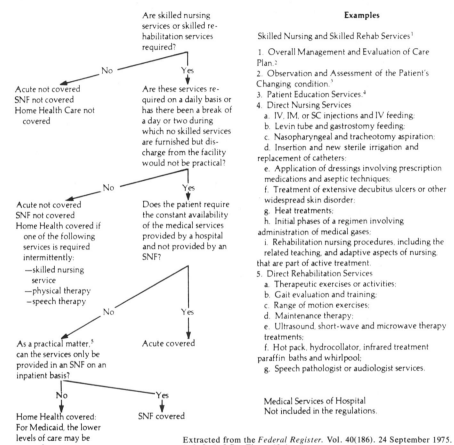

Are skilled nursing services or skilled rehabilitation services required?

No — Yes

Acute not covered
SNF not covered
Home Health Care not covered

Are these services required on a daily basis or has there been a break of a day or two during which no skilled services are furnished but discharge from the facility would not be practical?

No — Yes

Acute not covered
SNF not covered
Home Health covered if one of the following services is required intermittently:
—skilled nursing service
—physical therapy
—speech therapy

Does the patient require the constant availability of the medical services provided by a hospital and not provided by an SNF?

No — Yes

As a practical matter,[5] can the services only be provided in an SNF on an inpatient basis?

Acute covered

No — Yes

Home Health covered:
For Medicaid, the lower levels of care may be covered.

SNF covered

**Examples**

Skilled Nursing and Skilled Rehab Services[1]

1. Overall Management and Evaluation of Care Plan.[2]
2. Observation and Assessment of the Patient's Changing condition.[3]
3. Patient Education Services.[4]
4. Direct Nursing Services
   a. IV, IM, or SC injections and IV feeding;
   b. Levin tube and gastrostomy feeding;
   c. Nasopharyngeal and tracheotomy aspiration;
   d. Insertion and new sterile irrigation and replacement of catheters;
   e. Application of dressings involving prescription medications and aseptic techniques;
   f. Treatment of extensive decubitus ulcers or other widespread skin disorder;
   g. Heat treatments;
   h. Initial phases of a regimen involving administration of medical gases;
   i. Rehabilitation nursing procedures, including the related teaching, and adaptive aspects of nursing, that are part of active treatment.
5. Direct Rehabilitation Services
   a. Therapeutic exercises or activities;
   b. Gait evaluation and training;
   c. Range of motion exercises;
   d. Maintenance therapy;
   e. Ultrasound, short-wave and microwave therapy treatments;
   f. Hot pack, hydrocollator, infrared treatment paraffin baths and whirlpool;
   g. Speech pathologist or audiologist services.

Medical Services of Hospital
Not included in the regulations.

Extracted from the *Federal Register*. Vol. 40(186). 24 September 1975.
1, 2, 3, 4, 5 See Figure 12.4

issue, the Central Office examines it individually—as it arises—by determining whether the service in question is ordinarily rendered by hospitals as a class and/or by skilled nursing facilities as a class.

This explanation is not very helpful, because hospitals as a class do not provide the same services—ambulatory surgery is a good example; and SNFs as a class do not provide the same services— intravenous therapy is a good example. It is important, therefore, for hospital UR Committees to develop new criteria that specify

## Figure 12.4

### Clarifying Concepts for Medicare Levels of Care Criteria

(Numbers refer to footnotes in Figure 12.3)

1. Skilled Nursing or Skilled Rehabilitation Services

    Is the inherent complexity of a service prescribed for a patient such that it can be safely and/or effectively performed only by or under the supervision of technically or professionally trained nursing or rehabilitation personnel (e.g., registered nurse, licensed practical (vocational) nurse, physical therapist, occupational therapist, speech pathologist, audiologist)?

2. Overall Management and Evaluation of Care Plan

    Does the patient's overall physical or mental condition support a finding that his recovery and/or safety could be assured only if the total care he/she requires (including only a variety of unskilled services) is planned or managed by nursing or rehabilitation personnel?

3. Observation and Assessment of the Patient's Changing Condition

    Are the skills of a nurse or other professional person (rehabilitation, psychiatric) required to identify and evaluate the patient's need for possible modification of treatment and the initiation of additional medical procedures?

4. Patient Education Services

    Are technically or professionally trained nursing or rehabilitation personnel required to teach a patient self-maintenance?

5. Practical Matter

    Is the needed skilled service not available in the area in which the patient resides, and would it be an excessive physical hardship to transport him/her to the closest facility furnishing such services?

    Is it more economical or more efficient to provide skilled services in the institutional setting?

    Note: The availability of funds to pay for the services furnished by available alternative facilities is not a factor to be used in deciding whether, as a practical matter, the service can only be provided on an inpatient basis.

SOURCE: *Federal Register,* Vol. 40 (186), September 24, 1975.

the services their hospitals provide that are not provided in available SNFs.

**Problem:** A UR Committee has decided to develop its own facility-specific criteria. What process should the Committee use to generate the criteria?

To illustrate the use of the nominal group and delphi techniques discussed in Chapter 9, we will describe the development of explicit levels of care criteria in three California hospitals.* For two of the committees, the process was accomplished by the delphi technique,

*This study was first reported in Holloway, D. C., et al., "Development of Hospital Levels of Care Criteria," *Health Care Management Review,* Summer 1976.

which procured physician opinion by mail without requiring time-consuming meetings. For the third committee, the nominal group technique was used, in which each member attending the meeting acted silently and independently and was forced to withhold his evaluations of the criteria until all criteria were recorded. Texts of letters used in the delphi technique appear in Figures 12.5, 12.6 and 12.7.

In the first round at each of the three hospitals, each UR physician was asked, What services should a patient be receiving or have available in order to justify acute hospitalization? Facility-specific levels-of-care criteria and diagnosis/problem-specific criteria were clearly distinguished for the participants. It was indicated that levels-of-care-criteria specify those services a patient is or will be receiving that require *location* in an acute hospital; diagnostic/problem-specific criteria specify those services or care elements a patient *should receive* as a function of diagnosis and medical problem. Physicians on the committee were asked to assume that patients were receiving appropriate services for their diagnosis/problem, and to concentrate on which of those services require the patient to be in an acute facility.

The responses to the questions, compiled into a master list, were briefly discussed at the next regular UR Committee meeting. The master list was then returned to the physicians on the Committee so that they could add or delete from the list. Thus, they had feedback on the criteria their peers considered important, and they also had an opportunity to submit criteria they may have overlooked during the first round.

The responses and comments of the previous round were again collected in the third round and compiled into a second master list. This list was discussed at the next UR Committee meeting and returned to the physicians for their revision.

The fourth round entailed collecting the responses from round three and gathering the physicians together for a meeting, during which their responses, which composed the third and final master list, were thoroughly discussed. The end product at each of the three hospitals was an aggregated list of explicit criteria that provided the basis for justification of acute hospitalization. Figure 12.8 presents the explicit criteria lists for the three hospitals.

The three sets of hospital-developed criteria are remarkably similar. For example, under physician services, each hospital indicated, although it was stated somewhat differently, that one criterion for hospitalization in an acute facility was frequent physician visits. Under medical services available only in an acute facility, all three hospitals mentioned the operating room and surgical procedures. Also,

## Figure 12.5

### Example of First-Round Delphi Letter

Dear Doctor:

At the meeting of May 10, it was decided that an effort should be mounted to develop criteria outlining appropriate hospital utilization, and that in order to streamline this effort a process called the *delphi technique* should be used.

The delphi technique was developed several years ago as a method for obtaining the opinion of a group of experts on a particular matter without requiring time-consuming meetings. Additionally, it has been empirically demonstrated that the technique produces more comprehensive criteria than unstructured face-to-face meetings produce.

The first step of the delphi technique is sending this letter and the attached questionnaire. Its purpose is to obtain criteria from you that you feel are important in deciding whether or not a patient should be admitted or continued in an acute facility. In this regard, it is important that the distinction between utilization review criteria and medical audit criteria be clearly understood. U.R. criteria should specify those services that a patient is or will be receiving that require him to be in the acute hospital. Medical audit criteria specify those services or care elements a patient should receive as a function of his diagnosis and medical problem. Since the emphasis of this committee is on U.R., you should assume that patients are receiving appropriate services and should concentrate on which of these services require the patient to be in an acute facility.

The second step of the delphi technique will take place after we receive your responses to this round. Your individual lists of criteria will be combined into a single master list and resubmitted to you for your consideration and the opportunity to add or delete items that in your judgment should or should not be included. This will provide you with feedback on the first round and allow you the opportunity to submit criteria which you may have initially overlooked. The amended lists will be returned to us and we will again combine individual responses and return a new master list to you. The third step of the delphi technique will be to reconsider the list. After this, the committee will reconvene and discuss the results.

This round-robin process generates criteria that are an aggregate of committee members' best judgment. However, it requires your best effort and prompt response. For this reason, please complete the attached questionnaire and return it by Monday, June 4th. If it is easier for you, you may dictate it to central dictating.

We hope this technique meets with your approval and invite you to contact us if you have any questions.

Sincerely,

although there do exist several criteria that are not identical on all hospitals' lists, the basic facility-specific concepts are present in each. Developing levels-of-care criteria in this manner highlighted and made explicit the specific services which cause disagreement about the appropriate level of care for patients.

The three sets of criteria presented are real products of functioning hospital UR committees. These criteria represent a significant improvement over the general levels-of-care framework of the Medicare

## *Figure 12.6*

## *Example of Second-Round Delphi Letter*

Dear Doctor:

The attached sheets comprise the second round of the delphi process to generate "Criteria for Acute Hospitalization." On the first round, you were asked to list criteria that the Utilization Review Committee should use in deciding whether a patient requires an acute facility or could be cared for elsewhere. The response rate to the first round was 60% and after duplicate responses were eliminated the yield was 30 tentative criteria.

After analyzing these tentative criteria we found that they seemed to fall naturally into four basic categories related to (1) physician services (2) nursing services (3) hospital facilities and (4) barriers to transferring or discharging patients. In preparing round two, we felt it appropriate to pursue the generation of criteria within that framework. On the attached sheets you will notice that a new question has been formulated for each of these categories, and that your responses to round one have been transformed into declarative statements and arrayed under the appropriate question. To make sure we have not misrepresented your thoughts in this transformation, please use the comments column to make corrections.

Given this categorization, you are now asked to add, delete, or modify criteria for each category. Since some of the criteria did not fit nicely into one of these four categories, and since you may have a criterion that you don't think fits into one of these four, the last page provides a list of the other criteria for you to add to, subtract from, or modify.

We feel that a major reason for the low response rate to the first round was confusion as to how, where, and when you were to respond. For this reason, we ask that you send responses to the Utilization Review Coordinator by placing them in the enclosed envelope. Please respond by Friday, June 29, so that we may analyze the results of this questionnaire in time for the next meeting of this special committee. A more immediate response, if it is possible, would help us even more.

Thank you for your participation.

Sincerely,

criteria because they provide the specificity necessary to make consistent decisions in concurrent UR. This ability to make consistent decisions, based on good criteria, will make it easier for UR committee physicians when defending difficult decisions to their peers or to fiscal intermediaries, and will provide a broader decision-making base than committee members' personal judgment.

Furthermore, UR physicians and UR coordinators who use facility-specific criteria indicate that diagnosis-specific criteria will have to include criteria for admission and continued stays in SNFs and home health agencies, as well as hospitals, or reviewers will be forced to apply their own *implicit* levels-of-care criteria.

## Figure 12.7

### Example of Third-Round Delphi Letter

Dear Doctor:

During our meeting of July 17, the Special Utilization Review Committee decided to comment once more on the proposed screening criteria. Accordingly, enclosed is another copy of these criteria. Please note that the comments elicited from the last round of the delphi process appear in summary form in the comments column. We thought these summaries would be helpful to you in responding during this third round. Since many of the criteria have conflicting comments, we are particularly interested in how you would resolve those conflicts.

In addition, two important points were agreed upon during our July 17 meeting which may bear on your responses to this round.

1. These criteria are *screening* criteria to be used by the UR Coordinator in determining which cases to bring to the attention of the utilization review physician; however, the ultimate responsibility for deciding whether a patient is in the appropriate location belongs to the physician.

2. Once the screening criteria are finalized, the UR coordinator will use them to review a sample of patients, not for decision-making purposes, but to evaluate the criteria by identifying the reason for and frequency of exceptions to the criteria.

We are certainly gratified by the exceptionally high number of responses to the last round in the delphi process and hope that you will continue your interest in and support of this important matter.

I am enclosing an envelope, addressed to the UR Coordinator, for you to use in returning your comments. Please send your responses by Friday, July 27.

Sincerely,

## Figure 12.8

### Committee-Developed Levels of Care Criteria for Acute Facility

| | | Hospital 1 | Hospital 2 | Hospital 3 |
|---|---|---|---|---|
| I. | Physician Services | 1. Frequent physician attendance and decision making | 1. Specific requirement for daily visits, e.g., situations requiring physician skills to observe, evaluate & adjust orders | 1. Daily or frequent physician visits & observation |
| | | | 2. Examinations & orders for treatment during pre-operative period of stay | |
| II. | Skilled Nursing Services | 1. Continuous availability of nurses for decision making & intermittent observation, incl. but not limited to: | | 1. Observing patients' unstable (or potentially unstable) conditions, such as but not limited to: |

## *Figure 12.8 (Continued)*

| Hospital 1 | Hospital 2 | Hospital 3 |
|---|---|---|
| a. where potentially dangerous drugs or drug combinations are being used | | a. uncontrolled diabetes |
| b. where patient is acutely ill | 1. Observe and control bleeding | b. uncontrolled hypertension requiring changing medications and/or monitoring |
| c. where complex diagnostic or therapeutic procedures are being done | 2. Treatment services requiring frequent or repeated observation of vital signs and/or signs of progress | |
| d. where pre- and post-surgical management is provided | 3. Observation during pre-operative period of stay | |
| | 4. Post-operative nursing care | |
| | | c. correction of electrolyte imbalance (acute) |
| | | d. injuries coupled with any other criteria |
| | | e. infections coupled with any other criteria |
| 2. Frequent skilled nursing services including, but not limited to: | | 2. Diagnostic & therapeutic procedures for unstable (or potentially unstable) conditions such as: |
| a. IM medications | 5. Administration (oral or parenteral) of medications that require observations for severe side-effects, reactions, allergies | a. parenteral medications |
| b. inhalation therapy & urgent administration of oxygen | | |
| c. IV therapy | 6. Transfusions & IVs with medication | b. intravenous fluids |
| | | c. blood transfusions requiring observation |
| d. teaching management of post-surgical appliances, medication regiments, & special diets | 7. Teaching procedures for self-care to patients | d. patient education when frequent or complicated instruction required, e.g., inhalation therapy, special diets, diabetes |
| e. specialized procedures, e.g., suctioning, postural drainage, compresses, frequent dressing changes, etc. | 8. Therapeutic catheterization<br>9. Assisted ventilation<br>10. Respiratory therapy (e.g., postural drainage & PT of chest) | e. endotracheal airway & pulmonary assistance |

*Figure 12.8 (Continued)*

| | Hospital 1 | Hospital 2 | Hospital 3 |
|---|---|---|---|
| | f. cardiac resuscitation<br>g. pulmonary therapy (when done by nurse) | 11. Intensive care or coronary care nursing<br>12. Specialized nursing care (e.g., cardiac, rehab., dialysis) | f. ICU<br>g. CCU<br>h. respiratory ICU<br><br>3. Obstetrical care:<br>a. antenatal complications<br>b. delivery<br>c. post partum care<br>d. newborn care |
| III. Medical Services Only Available in Acute Facility | 1. Surgical procedures usually (agreed upon by committee) performed in acute hospital operating room<br><br>2. Medical procedures usually (agreed upon by committee) performed in acute hospital | 1. Operating room & equipment<br><br>2. Specialized procedures, e.g., surgery, cut-down<br><br>3. Infectious disease procedure-isolation & reverse isolation<br>4. Diagnostic services that are complicated & require skilled observation or procedures by physician (e.g., liver biopsy) | 1. Surgery or major anesthesia (general or spinal)<br><br>2. Diagnostic tests, therapeutic procedures & medications which are dangerous (or potentially dangerous) such as:<br>a. heavy sedation<br>b. monitoring<br>c. antagonistic drugs |
| | 3. Group of diagnostic tests or procedures that would take too long to perform on outpatient basis for reasons such as, but not limited to:<br><br>a. group of tests & procedures are too complex | 5. Diagnostic services that are complicated or prolonged if performed by outpatient department-cases that make access to post-test bed rest & observation mandatory or cases which require special continued assistance by nurses or physician (e.g., cardiac catheterization) | 3. Multiple diagnostic procedures requiring scheduling too intense & complexity too great for outside hospital, e.g., carotid, lumbar, & femoral arteriography; pneumoencephalography |
| | b. patient's condition is fragile & complications would be likely to occur | 6. Observation for change in physical or behavioral state that would pose a threat to patient or others & would require availability of immediate response by emergency team (e.g., code blue) | |

## Figure 12.8 (Continued)

| | Hospital 1 | Hospital 2 | Hospital 3 |
|---|---|---|---|
| | c. adequate diagnostic testing of present disease process | | |
| | d. patient's condition is too fragile for conducting diagnostic tests as outpatient because complications would be likely to occur | | 4. Radiation therapy for unstable patients<br>5. Daily laboratory work on unstable conditions<br>6. Traction for acute condition or acute exacerbation of chronic problem |
| | 4. Test or procedures that cannot be performed outside acute hospital (machinery or personnel not available) | | |
| IV. Rehabilitation Services | | 1. Rehabilitation requiring a multidisciplinary approach<br>2. Intensive therapy or rehabilitation-two or more sessions daily | 1. Initial rehabilitation efforts |
| V. Psychiatric Services | 1. Patient requires a combination of two of the following:<br>a. psychotherapy by the attending physician<br>b. hospital drug management, e.g., Tricyclics, Phenothiazines, or lithium<br>c. shock therapy<br>d. intensive group therapy<br>2. Patient requires services for the purpose of diagnostic study and/or services to reduce or control the patient's psychotic or neurotic symptoms necessitating hospitalization | 1. Environmental control for patients with acute problem (psych.) | 1. Acute psychiatric care, overdose, self-inflicted injuries, conversion reaction, psychiatric problems which present as organic problems |
| VI. Barriers to Above Criteria | 1. Acute hospital environment for reasons such as, but not limited to:<br>a. patient must be removed from social environment | | 1. Social & environmental factors:<br><br>a. condition requiring more complete bedrest than at home |

*Figure 12.8 (Continued)*

| Hospital 1 | Hospital 2 | Hospital 3 |
|---|---|---|
| b. patient is un-cooperative with diagnostic or therapeutic program | | b. patient uncoop-erative on outside |
| a. condition requir-ing more com-plete bedrest than at home | | c. outpatient pre-supposes stable home environment |
| b. patient uncoop-erative on outside | | |
| c. outpatient pre-supposes stable home environ-ment | | |
| 2. Socio-economic factors inhibit dis-charge or transfer, including, but not limited to: | | |
| a. type of insurance coverage | | |
| b. unable to cope by self in facili-ties other than acute hospital | | |
| c. no beds available elsewhere | | |
| d. family unable to care for patient | | |
| e. hospitalization necessary be-cause of 3-day rule prior to transfer to a skilled nursing facility | | |
| 3. Patient is terminal and it is appropri-ate to keep him/her in the acute facility for at most 14 days for humanitarian reasons | | |
| 4. The number of skilled nursing hours needed per patient is a number available in a hospi-tal, but not in an SNF, to perform di-rect services, ob-servation, and decision making | | |
| 5. Patient is conva-lescing from an ill-ness and it is anticipated that his/her stay in a skilled nursing facility would be less than 72 hours | | |

## 12.6 BARRIERS TO PLACING PATIENTS IN APPROPRIATE LEVELS OF CARE

According to the cybernetic control framework, once a discrepancy between a patient's desirable level of care, using criteria like those described above, and his actual level of care is discovered, the cause of the discrepancy needs to be identified. How often are patients not placed in the desired level of care for their needs? What types of barriers to placing patients in desired levels of care occur? How often is the patient, physician, facility, or environment responsible for inappropriate placement of patients? We will illustrate possible answers to these questions by reporting results obtained by studying a random sample of patients in one hospital (first reported in Restuccia and Holloway: see Additional Reading). The method illustrates an approach any hospital can take.

Answers to these questions help establish priorities in allocating resources within a facility for reducing the discrepancy between actual and desired placement of patients. Feedback could be given to the attending physician and/or patient, resulting in their solving the problem; or back-up support could be provided by the administrator so that facility-related problems can be solved; or the physician and administrator could work at changing the environment and/or at understanding and anticipating change in the environment if they cannot change it.

If PROs expect to meet their objective of assuring the appropriate use of health resources, they must be able to determine when and why health resources are misutilized so that corrective action may be taken. Since knowing if and why health resources are being misutilized is necessary for planning additional services, planning agencies could also use this information to assist in determining the need for additional facilities.

A basis for seeing the interrelationship between level-of-care decisions and health facilities management is evident from the first chapter, Section 1.4. The size of the acute facility, acute-based SNF, etc., will effect the ability of physicians to place patients in the most economical level of care. An overbedded acute facility and underbedded SNF will result in overutilization of the acute facility (from the community systems' view), while an underbedded acute facility and overbedded SNF will result in underutilization of the acute facility.

Likewise, the types, quantity, and intensity of the services each level of care decides to provide affects the physicians' placement of patients. For example, some SNFs are not equipped to provide intravenous therapy, even though they theoretically (according to Medicare and Medicaid guidelines) are able to render this skilled nursing service. If this therapy were required, the physician would most likely not transfer a patient to such an SNF. Also, the amount of nursing time available per patient may be much less than the patient requires. This may mean the patient is receiving a lower level of care than the facility should be able to provide.

The location of the facilities also affects the level-of-care decision. A physician's willingness to transfer a patient to an SNF is naturally greater if it is located within the acute facility than if it is twenty miles away.

Scheduling of patients and personnel is also crucial to levels-of-care decisions. If the level of care decision is thought of as being made each day of a patient's acute stay, some days may be "underutilized" because of poor scheduling. A misscheduled patient, an inpatient unable to be seen because of scheduling conflicts with outpatients, a cancelled surgical schedule, poorly scheduled diagnostic tests, etc., are all potential causes of misutilization.

> **Problem:** A UR committee wants to identify the barriers to placing patients at the desired level of care and the frequency with which the barriers occur. What process should be used to obtain this information?

We will report on a study that attempted to identify how often these barriers to appropriate levels of care occurred in one hospital. According to the control framework (Control Requirement 5: Learn About Environment) such a study is required in any hospital that hopes to increase the economical placement of patients. The study was conducted at a medium-sized community hospital located in California. The hospital employed a UR nurse coordinator who concurrently reviewed patients in the hospital to determine, for each day of stay, whether a patient could be appropriately located at a subacute level of care, i.e., in an SNF, at home with home health care, or at home with outpatient or no care. Data were collected by the nurse coordinator between October 15, 1973, and August 15, 1974, on a random sample of 218 patients covered by Medicare and/or Medicaid. Each patient was followed throughout his course of hospitalization, irrespective of length of stay. Medicare levels-of-care criteria (Figure 12.3) were applied each day. When these criteria indicated that the patient did not need the acute facility, the nurse coordinator determined why the patient was not discharged or transferred (barrier to transfer), or why the patient was not receiving services ordered by the physician (barrier to efficient delivery of services).

A "barrier" to appropriate utilization is the reason for a patient's remaining in the acute hospital despite the determination that, according to the Medicare levels-of-care criteria, the patient could be appropriately cared for at a lower level of care. Thus, a barrier indicates the factor causing the failure to meet the criteria on a particular day.

An a priori list of barriers to appropriate utilization (Table 12.1) was developed after interviewing nine UR nurse coordinators, eleven discharge planners, three physicians, and three hospital administrators. Collectively representing five hospitals, the interviewed individuals were asked to provide examples of barriers which they knew to have occurred at their hospital. The list was made as comprehensive as possible so as to include all potential barriers, with no prior judgment made regarding their significance.

The barriers were classified according to areas of responsibility, i.e., to whose action or inaction a particular barrier could be attributed. The four responsibility classifications, along with a general description of the type of barriers each included, were as follows:

1. *Physician Responsibility* included barriers which fall within the scope of the physicians' knowledge and their own availability to render professional services to the patient. These barriers typically applied to the patient's attending physician, but also included barriers attributed to any physician(s) directly participating in the medical treatment of a patient, e.g., a hospital-based specialist, a consultant, a house staff member, etc.

2. *Hospital Responsibility* included barriers which related to the organization's operating systems and its employees.

3. *Patient or Family Responsibility* included barriers which related to the patient's or family's participation in the patient's therapeutic program.

4. *Environmental Responsibility* included barriers which were viewed as exogenous variables in locating patients appropriately; they are beyond the immediate scope of influence of the physician, hospital, patient and his or her own family. Barriers related to insurance coverage, alternative health care facilities and the social and economic constraints on the patient were classified as environmental.

## Table 12.1

## List of Potential Barriers

Barriers: Physician Responsibility

1. Patient is admitted for problem outside the area of competency of attending physician (e.g. should have referred patient to physician in different specialty).
2. Some or all of work-up could have been done on an outpatient rather than inpatient basis; e.g. preadmission work-up prior to surgery is inadequate. (Preoperative day, however, is to be regarded as appropriate unless clearly inappropriate.)
3. Physician admits patient to hold bed (for possible future patient).
4. "Political admission," as with VIP. (Please comment.)
5. Physician admits patient for acute condition, then decides to work-up patient for chronic condition, causing delay.
6. Physician delays scheduling of test or procedure.
7. Unavailability of physician causes delay in performing a procedure, (e.g. surgery which could have been performed on a Wednesday is delayed until Thursday because the physician is unavailable on Wednesday).
8. Test sequencing is inadequate, i.e., ordering test in the wrong sequence causes delay in diagnosis and/or treatment. (Please comment.)
9. Physician requests consultation—delay in carrying out consultation or in receiving report of consultation.
10. Failure of attending physician to provide patient (or family) with necessary information for informed consent causes delay.
11. Failure of other physician (e.g. anesthesiologist) to provide patient (or family) with necessary information for informed consent causes delay.
12. Physician is not visiting the patient.
13. UR review physician is not forceful enough in supporting UR function.
14. Physician has legal problem with patient, i.e., malpractice threat or involvement with an attorney.
15. Physician's medical management of patient is conservative.
16. Physician delays decision regarding further treatment of the patient because of the complex medical nature of the case, yet does not request a consultation.
17. Patient is kept in hospital because it is easier for his/her physician to have all patients in one facility. (Please comment.)
18. Physician refuses alternative facility because "it's too far away" for him/her to visit patient there.
19. Physician delays transfer or discharge of patient because, "I want to watch him/her for a few more days myself."
20. Physician has no confidence in quality of services available at SNF.
21. "Interesting case" is kept in hospital for teaching purposes.
22. Patient's transfer is delayed because of late date at which physician writes order.
23. Physician does not want to use SNF on prolonged case because "Then Blue Cross will expect this treatment on all cases like this," (e.g., orthopedic problem which could be treated in several different ways).
24. Other. (Please comment.)

Barriers: Hospital Responsibility

25. Problem in hospital scheduling for test or procedure causes delay.
26. Failure of nursing service to obtain consent for a procedure causes delay.
27. Return of test results is delayed, causing delay in diagnosis or treatment. (Please specify type of test.)
28. Scheduling or transfer of patient to another institution to perform a special procedure causes delay.
29. Communications failure, e.g., missed doctor's order. (Please comment.)
30. Hospital has legal problem with patient, i.e., malpractice threat or involvement with an attorney.
31. Lack of administrative support contributes to inappropriate utilization, (e.g., inadequate clerical support creates excessively heavy workload for coordinator). (Please comment.)

## Table 12.1 *(Continued)*

32. Patient's transfer or discharge is delayed because of inadequate discharge planning on the part of hospital personnel.
33. Other. (Please comment.)

Barriers: Patient or Family Responsibility

34. Patient or family insists on admission to hospital.
35. Patient is admitted because he/she is uncooperative with therapeutic or diagnostic program outside the hospital.
36. Indecisiveness of patient (or family) regarding a procedure (despite provision of adequate information by physician and hospital personnel) causes delay.
37. Patient is uncooperative with therapeutic program in the hospital, causing delay.
38. Patient or family refuses alternative facility because it is too far away.
39. Patient or family insists on patient remaining in hospital.
40. Family member (or friend) is unwilling to care for patient after discharge.
41. Other. (Please comment.)

Barriers: Environmental Responsibility

42. Insurance coverage for *diagnostic* procedures is more complete on an inpatient than on an outpatient basis.
43. Insurance coverage for *therapeutic* procedures is more complete on an inpatient than on an outpatient basis.
44. Medicare requires three-day acute hospitalization prior to SNF coverage.
45. Patient must be admitted to remove him from environment adverse to health, e.g., unavailability of family or friends to provide care. (Please comment.)
46. Terminal patient might die in transit to alternative facility.
47. Patient from unhealthy environment (e.g., home environment) is kept until environment becomes acceptable or alternative facility is found.
48. Patient is convalescing from an illness and it is anticipated that his/her stay in an alternative facility would be less than 72 hours.
49. Patient is terminal and stable, yet is kept in the acute hospital for humanitarian reasons. (Please comment.)
50. Patient is kept in hospital for short period of time (at end of hospitalization) because patient or family needs to be taught self-care, (as with illeostomy).
51. Patient's insurance coverage is more complete in an acute hospital than in an alternative facility or home health care program.
52. Unavailability of SNF bed.
53. Unavailability of sub-SNF level of care facility (e.g., nursing home, boarding house, etc.).
54. Unavailability of SNF with ability to provide the necessary *type* of skilled *nursing* services. (Please specify type of service.)
55. Patient is Medicare-Medicaid "crossover." Either no alternative facility is available or is willing to incur financial risk with patient having both Medicare and Medicaid coverage. Medicaid requires that Medicare be billed first and that Medicare gives confirmation that it does not cover certain patient services before Medicaid will assume coverage of those services.
56. Unavailability of SNF with ability to provide the necessary *amount* of (all types of) *nursing* services. (Please specify amount of service.)
57. Unavailability of SNF with necessary *ancillary* service(s). (Please specify type of service.)
58. Awaiting financial clearance from alternative facility for transfer.
59. Awaiting medical clearance from alternative facility for transfer.
60. Awaiting financial clearance from insurance program for transfer to alternative facility.
61. Family member (or friend) is not available to transport patient from the hospital.
62. Family member (or friend) is not available to care for patient after discharge.
63. Other. (Please comment.)

SOURCE: Restuccia and Holloway (see Additional Reading).

If the UR coordinator decided that a patient did not meet the Medicare levels-of-care criteria, using the list of potential barriers, she identified the area of responsibility and the particular barrier within the area that caused the patient to remain in the hospital or caused services to be delivered inefficiently. If two barriers existed for any day of stay and if, in her opinion, either barrier in the absence of the other could have caused the day to be inappropriate, both barriers were listed as contributing to the inappropriate day. If a description of the barrier was requested on the barrier list or if an unlisted barrier was occurring, the nurse coordinator recorded that information as well. Thus, each day determined to be "inappropriate acute" was associated with a particular barrier or barriers.

The UR coordinator used the patient's medical record to identify both misutilization and barriers. Moreover, whenever it seemed necessary, the UR coordinator sought additional information from nursing personnel on the patient's floor, the attending physician, discharge planners, or other hospital personnel.

For the 218 patients sampled, the number of days judged inappropriate was 201 (10.6 percent) of the 1,902 total days of hospitalization. Fifty-three (26 percent) of the 218 patients had at least one inappropriate day of stay, with an average of 3.8 inappropriate days for these patients. It is likely, then, that a day determined to be inappropriate will be followed by other inappropriate days. This assertion is supported by the fact that 43 (81 percent) of the 53 patients having at least one inappropriate day had a second, consecutive inappropriate day.

In examining the relationship between length of patient stay and the proportion of misutilization as determined by the UR coordinator's application of Medicare levels-of-care criteria, several methods of analysis are relevant. Of the 201 inappropriate days, 85 (42 percent) occurred before the average length of stay of 8.7 days for the sampled patients. A more important relationship, however, is the proportion of misutilization occurring before and after the 50th and 75th percentiles of length of stay by diagnosis, since these "checkpoints" are commonly used as criteria to determine when to perform a review. Using regionalized data published by the Commission on Professional and Hospital Activities (PAS-MAP) and adjusting for patient age and multiple diagnoses at admission, we find that 43 (21 percent) of the 201 inappropriate days occurred before the 50th percentile of length of stay by diagnosis while 74 inappropriate days (37 percent) occurred before the 75th percentile.

The results call into question the use of average length of stay as the screening criteria for deciding when to review a patient, since a significant amount of misutilization occurred before it would have been applied. This finding supports similar conclusions of other studies. Use of median length of stay by diagnosis proved to be a more discriminating criterion, although it still would "miss" over one-fifth of inappropriate days.

The distribution of inappropriate days over the various days of patient stay indicates a decreasing trend in the number of inappropriate days as length of stay increases (see Figure 12.9). However, since the total number of patient days in each day of stay rapidly decreases over time (see Table 12.2), there is a generally increasing trend in inappropriate days as a percentage of the number of total patient days per day of stay, particularly through the first three weeks (see Figure 12.10). Thus, the total number of inappropriate days is inversely related to length of stay, while the probability of an inappropriate day occurring in any given week is, in general, directly related to length of stay.

The insignificant amount of misutilization occurring on the day of admission demonstrates that a system to screen patients for appropriate location *prior* to admission would have little impact in reducing misutilization at the study hospital. Substantially the same results regarding misutilization of the day of admission have been found in other hospitals.

In order to represent the point in a patient's stay at which barriers are most likely to occur, irrespective of length of stay, the classification *stage of stay* was developed. The three stages of stay are differentiated by the sequence of appropriate and inappropriate days in the patient's total stay as follows:

1. *Initial stage*—inappropriate day(s) followed by appropriate day(s) and/or discharge;

2. *Mid-stage*—appropriate day(s) followed by inappropriate day(s) followed by appropriate day(s) until discharge; and

3. *End-stage*—appropriate day(s) followed by inappropriate day(s) until discharge.

For example, a patient admitted to the hospital appropriately, inappropriately located on the fifth and sixth days of hospitalization, and discharged on the seventh day represents end-stage misutilization.

The distribution of barriers by stage of stay indicates that end-stage misutilization was far more likely to occur than initial-

*Figure 12.9*

*Number of Inappropriate Days in Each Day of Stay*

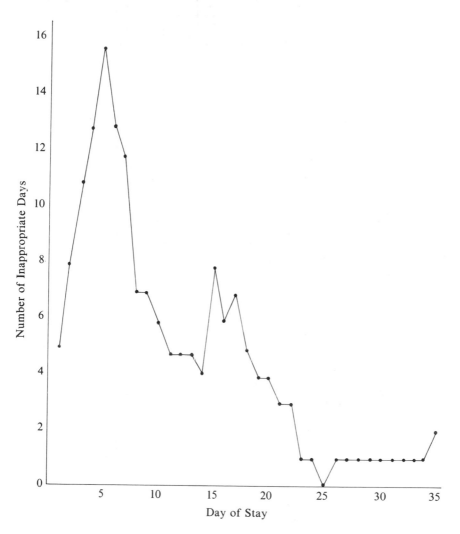

or mid-stage misutilization. In fact, 65 percent of barrier days were classified as end-stage (see Figure 12.11). This pattern was consistent within each responsibility area.

The prevalence of end-stage misutilization and misutilization appropriate for SNF level of care indicates a significant proportion of the barriers which occurred are related to discharge problems. This hypothesis is supported by the fact that, of the 25 barriers identified at least once, 10 are concerned exclusively with discharge

### Table 12.2

#### Percentage of Misutilized Days in Each Day of Stay

| DAY OF STAY | 1 | 2 | 3 | 4 | 5 | 6 | 7 | 8 | 9 | 10 | 11 | 12 | 13 | 14 | 15 | 16 | 17 | 18 | 19 | 20 | 21 | 22 | 23 | 24 | 25 | 26 | 27 | 28 | 29 | 30 | 31 | 32 | 33 | 34 | 35 |
|---|---|---|---|---|---|---|---|---|---|---|---|---|---|---|---|---|---|---|---|---|---|---|---|---|---|---|---|---|---|---|---|---|---|---|---|
| A) TOTAL PATIENT DAYS | 218 | 196 | 174 | 151 | 126 | 104 | 87 | 74 | 63 | 56 | 48 | 44 | 40 | 39 | 36 | 35 | 31 | 25 | 24 | 22 | 19 | 19 | 18 | 16 | 14 | 12 | 12 | 12 | 11 | 9 | 8 | 8 | 8 | 8 | 8 |
| B) MISUTILIZED DAYS | 5 | 8 | 11 | 13 | 16 | 13 | 12 | 7 | 7 | 6 | 5 | 5 | 5 | 4 | 8 | 6 | 7 | 5 | 4 | 4 | 3 | 3 | 1 | 1 | 0 | 1 | 1 | 1 | 1 | 1 | 1 | 1 | 1 | 1 | 2 |
| C) % OF THAT DAY $C = B \div A$ | 2.3 | 4.1 | 6.3 | 8.6 | 12.7 | 12.5 | 13.8 | 9.5 | 11.1 | 10.7 | 10.4 | 11.4 | 12.5 | 10.3 | 22.2 | 17.1 | 22.6 | 20.0 | 16.7 | 18.2 | 15.8 | 15.8 | 5.6 | 6.3 | 0 | 8.3 | 8.3 | 8.3 | 9.1 | 11.1 | 12.5 | 12.5 | 12.5 | 12.5 | 25.0 |

SOURCE: Restuccia and Holloway (see Additional Reading).

*Figure 12.10*

Inappropriate Days as a Percentage of Total Patient Days in Each Day of Stay (•————•————•) and as a Percentage of Total Patient Days in Each Week of Stay (————). Total Patient Days = 1,902; Total Inappropriate Days = 201.

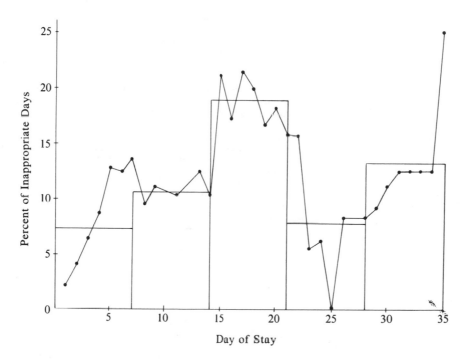

problems (see Table 12.3). Collectively, these barriers represent 63 percent of all barrier days. Thus, the proportion of misutilization caused by discharge-related barriers, cutting across responsibility classifications, provides another area of focus in attempting to reduce misutilization.

Of the 63 potential barriers contained on the barrier list, 25 were identified as causes of misutilization at the study hospital. Barriers occurred 229 times in the 201 inappropriate days. Further, 28 inappropriate days (229 less 201) were caused by two barriers occurring at the same time, and 11 of the 53 patients experiencing misutilization had two or more barriers occur.

The majority of barriers came from Physician Responsibility and Environmental Responsibility classifications, each one accounting for 41.5 percent of all barriers (see Table 12.3). Misutilization

## Table 12.3

### Distribution of Barriers

| Area of Responsibility | Barrier Number | Summary Description of Barrier | Number of Occurrences |
|---|---|---|---|
| PHYSICIAN | 7 | Physician is unavailable to perform a procedure | 5 |
| | 8 | Sequence of diagnostic tests is inadequate | 3 |
| | 9 | Consultation or consult report is delayed | 2 |
| | 12 | Physician is not visiting patient | 5 |
| | 14 | Physician has legal problem with patient | 4 |
| | 15 | Physician's medical management of patient is conservative | 37 |
| | 16 | Treatment is delayed due to failure to request consultation | 13 |
| | *19 | Physician delays transfer to observe patient's condition | 17 |
| | *22 | Late date of order for transfer causes delay | 2 |
| | *23 | Physician refuses SNF use due to belief that intermediary will expect all patients with same diagnosis to be transferred | 7 |
| HOSPITAL | 25 | Problem in hospital schedule for test or procedure | 9 |
| | *32 | Inadequate discharge planning by hospital | 8 |
| | | Sub-Total | 17 |
| PATIENT OR FAMILY | 36 | Patient is indecisive about performance of a procedure | 5 |
| | 37 | Patient is uncooperative with therapeutic program | 8 |
| | *39 | Patient insists on remaining in hospital | 6 |
| | 41 | Other problem with patient | 3 |
| | | Sub-Total | 22 |
| ENVIRONMENT | 43 | Insurance coverage for therapeutic procedure is more complete as inpatient | 1 |
| | 44 | Medicare requires three days in hospital before SNF is covered | 6 |
| | *48 | Patient needs SNF for less than 72 hours | 5 |
| | *49 | Terminal patient not transferred due to humanitarian reasons | 15 |
| | *52 | Unavailability of SNF bed | 7 |
| | *54 | Unavailability of SNF with necessary type of nursing service | 3 |
| | *56 | Unavailability of SNF with necessary amount of nursing services | 54 |
| | *62 | Unavailability of someone to care for patient at home | 2 |
| | 63 | Other | 2 |
| | | Sub-Total | 95 |
| | | TOTAL | 229 |

*Asterisk denotes discharge-related barriers
SOURCE: Restuccia and Holloway (see Additional Reading).

*Figure 12.11*

## Percent of Inappropriate Days by Stage of Stay
## (Total Inappropriate Days = 201)

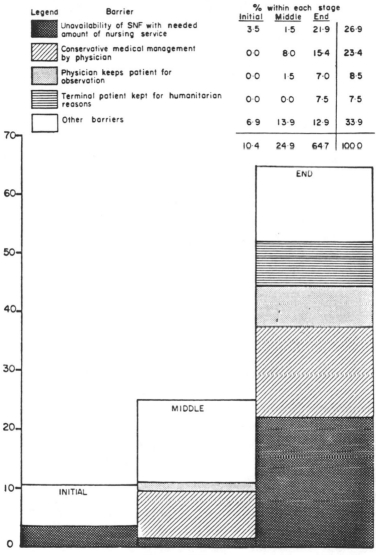

Stage of Stay

associated with the hospital and the patient or family was comparatively insignificant, with 7 percent of all barriers in the former
classification and 10 percent in the latter.

The predominance of barriers in the areas of Physician and

Environmental Responsibility would indicate that resources allocated to the reduction of misutilization *at the study hospital* should be concentrated in these areas. Of particular significance is the fact that only *four* barriers, two attributed to the physician and two to the environment, accounted for 54 percent of total barriers. These barriers, with their respective number of barrier days, are the following:

—Physician's medical management of the patient is conservative (to the extent that the services received by the patient do not justify an acute location according to the Medicare levels-of-care criteria), accounting for 37 barrier days.

—Physician delays transfer or discharge of the patient because, "I want to watch him/her for a few more days myself" (i.e. for purposes of observing), accounting for 17 barrier days.

—The patient is terminal and stable, yet is kept in the acute hospital for humanitarian reasons, accounting for 15 barrier days.

—Skilled nursing facility with ability to provide the necessary amount of nursing services is unavailable, accounting for 54 barrier days.

These barriers are perhaps the most difficult ones to be dealt with by an individual hospital. By definition, the two environmental barriers are beyond the scope of influence of the hospital and its medical staff, at least in the short run. The two physician-related barriers would also be difficult to deal with since (1) attempts at correcting them may be interpreted as intrusion into the closely-guarded realm of professional medical judgment, and (2) a case could be made that subtle socio-economic, psychological, and/or environmental factors enter into a physician's decision to keep a patient hospitalized, and thus these factors enter into the realm of "medical judgment" and cannot be subject to a set of objective standards such as the Medicare levels-of-care criteria.

It is evident, however, that certain measures can be taken to eliminate or at least reduce barriers to appropriate utilization. Systems studies could certainly reduce misutilization caused by barriers within the Hospital Responsibility category. Barriers attributable to patients or their families may be reduced (1) by providing sufficient information regarding the extent and limitations of insurance coverage, and (2) by intensifying the efforts of attending physicians, social workers, and discharge planners to find an alternative location acceptable to the patients and their families. Physician barriers should be made the subject of professional consideration by UR, medical audit, and other medical staff committees. Action should be taken to address physician barriers through concurrent review and medical care evaluation studies.

In the study hospital, the predominance of both end-stage and SNF-level misutilization resulted in efforts to reduce these barriers. Among these efforts were an expanded role for social services and discharge planning, education of physicians and patients in the appropriate utilization of health care facilities, and a decision to establish a hospital-based SNF. Moreover, a study of similar barrier patterns—environmental barriers in particular—at hospitals with overlapping service areas may reveal problems that can be alleviated by allocating resources on a community-wide or higher level, by modifying insurance benefit structures and providing reimbursement to encourage such allocations.

## 12.7 EVALUATION OF THE CYBERNETIC UTILIZATION REVIEW SYSTEM

With the above section as background, we ask whether concurrent review systems can reduce the number of inappropriate days (days when patients in acute facilities could be at a lower level of care). Does it matter whether the cybernetic control framework is used, or would bureaucratic rules and procedures work just as well? Naturally, we do not expect inappropriate days due to environmental barriers, or possibly even hospital-related barriers, to be reduced by concurrent feedback. Attending physicians cannot control their environment. However, physicians accounted for 32 percent of the 201 inappropriate days in the study hospital of the previous section, so we would expect some of those days to be eliminated by a well-designed system of concurrent feedback.

In contrast to a concurrent UR system designed on cybernetic control principles, current federal UR regulations require that control be attempted through bureaucratic rules and procedures. For example, PSRO regulations limited UR coordinators' roles to that of a screening function. If they found a questionable admission or continued stay, coordinators were required to seek the intervention of a UR physician, who was then responsible for further review and for providing any information that might be fed back to the attending physician. Thus, the rules prevent coordinators from providing feedback directly to attending physicians and from providing assistance in resolving the utilization problem. Even though these rules may be changed under the PRO program, they provide a good illustration of an alternative to the cybernetic control process. We would anticipate this alternative system to be less effective in reducing inappropriate days.

In order to compare the effectiveness of a cybernetic UR system and a bureaucratic UR system such as that mandated under federal UR regulations, a study was conducted at four hospitals in the San Francisco Bay Area, focusing upon the importance of feedback in achieving effective control. (See Restuccia in Additional Reading.) In each of the four hospitals, UR nurse coordinators were asked to provide different types of feedback to physicians about patients randomly assigned to one of four feedback strategies (including no feedback). The four strategies varied according to the channel used to provide feedback to the attending physician and the amount of discretion accorded the coordinator in deciding whether, when, and to whom feedback was provided. In each strategy, this feedback decision was triggered by the coordinator's detection of a patient inappropriately located (on the basis of Medicare levels-of-care criteria in Figure 12.3). The four strategies were as follows:

1. *Direct Feedback.* The UR coordinator directly informed the attending physician that his or her patient was inappropriately located.

2. *Indirect Feedback.* The UR coordinator informed a UR physician that a patient was inappropriately located. It then became the UR physician's responsibility to decide whether to contact the patient's attending physician (current federal regulation).

3. *No Feedback.* Neither the attending physician nor a UR physician was informed that a patient was inappropriately located.

4. *Judgmental Feedback.* The UR coordinator was permitted to decide whether and in what order to inform the attending physician, a UR physician, both, or neither physician. Thus, this category included any one or combination of the three categories above, depending upon the discretion of the UR coordinator (cybernetic control system).

The judgmental feedback strategy was designed to represent cybernetic control while the indirect feedback strategy represents bureaucratic control. The direct feedback strategy is in between the two, allowing coordinators to provide information directly to the attending physician but restricting their discretion over the feedback decision (i.e. coordinators were not allowed to contact a UR physician or to provide no feedback). The strategy in which no feedback was provided serves as a control group since no concurrent action was taken by the coordinator for inappropriately located patients in this group.

The measure of performance (the dependent variable) was the same as discussed in Section 12.4: the number of inappropriate patient days occurring for patients using each feedback strategy. The null hypothesis tested was that there is no difference in the average number of inappropriate patient days resulting from each strategy. However, on the basis of cybernetic theory, we would expect better performance in cases where feedback is more direct and discretionary. Thus, we would predict that the smallest number of inappropriate days would occur in the judgmental feedback strategy, followed in order by the direct, indirect, and no feedback strategies.

In the four participating hospitals, the UR coordinators reviewed a total of 1,385 patients over a two-month period. Of these, 333 patients (24 percent) were found to have at least one inappropriate day with an average of 2.85 inappropriate days for each of these 333 patients.

The average number of inappropriate days per patient for each of the four feedback strategies supports the hypothesized results.

### Table 12.4

### Average Number of Inappropriate Days per Patient by Type of Feedback

| Feedback Strategy | All Patients ($N = 333$) | All Patients But Truncated Dependent Variable ($N = 333$) | Excluding Patients With Environmental Barriers ($N = 180$) |
|---|---|---|---|
| Judgemental Feedback | 2.63 | 2.24 | 2.19 |
| Direct Feedback | 2.75 | 2.20 | 2.83 |
| Indirect Feedback | 3.18 | 2.70 | 3.48 |
| No feedback | 3.21 | 2.77 | 3.48 |
| ALL STRATEGIES | 2.85 | 2.40 | 2.77 |
| Significance Level | .020 | .002 | .001 |

SOURCE: J. D. Restuccia (see Additional Reading).

The average number of inappropriate days was smallest with the judgmental feedback strategy, followed by the direct feedback, indirect feedback, and no feedback strategies, in that order (see Table 12.4, first column). To determine the statistical significance of these differences in means, an analysis of variance was conducted on the results (see Freund and Williams for a discussion of analysis of variance). The result of this analysis indicated that the differences in means among different types of feedback are significant at the 2 percent level (i.e., $p = .020$). Stated another way, these differences had only a 2 percent probability of occurring by chance.

A second analysis of variance was conducted with the dependent variable—the number of inappropriate days per patient—truncated at a maximum of five days (i.e., inappropriate days in excess of five per patient were not included in the dependent variable). This second analysis of variance was performed because the UR coordinators had the option of switching to the judgemental type of feedback for patients in the direct feedback, indirect feedback, and control groups when four consecutive inappropriate days were experienced by a patient. (This was a limitation imposed on the study so that the hospitals would not experience misutilization to an extent that would jeopardize their Medicare reimbursement.) If, as hypothesized, judgemental feedback was the most effective type provided, truncating the dependent variable would indicate a higher level of significance than found in the analysis of variance with no truncation. This result did occur with the second analysis of variance, indicating significance at a level of 0.2 percent (i.e., $p = .002$). The second column of Table 12.4 contains the mean number of inappropriate days per patient truncated at five days for each feedback strategy.

A third analysis of variance was conducted to help determine the extent to which environmental barriers prevented the UR systems from functioning effectively. In this analysis, patients having inappropriate days associated with barriers identified by the UR coordinators as *beyond* the immediate control of the hospital, attending physician, and patient (or the patient's family) were excluded. If such barriers did decrease the UR systems' control over reducing misutilization, we would expect that this analysis would indicate a higher level of significance than did the first analysis of variance. Again, this was in fact the case, with significance found at the 0.1 percent level ($p = .001$). The third column of Table 12.4 summarizes the results of the third analysis of variance.

A fourth analysis of variance was conducted upon another dependent variable—patients' length of stay—in each of the four

## Table 12.5

### Average Length of Stay

| Feedback strategy | Average Length of Stay |
|---|---|
| Judgemental Feedback | 12.25 |
| Direct Feedback | 14.25 |
| Indirect Feedback | 15.06 |
| No Feedback | 14.98 |
| ALL STRATEGIES | 13.62 |
| Significance Level | .010 |

SOURCE: J. D. Restuccia (see Additional Reading).

feedback strategies. While length of stay is a less sensitive measure of performance of the control exerted by a UR system, it would still be expected to reflect differences in the feedback strategies. The mean length of stay for patients assigned to each feedback strategy is shown in Table 12.5. The analysis of variance on length of stay indicated differences at the 1 percent level of significance ($p = .010$).

The results of this study indicate that cybernetic feedback in these four hospitals reduced inappropriate days by .58 days compared to no feedback. In addition, lengths of stay for patients having inappropriate days were significantly lowered when using the cybernetic control system. This provides supporting evidence that concurrent review systems can reduce the number of inappropriate days and that the cybernetic control framework performs better than the bureaucratic rules, in this application.

We have summarized the results of applying the cybernetic control framework to the design of a concurrent utilization review system. Although we limited our discussion to explicit criteria for levels-of-care decisions, the methods are similar when developing criteria for deciding appropriate services (i.e., services that are medically necessary and consistent with professionally recognized standards of care). Likewise, although the barrier study we described was conducted to discover the reasons that levels-of-care criteria were not being met, a similar study would be required to determine the reason that appropriate services were not being delivered. And finally, although the study to evaluate four feedback strategies found that nurse coordinators should be allowed to decide whether, when, and to whom to provide feedback when levels-of-care criteria were not met, we would anticipate similar results if the study were conducted in a situation where appropriate services criteria were not being met.

We would also anticipate, however, that because of the complexity and uncertainty of deciding on the appropriate services for a patient, the nurse coordinators would choose not to provide concurrent feedback to the attending physician about inappropriate services as often as they would about inappropriate levels of care. Retrospective medical care evaluation studies would have to be used to follow up on suspected inappropriate services.

## Exercises

12.1 After working in a 400-bed community hospital for six months as assistant administrator in charge of medical audit and utilization review (in addition to other areas of responsibility), you are asked by the chief of staff to do a study to determine how fast cardiac patients are being connected to monitors. About two years ago, your former chief of staff "railroaded through" (the present chief's term) a policy of having cardiac patients on monitors within 45 minutes of arrival, and kept on them at least 24 hours.

You do a study over a period of one month (148 patients) and find that less than half of the cardiac patients' treatment meets this policy. The present chief of staff said he "thought so," when you reported the findings, and further says he's not sure it's such a good policy anyway. He asks you to set up an agenda for him and a small subcommittee (including you) to "look at this policy and why it's not being met." This is your chance to show your stuff, as you realize that he's talking about a general agenda for looking at policies of this kind.

Develop a 1–3 page agenda for this meeting. (Hint: review Chapters 1 and 2.)

In each of the remaining exercises, two alternatives are presented for the design of a concurrent UR system. Select the alternative that you believe should be implemented and justify your selection, applying the six structural requirements and/or the process of cybernetic control.

12.2 a. For concurrent utilization review, an admitting clerk would compare the admission diagnosis with a set of explicit criteria, and if the admission met the criteria, would assign a length of stay for future review.

b. For concurrent utilization review, a nurse would review the face sheet with explicit criteria and decide when to make another review.

12.3 a. For concurrent utilization review, a nurse reviews a patient on the seventh day and, without criteria, reports to the attending physician that the patient no longer appears to require hospitalization.

b. For concurrent utilization review, a nurse reviews a patient and, applying the levels-of-care criteria, reports to the physician that the patient could be located in an alternative facility (SNF) to receive the same services.

12.4 a. In concurrent utilization review, when the nurse reviewer detects a deviation from the explicit criteria, he reports to the utilization review physician who contacts the attending physician.

b. In concurrent utilization review, when the nurse reviewer detects a deviation from the explicit criteria, he contacts the attending physician and points out the discrepancy.

12.5 a. The nurse reviews a patient and, on the basis of facility-specific levels-of-care criteria, determines that the patient could be located in an alternate facility to receive the same services.

b. The nurse reviews the patient on the basis of diagnosis-specific levels-of-care criteria and indicates to the physician that the patient no longer requires the acute facility because he has been in the hospital as long as the average patient with that diagnosis.

12.6 a. The nurse identifies a delay in the delivery of physical therapy and contacts the attending physician and the physical therapist to explain the consequences of the delay.

b. The nurse identifies a delay in the delivery of physical therapy and contacts the UR physician to explain the consequences of the delay.

12.7 A common problem in hospital operating rooms is the amount of delay in starting scheduled operations because surgeons arrive late. Consider the analogies between this problem and that of utilization review; design a system (either concurrent or retrospective), based on the cybernetic control framework, for reducing the amount of delay time in starting scheduled operations.

## Additional Reading

Brian, E. W. "Government Control of Hospital Utilization—A California Experience." *New England Journal of Medicine* 286 (1972): 1340.

Brian, E. W. "Foundation for Medical Care Control of Hospital Utilization: CHAP—a PSRO Prototype." *New England Journal of Medicine* 288 (1973): 878.

Commission on Professional and Hospital Activities. *Length of Stay in PAS Hospitals, United States, Western Region, 1973.* Ann Arbor, Michigan, 1974.

"Conditions of Participation—Hospitals and Nursing Facilities, Utilization Review." Social Security Administration, DHEW. 30 *Federal Register* 41604 (November 29, 1974).

Cunningham, R. M., Contributing Editor. "PSRO: Around the Nation." *PSRO Letter* 42 (May 1975): 5.

Dalkey, N. D. *The Delphi Method: An Experimental Study of Group Opinion.* RAND Corporation, RM-5868-PR, June 1969.

Dalkey, N. and Helmer, O. "An Experimental Application of the Delphi Method to the Use of Experts." *Management Science* 9 (1963): 458.

Delbecq, A. L. and Van de Ven, A. H. "A Group Process Model for Problem Identification and Program Planning." *Journal of Applied Behavioral Science* 7 (July/August 1971).

Donabedian, A. "Evaluating the Quality of Medical Care." *Milbank Memorial Fund Quarterly* (July 1966).

Eddy, D. M. "Clinical Policies and the Quality of Clinical Practice." *New England Journal of Medicine* 307 (August 5, 1982): 343–347.

Flynn, P. F. "Criteria for Levels of Care Evaluation under Medicare." *California Medicine* 119 (1973): 80.

Freund, J. E. and Williams, F. J. *Elementary Business Statistics.* Englewood Cliffs, N.J.: Prentice-Hall, 1972.

Gertman, P. M. and Bucher, B. M. "Inappropriate Hospital Bed Days and Their Relationship to Length of Stay Parameters." Presented at the Medical Care Section, 99th Annual Meeting of the American Public Health Association, Minneapolis, Minnesota, October 11, 1969.

Goldberg, G. A. and Holloway, D. C. "Emphasizing 'Level of Care' over 'Length of Stay' in Hospital Utilization Review." *Medical Care* 12 (June 1975): 474.

Goran, M. J., et al. "The PSRO Hospital Review System." *Medical Care* Supplement 12 (April 1975): 1.

"Guidelines for Hospital Patient Care Evaluation: Patient Care Audit and Utilization Review" (draft). California Medical Association and California Hospital Association, January 23, 1975.

Hage, J. *Communication and Organizational Control: Cybernetics in Health and Welfare Settings.* New York: John Wiley and Sons, 1974.

*Health Insurance for the Aged, Hospital Manual.* Department of Health, Education, and Welfare, Social Security Administration, HIM-10.

*Health Insurance for the Aged, Extended Care Facility Manual.* Department of Health, Education, and Welfare, Social Security Administration, HIM-12.

"HEW Prepared New UR Guidelines as Regs' Effective Date Nears." *PSRO Letter* 42 (May 1, 1975): 3.

Holloway, D. C. and Holton, J. "Mechanisms for Evaluation of a Utilization and Audit System." *PSRO Utilization and Audit in Patient Care.* Edited by Sharon Davidson. St. Louis, Mo.: The C. V. Mosby Co., 1976.

Holloway, D. C., Holton, J., Goldberg, G. A., and Restuccia, J. D. "Development of Hospital Levels of Care Criteria." *Health Care Management Review* 1 (Summer 1976): 61–72.

Holloway, D. C., Restuccia, J. D., Goldberg, G. A. and Fuhrer, R. "Determining the Appropriate Level of Care for Patients." *Proceedings of the Conference on Measure of Quality of Care.* Atlanta, Ga.: National Cooperative Services Center for Hospital Management Engineering, March 1975.

Holloway, D. C., Wiczai, L. J. and Carlson, E. T. "Evaluating an Information System for Medical Care Evaluation Studies." *Medical Care* 13 (April 1975): 329–40.

*Hospital Utilization Project.* Hospital Utilization Project, 400 Penn Central Boulevard, Pittsburgh, Pennsylvania, 1974.

Jeffrey, I. J. and Barr, A. "A Method of Evaluating the Use Made of Hospital Beds." *International Journal of Health Services* 3 (1973): 245.

McDowell, W. "The Nurse-Patient-Physician Triad As a Self-Regulating Mechanism: A Homeostatic Model for Measuring Patient Care." Ph.D dissertation, University of Michigan, 1968.

McKay–Dee Hospital Center. *Multilevel Care.* 3939 Harrison Boulevard, Ogden, Utah 84402, undated.

"Medicaid, Utilization Control of Care and Services." Social and Rehabilitation Service, DHEW. 39 *Federal Register* 41610 (November 29, 1974).

*Medicare Hospital Manual,* Section 290–296. U.S. Department of Health, Education, and Welfare, Social Security Administration, 1972.

Murnaghan, J. H. "Health-Services Information System in the United States Today." *New England Journal of Medicine* 290 (1974): 603.

Payne, B. C. *Hospital Utilization Review Manual.* Ann Arbor, Michigan: University of Michigan Medical School, Department of Postgraduate Medicine, 1968.

Payne, B. C. and Lyons, T. F. *Methods of Evaluating and Improving Personal Medical Care Quality: Episode of Illness Study for Hawaii Medical Association.* Ann Arbor, Michigan: University of Michigan School of Medicine, 1972.

Performance Evaluation Program, Joint Commission on Hospital Accreditation.

*Pre-PAS, A Medical Record Information System.* Ann Arbor, Michigan: Commission on Professional and Hospital Activities, 1972.

*Professional Activity Study—Medical Audit Program.* Ann Arbor, Michigan: Commission on Professional and Hospital Activities, 1972.

*PSRO Program Manual.* Washington, D.C.: U.S. Department of Health, Education, and Welfare, Office of Professional Standards Review, 1974.

*Quality Assurance Program for Medical Care in the Hospital.* Chicago: American Hospital Association, 1972.

Restuccia, J. D. "The Effects of Feedback on Physicians' Levels of Care Decisions." Dr. P. H. dissertation, University of California–Berkeley, 1977.

Restuccia, J. D. and Holloway, D. C. "Barriers to Appropriate Utilization of Acute Facility." *Medical Care* 19 (July 1976): 559–73.

Rosenfeld, L. S. F., Goldmann, F. and Kaprio, L. A. "Reasons for Prolonged Hospital Stay." *Journal of Chronic Diseases* 6 (August 1957): 341.

Sanazaro, P. J., Goldstein, R. L., Roberts, J. S. et al. "Research and Development in Quality Assurance—The Experimental Medical Care Review Organization Program." *New England Journal of Medicine* 287 (1972): 1125.

Smits, H. L. "The PSRO in Perspective." *New England Journal of Medicine* 305 (1981): 253–259.

Stuart, B. and Stockton, R. "Control Over the Utilization of Medical Services." *Milbank Memorial Fund Quarterly* 51 (1973): 341.

U.S. Department of Health, Education, and Welfare, Office of Nursing Home Affairs. *Long Term Care Facility Survey (Interim Report)*. Rockville, Maryland: U.S. Dept. of Health, Education, and Welfare, March 1975.

Zimmer, J. G. "An Evaluation of Observer Variability in a Hospital Bed Utilization Study." *Medical Care* 5 (1967): 221.

Zimmer, J. G. and Groomes, E. W. "An Observer Reliability Study of Physicians' and Nurses' Decisions in Utilization Review in Chronic-Care Facilities." *Medical Care* 7 (1969): 14.

Zimmer, J. G. "Length of Stay and Hospital Bed Misutilization." *Medical Care* 12 (1974): 453.

# Appendix

## Table I

### Areas under the Normal Curve

An entry in the table below is the area under the standard normal curve bounded on the left by a vertical line at the mean and on the right by a vertical line z standard deviations from the mean, where z is indicated on the table by adding an entry's column label to its row label.

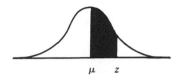

$\mu \quad z$

Example: The area between the mean and 1.44 standard deviations from the mean is .4251.

Example: A random variable is normally distributed with mean 25 and standard deviation 10. The probability that it will take on a value between 35 and 45 (i.e. between 1 and 2 standard deviations above the mean) is .4772 − .3413 = .1359 (the table entry for 2.00 less the entry for 1.00).

| z | 0.00 | 0.01 | 0.02 | 0.03 | 0.04 | 0.05 | 0.06 | 0.07 | 0.08 | 0.09 |
|---|------|------|------|------|------|------|------|------|------|------|
| 0.0 | 0.0000 | 0.0040 | 0.0080 | 0.0120 | 0.0160 | 0.0199 | 0.0239 | 0.0279 | 0.0319 | 0.0359 |
| 0.1 | 0.0398 | 0.0438 | 0.0478 | 0.0517 | 0.0557 | 0.0596 | 0.0636 | 0.0675 | 0.0714 | 0.0753 |
| 0.2 | 0.0793 | 0.0832 | 0.0871 | 0.0910 | 0.0948 | 0.0987 | 0.1026 | 0.1064 | 0.1103 | 0.1141 |
| 0.3 | 0.1179 | 0.1217 | 0.1255 | 0.1293 | 0.1331 | 0.1368 | 0.1406 | 0.1443 | 0.1480 | 0.1517 |
| 0.4 | 0.1554 | 0.1591 | 0.1628 | 0.1664 | 0.1700 | 0.1736 | 0.1772 | 0.1808 | 0.1844 | 0.1879 |
| 0.5 | 0.1915 | 0.1950 | 0.1985 | 0.2019 | 0.2054 | 0.2088 | 0.2123 | 0.2157 | 0.2190 | 0.2224 |
| 0.6 | 0.2257 | 0.2291 | 0.2324 | 0.2357 | 0.2389 | 0.2422 | 0.2454 | 0.2486 | 0.2518 | 0.2549 |
| 0.7 | 0.2580 | 0.2612 | 0.2642 | 0.2673 | 0.2704 | 0.2734 | 0.2764 | 0.2794 | 0.2823 | 0.2852 |
| 0.8 | 0.2881 | 0.2910 | 0.2939 | 0.2967 | 0.2995 | 0.3023 | 0.3051 | 0.3078 | 0.3106 | 0.3133 |
| 0.9 | 0.3159 | 0.3186 | 0.3212 | 0.3238 | 0.3264 | 0.3289 | 0.3315 | 0.3340 | 0.3365 | 0.3389 |
| 1.0 | 0.3413 | 0.3438 | 0.3461 | 0.3485 | 0.3508 | 0.3531 | 0.3554 | 0.3577 | 0.3599 | 0.3621 |
| 1.1 | 0.3643 | 0.3665 | 0.3686 | 0.3708 | 0.3729 | 0.3749 | 0.3770 | 0.3790 | 0.3810 | 0.3830 |
| 1.2 | 0.3849 | 0.3869 | 0.3888 | 0.3907 | 0.3925 | 0.3944 | 0.3962 | 0.3980 | 0.3997 | 0.4015 |
| 1.3 | 0.4032 | 0.4049 | 0.4066 | 0.4082 | 0.4099 | 0.4115 | 0.4131 | 0.4147 | 0.4162 | 0.4177 |
| 1.4 | 0.4192 | 0.4207 | 0.4222 | 0.4236 | 0.4251 | 0.4265 | 0.4279 | 0.4292 | 0.4306 | 0.4319 |
| 1.5 | 0.4332 | 0.4345 | 0.4357 | 0.4370 | 0.4382 | 0.4394 | 0.4406 | 0.4418 | 0.4429 | 0.4441 |
| 1.6 | 0.4452 | 0.4463 | 0.4474 | 0.4484 | 0.4495 | 0.4505 | 0.4515 | 0.4525 | 0.4535 | 0.4545 |
| 1.7 | 0.4554 | 0.4564 | 0.4573 | 0.4582 | 0.4591 | 0.4599 | 0.4608 | 0.4616 | 0.4625 | 0.4633 |
| 1.8 | 0.4641 | 0.4649 | 0.4656 | 0.4664 | 0.4671 | 0.4678 | 0.4686 | 0.4693 | 0.4699 | 0.4706 |
| 1.9 | 0.4713 | 0.4719 | 0.4726 | 0.4732 | 0.4738 | 0.4744 | 0.4750 | 0.4756 | 0.4761 | 0.4767 |
| 2.0 | 0.4772 | 0.4778 | 0.4783 | 0.4788 | 0.4793 | 0.4798 | 0.4803 | 0.4808 | 0.4812 | 0.4817 |
| 2.1 | 0.4821 | 0.4826 | 0.4830 | 0.4834 | 0.4838 | 0.4842 | 0.4846 | 0.4850 | 0.4854 | 0.4857 |
| 2.2 | 0.4861 | 0.4864 | 0.4868 | 0.4871 | 0.4875 | 0.4878 | 0.4881 | 0.4884 | 0.4887 | 0.4890 |
| 2.3 | 0.4893 | 0.4896 | 0.4898 | 0.4901 | 0.4904 | 0.4906 | 0.4909 | 0.4911 | 0.4913 | 0.4916 |
| 2.4 | 0.4918 | 0.4920 | 0.4922 | 0.4925 | 0.4927 | 0.4929 | 0.4931 | 0.4932 | 0.4934 | 0.4936 |
| 2.5 | 0.4938 | 0.4940 | 0.4941 | 0.4943 | 0.4945 | 0.4946 | 0.4948 | 0.4949 | 0.4951 | 0.4952 |
| 2.6 | 0.4953 | 0.4955 | 0.4956 | 0.4957 | 0.4959 | 0.4960 | 0.4961 | 0.4962 | 0.4963 | 0.4964 |
| 2.7 | 0.4965 | 0.4966 | 0.4967 | 0.4968 | 0.4969 | 0.4970 | 0.4971 | 0.4972 | 0.4973 | 0.4974 |
| 2.8 | 0.4974 | 0.4975 | 0.4976 | 0.4977 | 0.4977 | 0.4978 | 0.4979 | 0.4979 | 0.4980 | 0.4981 |
| 2.9 | 0.4981 | 0.4982 | 0.4982 | 0.4983 | 0.4984 | 0.4984 | 0.4985 | 0.4985 | 0.4986 | 0.4986 |
| 3.0 | 0.4986 | 0.4987 | 0.4987 | 0.4988 | 0.4988 | 0.4989 | 0.4989 | 0.4989 | 0.4990 | 0.4990 |
| 3.1 | 0.4990 | 0.4991 | 0.4991 | 0.4991 | 0.4992 | 0.4992 | 0.4992 | 0.4992 | 0.4993 | 0.4993 |
| 3.2 | 0.4993 | 0.4993 | 0.4994 | 0.4994 | 0.4994 | 0.4994 | 0.4994 | 0.4995 | 0.4995 | 0.4995 |
| 3.3 | 0.4995 | 0.4995 | 0.4995 | 0.4996 | 0.4996 | 0.4996 | 0.4996 | 0.4996 | 0.4996 | 0.4997 |
| 3.4 | 0.4997 | 0.4997 | 0.4997 | 0.4997 | 0.4997 | 0.4997 | 0.4997 | 0.4997 | 0.4998 | 0.4998 |
| 3.5 | 0.4998 | 0.4998 | 0.4998 | 0.4998 | 0.4998 | 0.4998 | 0.4998 | 0.4998 | 0.4998 | 0.4998 |
| 3.6 | 0.4998 | 0.4998 | 0.4999 | 0.4999 | 0.4999 | 0.4999 | 0.4999 | 0.4999 | 0.4999 | 0.4999 |
| 3.7 | 0.4999 | 0.4999 | 0.4999 | 0.4999 | 0.4999 | 0.4999 | 0.4999 | 0.4999 | 0.4999 | 0.4999 |
| 3.8 | 0.4999 | 0.4999 | 0.4999 | 0.4999 | 0.4999 | 0.4999 | 0.4999 | 0.5000 | 0.5000 | 0.5000 |
| 3.9 | 0.5000 | 0.5000 | 0.5000 | 0.5000 | 0.5000 | 0.5000 | 0.5000 | 0.5000 | 0.5000 | 0.5000 |

## Table II

## The F Distribution with $v_1$ and $v_2$ Degrees of Freedom

Upper 5% points

| $v_2$ \ $v_1$ | 1 | 2 | 3 | 4 | 5 | 6 | 7 | 8 | 9 | 10 | 12 | 15 | 20 | 24 | 30 | 40 | 60 | 120 | ∞ |
|---|---|---|---|---|---|---|---|---|---|---|---|---|---|---|---|---|---|---|---|
| 1 | 161·4 | 199·5 | 215·7 | 224·6 | 230·2 | 234·0 | 236·8 | 238·9 | 240·5 | 241·9 | 243·9 | 245·9 | 248·0 | 249·1 | 250·1 | 251·1 | 252·2 | 253·3 | 254·3 |
| 2 | 18·51 | 19·00 | 19·16 | 19·25 | 19·30 | 19·33 | 19·35 | 19·37 | 19·38 | 19·40 | 19·41 | 19·43 | 19·45 | 19·45 | 19·46 | 19·47 | 19·48 | 19·49 | 19·50 |
| 3 | 10·13 | 9·55 | 9·28 | 9·12 | 9·01 | 8·94 | 8·89 | 8·85 | 8·81 | 8·79 | 8·74 | 8·70 | 8·66 | 8·64 | 8·62 | 8·59 | 8·57 | 8·55 | 8·53 |
| 4 | 7·71 | 6·94 | 6·59 | 6·39 | 6·26 | 6·16 | 6·09 | 6·04 | 6·00 | 5·96 | 5·91 | 5·86 | 5·80 | 5·77 | 5·75 | 5·72 | 5·69 | 5·66 | 5·63 |
| 5 | 6·61 | 5·79 | 5·41 | 5·19 | 5·05 | 4·95 | 4·88 | 4·82 | 4·77 | 4·74 | 4·68 | 4·62 | 4·56 | 4·53 | 4·50 | 4·46 | 4·43 | 4·40 | 4·36 |
| 6 | 5·99 | 5·14 | 4·76 | 4·53 | 4·39 | 4·28 | 4·21 | 4·15 | 4·10 | 4·06 | 4·00 | 3·94 | 3·87 | 3·84 | 3·81 | 3·77 | 3·74 | 3·70 | 3·67 |
| 7 | 5·59 | 4·74 | 4·35 | 4·12 | 3·97 | 3·87 | 3·79 | 3·73 | 3·68 | 3·64 | 3·57 | 3·51 | 3·44 | 3·41 | 3·38 | 3·34 | 3·30 | 3·27 | 3·23 |
| 8 | 5·32 | 4·46 | 4·07 | 3·84 | 3·69 | 3·58 | 3·50 | 3·44 | 3·39 | 3·35 | 3·28 | 3·22 | 3·15 | 3·12 | 3·08 | 3·04 | 3·01 | 2·97 | 2·93 |
| 9 | 5·12 | 4·26 | 3·86 | 3·63 | 3·48 | 3·37 | 3·29 | 3·23 | 3·18 | 3·14 | 3·07 | 3·01 | 2·94 | 2·90 | 2·86 | 2·83 | 2·79 | 2·75 | 2·71 |
| 10 | 4·96 | 4·10 | 3·71 | 3·48 | 3·33 | 3·22 | 3·14 | 3·07 | 3·02 | 2·98 | 2·91 | 2·85 | 2·77 | 2·74 | 2·70 | 2·66 | 2·62 | 2·58 | 2·54 |
| 11 | 4·84 | 3·98 | 3·59 | 3·36 | 3·20 | 3·09 | 3·01 | 2·95 | 2·90 | 2·85 | 2·79 | 2·72 | 2·65 | 2·61 | 2·57 | 2·53 | 2·49 | 2·45 | 2·40 |
| 12 | 4·75 | 3·89 | 3·49 | 3·26 | 3·11 | 3·00 | 2·91 | 2·85 | 2·80 | 2·75 | 2·69 | 2·62 | 2·54 | 2·51 | 2·47 | 2·43 | 2·38 | 2·34 | 2·30 |
| 13 | 4·67 | 3·81 | 3·41 | 3·18 | 3·03 | 2·92 | 2·83 | 2·77 | 2·71 | 2·67 | 2·60 | 2·53 | 2·46 | 2·42 | 2·38 | 2·34 | 2·30 | 2·25 | 2·21 |
| 14 | 4·60 | 3·74 | 3·34 | 3·11 | 2·96 | 2·85 | 2·76 | 2·70 | 2·65 | 2·60 | 2·53 | 2·46 | 2·39 | 2·35 | 2·31 | 2·27 | 2·22 | 2·18 | 2·13 |
| 15 | 4·54 | 3·68 | 3·29 | 3·06 | 2·90 | 2·79 | 2·71 | 2·64 | 2·59 | 2·54 | 2·48 | 2·40 | 2·33 | 2·29 | 2·25 | 2·20 | 2·16 | 2·11 | 2·07 |
| 16 | 4·49 | 3·63 | 3·24 | 3·01 | 2·85 | 2·74 | 2·66 | 2·59 | 2·54 | 2·49 | 2·42 | 2·35 | 2·28 | 2·24 | 2·19 | 2·15 | 2·11 | 2·06 | 2·01 |
| 17 | 4·45 | 3·59 | 3·20 | 2·96 | 2·81 | 2·70 | 2·61 | 2·55 | 2·49 | 2·45 | 2·38 | 2·31 | 2·23 | 2·19 | 2·15 | 2·10 | 2·06 | 2·01 | 1·96 |
| 18 | 4·41 | 3·55 | 3·16 | 2·93 | 2·77 | 2·66 | 2·58 | 2·51 | 2·46 | 2·41 | 2·34 | 2·27 | 2·19 | 2·15 | 2·11 | 2·06 | 2·02 | 1·97 | 1·92 |
| 19 | 4·38 | 3·52 | 3·13 | 2·90 | 2·74 | 2·63 | 2·54 | 2·48 | 2·42 | 2·38 | 2·31 | 2·23 | 2·16 | 2·11 | 2·07 | 2·03 | 1·98 | 1·93 | 1·88 |
| 20 | 4·35 | 3·49 | 3·10 | 2·87 | 2·71 | 2·60 | 2·51 | 2·45 | 2·39 | 2·35 | 2·28 | 2·20 | 2·12 | 2·08 | 2·04 | 1·99 | 1·95 | 1·90 | 1·84 |
| 21 | 4·32 | 3·47 | 3·07 | 2·84 | 2·68 | 2·57 | 2·49 | 2·42 | 2·37 | 2·32 | 2·25 | 2·18 | 2·10 | 2·05 | 2·01 | 1·96 | 1·92 | 1·87 | 1·81 |
| 22 | 4·30 | 3·44 | 3·05 | 2·82 | 2·66 | 2·55 | 2·46 | 2·40 | 2·34 | 2·30 | 2·23 | 2·15 | 2·07 | 2·03 | 1·98 | 1·94 | 1·89 | 1·84 | 1·78 |
| 23 | 4·28 | 3·42 | 3·03 | 2·80 | 2·64 | 2·53 | 2·44 | 2·37 | 2·32 | 2·27 | 2·20 | 2·13 | 2·05 | 2·01 | 1·96 | 1·91 | 1·86 | 1·81 | 1·76 |
| 24 | 4·26 | 3·40 | 3·01 | 2·78 | 2·62 | 2·51 | 2·42 | 2·36 | 2·30 | 2·25 | 2·18 | 2·11 | 2·03 | 1·98 | 1·94 | 1·89 | 1·84 | 1·79 | 1·73 |
| 25 | 4·24 | 3·39 | 2·99 | 2·76 | 2·60 | 2·49 | 2·40 | 2·34 | 2·28 | 2·24 | 2·16 | 2·09 | 2·01 | 1·96 | 1·92 | 1·87 | 1·82 | 1·77 | 1·71 |
| 26 | 4·23 | 3·37 | 2·98 | 2·74 | 2·59 | 2·47 | 2·39 | 2·32 | 2·27 | 2·22 | 2·15 | 2·07 | 1·99 | 1·95 | 1·90 | 1·85 | 1·80 | 1·75 | 1·69 |
| 27 | 4·21 | 3·35 | 2·96 | 2·73 | 2·57 | 2·46 | 2·37 | 2·31 | 2·25 | 2·20 | 2·13 | 2·06 | 1·97 | 1·93 | 1·88 | 1·84 | 1·79 | 1·73 | 1·67 |
| 28 | 4·20 | 3·34 | 2·95 | 2·71 | 2·56 | 2·45 | 2·36 | 2·29 | 2·24 | 2·19 | 2·12 | 2·04 | 1·96 | 1·91 | 1·87 | 1·82 | 1·77 | 1·71 | 1·65 |
| 29 | 4·18 | 3·33 | 2·93 | 2·70 | 2·55 | 2·43 | 2·35 | 2·28 | 2·22 | 2·18 | 2·10 | 2·03 | 1·94 | 1·90 | 1·85 | 1·81 | 1·75 | 1·70 | 1·64 |
| 30 | 4·17 | 3·32 | 2·92 | 2·69 | 2·53 | 2·42 | 2·33 | 2·27 | 2·21 | 2·16 | 2·09 | 2·01 | 1·93 | 1·89 | 1·84 | 1·79 | 1·74 | 1·68 | 1·62 |
| 40 | 4·08 | 3·23 | 2·84 | 2·61 | 2·45 | 2·34 | 2·25 | 2·18 | 2·12 | 2·08 | 2·00 | 1·92 | 1·84 | 1·79 | 1·74 | 1·69 | 1·64 | 1·58 | 1·51 |
| 60 | 4·00 | 3·15 | 2·76 | 2·53 | 2·37 | 2·25 | 2·17 | 2·10 | 2·04 | 1·99 | 1·92 | 1·84 | 1·75 | 1·70 | 1·65 | 1·59 | 1·53 | 1·47 | 1·39 |
| 120 | 3·92 | 3·07 | 2·68 | 2·45 | 2·29 | 2·17 | 2·09 | 2·02 | 1·96 | 1·91 | 1·83 | 1·75 | 1·66 | 1·61 | 1·55 | 1·50 | 1·43 | 1·35 | 1·25 |
| ∞ | 3·84 | 3·00 | 2·60 | 2·37 | 2·21 | 2·10 | 2·01 | 1·94 | 1·88 | 1·83 | 1·75 | 1·67 | 1·57 | 1·52 | 1·46 | 1·39 | 1·32 | 1·22 | 1·00 |

Upper 1% points

| $\nu_2$ \ $\nu_1$ | 1 | 2 | 3 | 4 | 5 | 6 | 7 | 8 | 9 | 10 | 12 | 15 | 20 | 24 | 30 | 40 | 60 | 120 | ∞ |
|---|---|---|---|---|---|---|---|---|---|---|---|---|---|---|---|---|---|---|---|
| 1 | 4052 | 4999·5 | 5403 | 5625 | 5764 | 5859 | 5928 | 5982 | 6022 | 6056 | 6106 | 6157 | 6209 | 6235 | 6261 | 6287 | 6313 | 6339 | 6366 |
| 2 | 98·50 | 99·00 | 99·17 | 99·25 | 99·30 | 99·33 | 99·36 | 99·37 | 99·39 | 99·40 | 99·42 | 99·43 | 99·45 | 99·46 | 99·47 | 99·47 | 99·48 | 99·49 | 99·50 |
| 3 | 34·12 | 30·82 | 29·46 | 28·71 | 28·24 | 27·91 | 27·67 | 27·49 | 27·35 | 27·23 | 27·05 | 26·87 | 26·69 | 26·60 | 26·50 | 26·41 | 26·32 | 26·22 | 26·13 |
| 4 | 21·20 | 18·00 | 16·69 | 15·98 | 15·52 | 15·21 | 14·98 | 14·80 | 14·66 | 14·55 | 14·37 | 14·20 | 14·02 | 13·93 | 13·84 | 13·75 | 13·65 | 13·56 | 13·46 |
| 5 | 16·26 | 13·27 | 12·06 | 11·39 | 10·97 | 10·67 | 10·46 | 10·29 | 10·16 | 10·05 | 9·89 | 9·72 | 9·55 | 9·47 | 9·38 | 9·29 | 9·20 | 9·11 | 9·02 |
| 6 | 13·75 | 10·92 | 9·78 | 9·15 | 8·75 | 8·47 | 8·26 | 8·10 | 7·98 | 7·87 | 7·72 | 7·56 | 7·40 | 7·31 | 7·23 | 7·14 | 7·06 | 6·97 | 6·88 |
| 7 | 12·25 | 9·55 | 8·45 | 7·85 | 7·46 | 7·19 | 6·99 | 6·84 | 6·72 | 6·62 | 6·47 | 6·31 | 6·16 | 6·07 | 5·99 | 5·91 | 5·82 | 5·74 | 5·65 |
| 8 | 11·26 | 8·65 | 7·59 | 7·01 | 6·63 | 6·37 | 6·18 | 6·03 | 5·91 | 5·81 | 5·67 | 5·52 | 5·36 | 5·28 | 5·20 | 5·12 | 5·03 | 4·95 | 4·86 |
| 9 | 10·56 | 8·02 | 6·99 | 6·42 | 6·06 | 5·80 | 5·61 | 5·47 | 5·35 | 5·26 | 5·11 | 4·96 | 4·81 | 4·73 | 4·65 | 4·57 | 4·48 | 4·40 | 4·31 |
| 10 | 10·04 | 7·56 | 6·55 | 5·99 | 5·64 | 5·39 | 5·20 | 5·06 | 4·94 | 4·85 | 4·71 | 4·56 | 4·41 | 4·33 | 4·25 | 4·17 | 4·08 | 4·00 | 3·91 |
| 11 | 9·65 | 7·21 | 6·22 | 5·67 | 5·32 | 5·07 | 4·89 | 4·74 | 4·63 | 4·54 | 4·40 | 4·25 | 4·10 | 4·02 | 3·94 | 3·86 | 3·78 | 3·69 | 3·60 |
| 12 | 9·33 | 6·93 | 5·95 | 5·41 | 5·06 | 4·82 | 4·64 | 4·50 | 4·39 | 4·30 | 4·16 | 4·01 | 3·86 | 3·78 | 3·70 | 3·62 | 3·54 | 3·45 | 3·36 |
| 13 | 9·07 | 6·70 | 5·74 | 5·21 | 4·86 | 4·62 | 4·44 | 4·30 | 4·19 | 4·10 | 3·96 | 3·82 | 3·66 | 3·59 | 3·51 | 3·43 | 3·34 | 3·25 | 3·17 |
| 14 | 8·86 | 6·51 | 5·56 | 5·04 | 4·69 | 4·46 | 4·28 | 4·14 | 4·03 | 3·94 | 3·80 | 3·66 | 3·51 | 3·43 | 3·35 | 3·27 | 3·18 | 3·09 | 3·00 |
| 15 | 8·68 | 6·36 | 5·42 | 4·89 | 4·56 | 4·32 | 4·14 | 4·00 | 3·89 | 3·80 | 3·67 | 3·52 | 3·37 | 3·29 | 3·21 | 3·13 | 3·05 | 2·96 | 2·87 |
| 16 | 8·53 | 6·23 | 5·29 | 4·77 | 4·44 | 4·20 | 4·03 | 3·89 | 3·78 | 3·69 | 3·55 | 3·41 | 3·26 | 3·18 | 3·10 | 3·02 | 2·93 | 2·84 | 2·75 |
| 17 | 8·40 | 6·11 | 5·18 | 4·67 | 4·34 | 4·10 | 3·93 | 3·79 | 3·68 | 3·59 | 3·46 | 3·31 | 3·16 | 3·08 | 3·00 | 2·92 | 2·83 | 2·75 | 2·65 |
| 18 | 8·29 | 6·01 | 5·09 | 4·58 | 4·25 | 4·01 | 3·84 | 3·71 | 3·60 | 3·51 | 3·37 | 3·23 | 3·08 | 3·00 | 2·92 | 2·84 | 2·75 | 2·66 | 2·57 |
| 19 | 8·18 | 5·93 | 5·01 | 4·50 | 4·17 | 3·94 | 3·77 | 3·63 | 3·52 | 3·43 | 3·30 | 3·15 | 3·00 | 2·92 | 2·84 | 2·76 | 2·67 | 2·58 | 2·49 |
| 20 | 8·10 | 5·85 | 4·94 | 4·43 | 4·10 | 3·87 | 3·70 | 3·56 | 3·46 | 3·37 | 3·23 | 3·09 | 2·94 | 2·86 | 2·78 | 2·69 | 2·61 | 2·52 | 2·42 |
| 21 | 8·02 | 5·78 | 4·87 | 4·37 | 4·04 | 3·81 | 3·64 | 3·51 | 3·40 | 3·31 | 3·17 | 3·03 | 2·88 | 2·80 | 2·72 | 2·64 | 2·55 | 2·46 | 2·36 |
| 22 | 7·95 | 5·72 | 4·82 | 4·31 | 3·99 | 3·76 | 3·59 | 3·45 | 3·35 | 3·26 | 3·12 | 2·98 | 2·83 | 2·75 | 2·67 | 2·58 | 2·50 | 2·40 | 2·31 |
| 23 | 7·88 | 5·66 | 4·76 | 4·26 | 3·94 | 3·71 | 3·54 | 3·41 | 3·30 | 3·21 | 3·07 | 2·93 | 2·78 | 2·70 | 2·62 | 2·54 | 2·45 | 2·35 | 2·26 |
| 24 | 7·82 | 5·61 | 4·72 | 4·22 | 3·90 | 3·67 | 3·50 | 3·36 | 3·26 | 3·17 | 3·03 | 2·89 | 2·74 | 2·66 | 2·58 | 2·49 | 2·40 | 2·31 | 2·21 |
| 25 | 7·77 | 5·57 | 4·68 | 4·18 | 3·85 | 3·63 | 3·46 | 3·32 | 3·22 | 3·13 | 2·99 | 2·85 | 2·70 | 2·62 | 2·54 | 2·45 | 2·36 | 2·27 | 2·17 |
| 26 | 7·72 | 5·53 | 4·64 | 4·14 | 3·82 | 3·59 | 3·42 | 3·29 | 3·18 | 3·09 | 2·96 | 2·81 | 2·66 | 2·58 | 2·50 | 2·42 | 2·33 | 2·23 | 2·13 |
| 27 | 7·68 | 5·49 | 4·60 | 4·11 | 3·78 | 3·56 | 3·39 | 3·26 | 3·15 | 3·06 | 2·93 | 2·78 | 2·63 | 2·55 | 2·47 | 2·38 | 2·29 | 2·20 | 2·10 |
| 28 | 7·64 | 5·45 | 4·57 | 4·07 | 3·75 | 3·53 | 3·36 | 3·23 | 3·12 | 3·03 | 2·90 | 2·75 | 2·60 | 2·52 | 2·44 | 2·35 | 2·26 | 2·17 | 2·06 |
| 29 | 7·60 | 5·42 | 4·54 | 4·04 | 3·73 | 3·50 | 3·33 | 3·20 | 3·09 | 3·00 | 2·87 | 2·73 | 2·57 | 2·49 | 2·41 | 2·33 | 2·23 | 2·14 | 2·03 |
| 30 | 7·56 | 5·39 | 4·51 | 4·02 | 3·70 | 3·47 | 3·30 | 3·17 | 3·07 | 2·98 | 2·84 | 2·70 | 2·55 | 2·47 | 2·39 | 2·30 | 2·21 | 2·11 | 2·01 |
| 40 | 7·31 | 5·18 | 4·31 | 3·83 | 3·51 | 3·29 | 3·12 | 2·99 | 2·89 | 2·80 | 2·66 | 2·52 | 2·37 | 2·29 | 2·20 | 2·11 | 2·02 | 1·92 | 1·80 |
| 60 | 7·08 | 4·98 | 4·13 | 3·65 | 3·34 | 3·12 | 2·95 | 2·82 | 2·72 | 2·63 | 2·50 | 2·35 | 2·20 | 2·12 | 2·03 | 1·94 | 1·84 | 1·73 | 1·60 |
| 120 | 6·85 | 4·79 | 3·95 | 3·48 | 3·17 | 2·96 | 2·79 | 2·66 | 2·56 | 2·47 | 2·34 | 2·19 | 2·03 | 1·95 | 1·86 | 1·76 | 1·66 | 1·53 | 1·38 |
| ∞ | 6·63 | 4·61 | 3·78 | 3·32 | 3·02 | 2·80 | 2·64 | 2·51 | 2·41 | 2·32 | 2·18 | 2·04 | 1·88 | 1·79 | 1·70 | 1·59 | 1·47 | 1·32 | 1·00 |

## Table III

## The $\chi^2$ Distribution with v Degrees of Freedom

Q is the area under the $\chi^2$ curve to the right of a vertical line at the table entry. For example, for 10 degrees of freedom, the area under the curve to the right of 23.2093 is .01.

| $\nu$ $\backslash$ Q | 0·995 | 0·990 | 0·975 | 0·950 | 0·900 | 0·750 | 0·500 |
|---|---|---|---|---|---|---|---|
| 1 | 392704·10⁻¹⁰ | 157088·10⁻⁹ | 982069·10⁻⁹ | 393214·10⁻⁸ | 0·0157908 | 0·1015308 | 0·454937 |
| 2 | 0·0100251 | 0·0201007 | 0·0506356 | 0·102587 | 0·210720 | 0·575364 | 1·38629 |
| 3 | 0·0717212 | 0·114832 | 0·215795 | 0·351846 | 0·584375 | 1·212534 | 2·36597 |
| 4 | 0·206990 | 0·297110 | 0·484419 | 0·710721 | 1·063623 | 1·92255 | 3·35670 |
| 5 | 0·411740 | 0·554300 | 0·831211 | 1·145476 | 1·61031 | 2·67460 | 4·35146 |
| 6 | 0·675727 | 0·872085 | 1·237347 | 1·63539 | 2·20413 | 3·45460 | 5·34812 |
| 7 | 0·989265 | 1·239043 | 1·68987 | 2·16735 | 2·83311 | 4·25485 | 6·34581 |
| 8 | 1·344419 | 1·646482 | 2·17973 | 2·73264 | 3·48954 | 5·07064 | 7·34412 |
| 9 | 1·734926 | 2·087912 | 2·70039 | 3·32511 | 4·16816 | 5·89883 | 8·34283 |
| 10 | 2·15585 | 2·55821 | 3·24697 | 3·94030 | 4·86518 | 6·73720 | 9·34182 |
| 11 | 2·60321 | 3·05347 | 3·81575 | 4·57481 | 5·57779 | 7·58412 | 10·3410 |
| 12 | 3·07382 | 3·57056 | 4·40379 | 5·22603 | 6·30380 | 8·43842 | 11·3403 |
| 13 | 3·56503 | 4·10691 | 5·00874 | 5·89186 | 7·04150 | 9·29906 | 12·3398 |
| 14 | 4·07468 | 4·66043 | 5·62872 | 6·57063 | 7·78953 | 10·1653 | 13·3393 |
| 15 | 4·60094 | 5·22935 | 6·26214 | 7·26094 | 8·54675 | 11·0365 | 14·3389 |
| 16 | 5·14224 | 5·81221 | 6·90766 | 7·96164 | 9·31223 | 11·9122 | 15·3385 |
| 17 | 5·69724 | 6·40776 | 7·56418 | 8·67176 | 10·0852 | 12·7919 | 16·3381 |
| 18 | 6·26481 | 7·01491 | 8·23075 | 9·39046 | 10·8649 | 13·6753 | 17·3379 |
| 19 | 6·84398 | 7·63273 | 8·90655 | 10·1170 | 11·6509 | 14·5620 | 18·3376 |
| 20 | 7·43386 | 8·26040 | 9·59083 | 10·8508 | 12·4426 | 15·4518 | 19·3374 |
| 21 | 8·03366 | 8·89720 | 10·28293 | 11·5913 | 13·2396 | 16·3444 | 20·3372 |
| 22 | 8·64272 | 9·54249 | 10·9823 | 12·3380 | 14·0415 | 17·2396 | 21·3370 |
| 23 | 9·26042 | 10·19567 | 11·6885 | 13·0905 | 14·8479 | 18·1373 | 22·3369 |
| 24 | 9·88623 | 10·8564 | 12·4011 | 13·8484 | 15·6587 | 19·0372 | 23·3367 |
| 25 | 10·5197 | 11·5240 | 13·1197 | 14·6114 | 16·4734 | 19·9393 | 24·3366 |
| 26 | 11·1603 | 12·1981 | 13·8439 | 15·3791 | 17·2919 | 20·8434 | 25·3364 |
| 27 | 11·8076 | 12·8786 | 14·5733 | 16·1513 | 18·1138 | 21·7494 | 26·3363 |
| 28 | 12·4613 | 13·5648 | 15·3079 | 16·9279 | 18·9392 | 22·6572 | 27·3363 |
| 29 | 13·1211 | 14·2565 | 16·0471 | 17·7083 | 19·7677 | 23·5666 | 28·3362 |
| 30 | 13·7867 | 14·9535 | 16·7908 | 18·4926 | 20·5992 | 24·4776 | 29·3360 |
| 40 | 20·7065 | 22·1643 | 24·4331 | 26·5093 | 29·0505 | 33·6603 | 39·3354 |
| 50 | 27·9907 | 29·7067 | 32·3574 | 34·7642 | 37·6886 | 42·9421 | 49·3349 |
| 60 | 35·5346 | 37·4848 | 40·4817 | 43·1879 | 46·4589 | 52·2938 | 59·3347 |
| 70 | 43·2752 | 45·4418 | 48·7576 | 51·7393 | 55·3290 | 61·6983 | 69·3344 |
| 80 | 51·1720 | 53·5400 | 57·1532 | 60·3915 | 64·2778 | 71·1445 | 79·3343 |
| 90 | 59·1963 | 61·7541 | 65·6466 | 69·1260 | 73·2912 | 80·6247 | 89·3342 |
| 100 | 67·3276 | 70·0648 | 74·2219 | 77·9295 | 82·3581 | 90·1332 | 99·3341 |
| X | −2·5758 | −2·3263 | −1·9600 | −1·6449 | −1·2816 | −0·6745 | 0·0000 |

# Table III (Continued)

| 0·250 | 0·100 | 0·050 | 0·025 | 0·010 | 0·005 | 0·001 |
|---|---|---|---|---|---|---|
| 1·32330 | 2·70554 | 3·84146 | 5·02389 | 6·63490 | 7·87944 | 10·828 |
| 2·77259 | 4·60517 | 5·99147 | 7·37776 | 9·21034 | 10·5966 | 13·816 |
| 4·10835 | 6·25139 | 7·81473 | 9·34840 | 11·3449 | 12·8381 | 16·266 |
| 5·38527 | 7·77944 | 9·48773 | 11·1433 | 13·2767 | 14·8602 | 18·467 |
| 6·62568 | 9·23635 | 11·0705 | 12·8325 | 15·0863 | 16·7496 | 20·515 |
| 7·84080 | 10·6446 | 12·5916 | 14·4494 | 16·8119 | 18·5476 | 22·458 |
| 9·03715 | 12·0170 | 14·0671 | 16·0128 | 18·4753 | 20·2777 | 24·322 |
| 10·2188 | 13·3616 | 15·5073 | 17·5346 | 20·0902 | 21·9550 | 26·125 |
| 11·3887 | 14·6837 | 16·9190 | 19·0228 | 21·6660 | 23·5893 | 27·877 |
| 12·5489 | 15·9871 | 18·3070 | 20·4831 | 23·2093 | 25·1882 | 29·588 |
| 13·7007 | 17·2750 | 19·6751 | 21·9200 | 24·7250 | 26·7569 | 31·264 |
| 14·8454 | 18·5494 | 21·0261 | 23·3367 | 26·2170 | 28·2995 | 32·909 |
| 15·9839 | 19·8119 | 22·3621 | 24·7356 | 27·6883 | 29·8194 | 34·528 |
| 17·1170 | 21·0642 | 23·6848 | 26·1190 | 29·1413 | 31·3193 | 36·123 |
| 18·2451 | 22·3072 | 24·9958 | 27·4884 | 30·5779 | 32·8013 | 37·697 |
| 19·3688 | 23·5418 | 26·2962 | 28·8454 | 31·9999 | 34·2672 | 39·252 |
| 20·4887 | 24·7690 | 27·5871 | 30·1910 | 33·4087 | 35·7185 | 40·790 |
| 21·6049 | 25·9894 | 28·8693 | 31·5264 | 34·8053 | 37·1564 | 42·312 |
| 22·7178 | 27·2036 | 30·1435 | 32·8523 | 36·1908 | 38·5822 | 43·820 |
| 23·8277 | 28·4120 | 31·4104 | 34·1696 | 37·5662 | 39·9968 | 45·315 |
| 24·9348 | 29·6151 | 32·6705 | 35·4789 | 38·9321 | 41·4010 | 46·797 |
| 26·0393 | 30·8133 | 33·9244 | 36·7807 | 40·2894 | 42·7956 | 48·268 |
| 27·1413 | 32·0069 | 35·1725 | 38·0757 | 41·6384 | 44·1813 | 49·728 |
| 28·2412 | 33·1963 | 36·4151 | 39·3641 | 42·9798 | 45·5585 | 51·179 |
| 29·3389 | 34·3816 | 37·6525 | 40·6465 | 44·3141 | 46·9278 | 52·620 |
| 30·4345 | 35·5631 | 38·8852 | 41·9232 | 45·6417 | 48·2899 | 54·052 |
| 31·5284 | 36·7412 | 40·1133 | 43·1944 | 46·9630 | 49·6449 | 55·476 |
| 32·6205 | 37·9159 | 41·3372 | 44·4607 | 48·2782 | 50·9933 | 56·892 |
| 33·7109 | 39·0875 | 42·5569 | 45·7222 | 49·5879 | 52·3356 | 58·302 |
| 34·7998 | 40·2560 | 43·7729 | 46·9792 | 50·8922 | 53·6720 | 59·703 |
| 45·6160 | 51·8050 | 55·7585 | 59·3417 | 63·6907 | 66·7659 | 73·402 |
| 56·3336 | 63·1671 | 67·5048 | 71·4202 | 76·1539 | 79·4900 | 86·661 |
| 66·9814 | 74·3970 | 79·0819 | 83·2976 | 88·3794 | 91·9517 | 99·607 |
| 77·5766 | 85·5271 | 90·5312 | 95·0231 | 100·425 | 104·215 | 112·317 |
| 88·1303 | 96·5782 | 101·879 | 106·629 | 112·329 | 116·321 | 124·839 |
| 98·6499 | 107·565 | 113·145 | 118·136 | 124·116 | 128·299 | 137·208 |
| 109·141 | 118·498 | 124·342 | 129·561 | 135·807 | 140·169 | 149·449 |
| +0·6745 | +1·2816 | +1·6449 | +1·9600 | +2·3263 | +2·5758 | +3·0902 |

## Table IV

### The Poisson Distribution

Entries are the probability that a Poisson process with mean λ will take on a value of N.

| N\λ | 0.1 | 0.2 | 0.3 | 0.4 | 0.5 | 0.6 | 0.7 | 0.8 | 0.9 | 1.0 | 1.1 | 1.2 | 1.3 | 1.4 | 1.5 | 1.6 | 1.7 | 1.8 | 1.9 | 2.0 |
|---|---|---|---|---|---|---|---|---|---|---|---|---|---|---|---|---|---|---|---|---|
| 0 | 0.905 | 0.819 | 0.741 | 0.670 | 0.607 | 0.549 | 0.497 | 0.449 | 0.407 | 0.368 | 0.333 | 0.301 | 0.273 | 0.247 | 0.223 | 0.202 | 0.183 | 0.165 | 0.150 | 0.135 |
| 1 | 0.090 | 0.164 | 0.222 | 0.268 | 0.303 | 0.329 | 0.348 | 0.359 | 0.366 | 0.368 | 0.366 | 0.361 | 0.354 | 0.345 | 0.335 | 0.323 | 0.311 | 0.298 | 0.284 | 0.271 |
| 2 | 0.005 | 0.016 | 0.033 | 0.054 | 0.076 | 0.099 | 0.122 | 0.144 | 0.165 | 0.184 | 0.201 | 0.217 | 0.230 | 0.242 | 0.251 | 0.258 | 0.264 | 0.268 | 0.270 | 0.271 |
| 3 | 0.000 | 0.001 | 0.003 | 0.007 | 0.013 | 0.020 | 0.028 | 0.038 | 0.049 | 0.061 | 0.074 | 0.087 | 0.100 | 0.113 | 0.126 | 0.138 | 0.150 | 0.161 | 0.171 | 0.180 |
| 4 | 0.000 | 0.000 | 0.000 | 0.001 | 0.002 | 0.003 | 0.005 | 0.008 | 0.011 | 0.015 | 0.020 | 0.026 | 0.032 | 0.039 | 0.047 | 0.055 | 0.064 | 0.072 | 0.081 | 0.090 |
| 5 | 0.000 | 0.000 | 0.000 | 0.000 | 0.000 | 0.000 | 0.001 | 0.001 | 0.002 | 0.003 | 0.004 | 0.006 | 0.008 | 0.011 | 0.014 | 0.018 | 0.022 | 0.026 | 0.031 | 0.036 |
| 6 | 0.000 | 0.000 | 0.000 | 0.000 | 0.000 | 0.000 | 0.000 | 0.000 | 0.000 | 0.000 | 0.001 | 0.001 | 0.002 | 0.003 | 0.004 | 0.005 | 0.006 | 0.008 | 0.010 | 0.012 |
| 7 | 0.000 | 0.000 | 0.000 | 0.000 | 0.000 | 0.000 | 0.000 | 0.000 | 0.000 | 0.000 | 0.000 | 0.000 | 0.000 | 0.001 | 0.001 | 0.001 | 0.001 | 0.002 | 0.003 | 0.003 |
| 8 | 0.000 | 0.000 | 0.000 | 0.000 | 0.000 | 0.000 | 0.000 | 0.000 | 0.000 | 0.000 | 0.000 | 0.000 | 0.000 | 0.000 | 0.000 | 0.000 | 0.000 | 0.000 | 0.000 | 0.001 |

| N\λ | 2.2 | 2.4 | 2.6 | 2.8 | 3.0 | 3.2 | 3.4 | 3.6 | 3.8 | 4.0 | 4.2 | 4.4 | 4.6 | 4.8 | 5.0 | 5.2 | 5.4 | 5.6 | 5.8 | 6.0 |
|---|---|---|---|---|---|---|---|---|---|---|---|---|---|---|---|---|---|---|---|---|
| 0 | 0.111 | 0.091 | 0.074 | 0.061 | 0.050 | 0.041 | 0.033 | 0.027 | 0.022 | 0.018 | 0.015 | 0.012 | 0.010 | 0.008 | 0.007 | 0.006 | 0.005 | 0.004 | 0.003 | 0.002 |
| 1 | 0.244 | 0.218 | 0.193 | 0.170 | 0.149 | 0.130 | 0.113 | 0.098 | 0.085 | 0.073 | 0.063 | 0.054 | 0.046 | 0.040 | 0.034 | 0.029 | 0.024 | 0.021 | 0.018 | 0.015 |
| 2 | 0.268 | 0.261 | 0.251 | 0.238 | 0.224 | 0.209 | 0.193 | 0.177 | 0.162 | 0.147 | 0.132 | 0.119 | 0.106 | 0.095 | 0.084 | 0.075 | 0.066 | 0.058 | 0.051 | 0.045 |
| 3 | 0.197 | 0.209 | 0.218 | 0.222 | 0.224 | 0.223 | 0.219 | 0.212 | 0.205 | 0.195 | 0.185 | 0.174 | 0.163 | 0.152 | 0.140 | 0.129 | 0.119 | 0.108 | 0.098 | 0.089 |
| 4 | 0.108 | 0.125 | 0.141 | 0.156 | 0.168 | 0.178 | 0.186 | 0.191 | 0.194 | 0.195 | 0.194 | 0.192 | 0.188 | 0.182 | 0.175 | 0.168 | 0.160 | 0.152 | 0.143 | 0.134 |
| 5 | 0.048 | 0.060 | 0.074 | 0.087 | 0.101 | 0.114 | 0.126 | 0.138 | 0.148 | 0.156 | 0.163 | 0.169 | 0.173 | 0.175 | 0.175 | 0.175 | 0.173 | 0.170 | 0.166 | 0.161 |
| 6 | 0.017 | 0.024 | 0.032 | 0.041 | 0.050 | 0.061 | 0.072 | 0.083 | 0.094 | 0.104 | 0.114 | 0.124 | 0.132 | 0.140 | 0.146 | 0.151 | 0.156 | 0.158 | 0.160 | 0.161 |
| 7 | 0.005 | 0.008 | 0.012 | 0.016 | 0.022 | 0.028 | 0.035 | 0.042 | 0.051 | 0.060 | 0.069 | 0.078 | 0.087 | 0.096 | 0.104 | 0.113 | 0.120 | 0.127 | 0.133 | 0.138 |
| 8 | 0.002 | 0.002 | 0.004 | 0.006 | 0.008 | 0.011 | 0.015 | 0.019 | 0.024 | 0.030 | 0.036 | 0.043 | 0.050 | 0.058 | 0.065 | 0.073 | 0.081 | 0.089 | 0.096 | 0.103 |
| 9 | 0.000 | 0.001 | 0.001 | 0.002 | 0.003 | 0.004 | 0.006 | 0.008 | 0.010 | 0.013 | 0.017 | 0.021 | 0.026 | 0.031 | 0.036 | 0.042 | 0.049 | 0.055 | 0.062 | 0.069 |
| 10 | 0.000 | 0.000 | 0.000 | 0.000 | 0.001 | 0.001 | 0.002 | 0.003 | 0.004 | 0.005 | 0.007 | 0.009 | 0.012 | 0.015 | 0.018 | 0.022 | 0.026 | 0.031 | 0.036 | 0.041 |
| 11 | 0.000 | 0.000 | 0.000 | 0.000 | 0.000 | 0.000 | 0.001 | 0.001 | 0.001 | 0.002 | 0.003 | 0.004 | 0.005 | 0.006 | 0.008 | 0.010 | 0.013 | 0.016 | 0.019 | 0.023 |
| 12 | 0.000 | 0.000 | 0.000 | 0.000 | 0.000 | 0.000 | 0.000 | 0.000 | 0.000 | 0.001 | 0.001 | 0.001 | 0.002 | 0.003 | 0.003 | 0.005 | 0.006 | 0.007 | 0.009 | 0.011 |
| 13 | 0.000 | 0.000 | 0.000 | 0.000 | 0.000 | 0.000 | 0.000 | 0.000 | 0.000 | 0.000 | 0.000 | 0.000 | 0.001 | 0.001 | 0.001 | 0.002 | 0.002 | 0.003 | 0.004 | 0.005 |
| 14 | 0.000 | 0.000 | 0.000 | 0.000 | 0.000 | 0.000 | 0.000 | 0.000 | 0.000 | 0.000 | 0.000 | 0.000 | 0.000 | 0.000 | 0.000 | 0.001 | 0.001 | 0.001 | 0.002 | 0.002 |
| 15 | 0.000 | 0.000 | 0.000 | 0.000 | 0.000 | 0.000 | 0.000 | 0.000 | 0.000 | 0.000 | 0.000 | 0.000 | 0.000 | 0.000 | 0.000 | 0.000 | 0.000 | 0.000 | 0.001 | 0.001 |

| N\λ | 6.5 | 7.0 | 7.5 | 8.0 | 8.5 | 9.0 | 9.5 | 10.0 | 10.5 | 11.0 | 11.5 | 12.0 | 13.0 | 14.0 | 15.0 | 16.0 | 17.0 | 18.0 | 19.0 | 20.0 |
|---|---|---|---|---|---|---|---|---|---|---|---|---|---|---|---|---|---|---|---|---|
| 0 | 0.002 | 0.001 | 0.001 | 0.000 | 0.000 | 0.000 | 0.000 | 0.000 | 0.000 | 0.000 | 0.000 | 0.000 | 0.000 | 0.000 | 0.000 | 0.000 | 0.000 | 0.000 | 0.000 | 0.000 |
| 1 | 0.010 | 0.006 | 0.004 | 0.003 | 0.002 | 0.001 | 0.001 | 0.000 | 0.000 | 0.000 | 0.000 | 0.000 | 0.000 | 0.000 | 0.000 | 0.000 | 0.000 | 0.000 | 0.000 | 0.000 |
| 2 | 0.032 | 0.022 | 0.016 | 0.011 | 0.007 | 0.005 | 0.003 | 0.002 | 0.002 | 0.001 | 0.001 | 0.000 | 0.000 | 0.000 | 0.000 | 0.000 | 0.000 | 0.000 | 0.000 | 0.000 |
| 3 | 0.069 | 0.052 | 0.039 | 0.029 | 0.021 | 0.015 | 0.011 | 0.008 | 0.005 | 0.004 | 0.003 | 0.002 | 0.001 | 0.000 | 0.000 | 0.000 | 0.000 | 0.000 | 0.000 | 0.000 |
| 4 | 0.112 | 0.091 | 0.073 | 0.057 | 0.044 | 0.034 | 0.025 | 0.019 | 0.014 | 0.010 | 0.007 | 0.005 | 0.003 | 0.001 | 0.001 | 0.000 | 0.000 | 0.000 | 0.000 | 0.000 |
| 5 | 0.145 | 0.128 | 0.109 | 0.092 | 0.075 | 0.061 | 0.048 | 0.038 | 0.029 | 0.022 | 0.017 | 0.013 | 0.007 | 0.004 | 0.002 | 0.001 | 0.000 | 0.000 | 0.000 | 0.000 |
| 6 | 0.157 | 0.149 | 0.137 | 0.122 | 0.107 | 0.091 | 0.076 | 0.063 | 0.051 | 0.041 | 0.033 | 0.025 | 0.015 | 0.009 | 0.005 | 0.003 | 0.001 | 0.001 | 0.000 | 0.000 |
| 7 | 0.146 | 0.149 | 0.146 | 0.140 | 0.129 | 0.117 | 0.104 | 0.090 | 0.077 | 0.065 | 0.053 | 0.044 | 0.028 | 0.017 | 0.010 | 0.006 | 0.003 | 0.002 | 0.001 | 0.001 |
| 8 | 0.119 | 0.130 | 0.137 | 0.140 | 0.138 | 0.132 | 0.123 | 0.113 | 0.101 | 0.089 | 0.077 | 0.066 | 0.046 | 0.030 | 0.019 | 0.012 | 0.007 | 0.004 | 0.002 | 0.001 |
| 9 | 0.086 | 0.101 | 0.114 | 0.124 | 0.130 | 0.132 | 0.130 | 0.125 | 0.118 | 0.109 | 0.098 | 0.087 | 0.066 | 0.047 | 0.032 | 0.021 | 0.014 | 0.008 | 0.005 | 0.003 |
| 10 | 0.056 | 0.071 | 0.086 | 0.099 | 0.110 | 0.119 | 0.124 | 0.125 | 0.124 | 0.119 | 0.113 | 0.105 | 0.086 | 0.066 | 0.049 | 0.034 | 0.023 | 0.015 | 0.009 | 0.006 |
| 11 | 0.033 | 0.045 | 0.059 | 0.072 | 0.085 | 0.097 | 0.107 | 0.114 | 0.118 | 0.119 | 0.118 | 0.114 | 0.101 | 0.084 | 0.066 | 0.050 | 0.036 | 0.025 | 0.016 | 0.011 |
| 12 | 0.018 | 0.026 | 0.037 | 0.048 | 0.060 | 0.073 | 0.084 | 0.095 | 0.103 | 0.109 | 0.113 | 0.114 | 0.110 | 0.098 | 0.083 | 0.066 | 0.050 | 0.037 | 0.026 | 0.018 |
| 13 | 0.009 | 0.014 | 0.021 | 0.030 | 0.040 | 0.050 | 0.062 | 0.073 | 0.083 | 0.093 | 0.100 | 0.106 | 0.110 | 0.106 | 0.096 | 0.081 | 0.066 | 0.051 | 0.038 | 0.027 |
| 14 | 0.004 | 0.007 | 0.011 | 0.017 | 0.024 | 0.032 | 0.042 | 0.052 | 0.063 | 0.073 | 0.082 | 0.090 | 0.102 | 0.106 | 0.102 | 0.093 | 0.080 | 0.065 | 0.051 | 0.039 |
| 15 | 0.002 | 0.003 | 0.006 | 0.009 | 0.014 | 0.019 | 0.027 | 0.035 | 0.044 | 0.053 | 0.063 | 0.072 | 0.088 | 0.099 | 0.102 | 0.099 | 0.091 | 0.079 | 0.065 | 0.052 |
| 16 | 0.001 | 0.001 | 0.003 | 0.005 | 0.007 | 0.011 | 0.016 | 0.022 | 0.029 | 0.037 | 0.045 | 0.054 | 0.072 | 0.087 | 0.096 | 0.099 | 0.096 | 0.088 | 0.077 | 0.065 |
| 17 | 0.000 | 0.001 | 0.001 | 0.002 | 0.004 | 0.006 | 0.009 | 0.013 | 0.018 | 0.024 | 0.031 | 0.038 | 0.055 | 0.071 | 0.085 | 0.093 | 0.096 | 0.094 | 0.086 | 0.076 |
| 18 | 0.000 | 0.000 | 0.000 | 0.001 | 0.002 | 0.003 | 0.005 | 0.007 | 0.010 | 0.015 | 0.020 | 0.026 | 0.040 | 0.055 | 0.071 | 0.083 | 0.091 | 0.094 | 0.091 | 0.084 |
| 19 | 0.000 | 0.000 | 0.000 | 0.000 | 0.001 | 0.001 | 0.002 | 0.004 | 0.006 | 0.008 | 0.012 | 0.016 | 0.027 | 0.041 | 0.056 | 0.070 | 0.081 | 0.089 | 0.091 | 0.089 |
| 20 | 0.000 | 0.000 | 0.000 | 0.000 | 0.000 | 0.001 | 0.001 | 0.002 | 0.003 | 0.005 | 0.007 | 0.010 | 0.018 | 0.029 | 0.042 | 0.056 | 0.069 | 0.080 | 0.087 | 0.089 |
| 21 | 0.000 | 0.000 | 0.000 | 0.000 | 0.000 | 0.000 | 0.000 | 0.001 | 0.002 | 0.002 | 0.004 | 0.006 | 0.011 | 0.019 | 0.030 | 0.043 | 0.056 | 0.068 | 0.078 | 0.085 |
| 22 | 0.000 | 0.000 | 0.000 | 0.000 | 0.000 | 0.000 | 0.000 | 0.000 | 0.001 | 0.001 | 0.002 | 0.003 | 0.006 | 0.012 | 0.020 | 0.031 | 0.043 | 0.056 | 0.068 | 0.077 |
| 23 | 0.000 | 0.000 | 0.000 | 0.000 | 0.000 | 0.000 | 0.000 | 0.000 | 0.000 | 0.000 | 0.001 | 0.002 | 0.004 | 0.007 | 0.013 | 0.022 | 0.032 | 0.044 | 0.056 | 0.067 |
| 24 | 0.000 | 0.000 | 0.000 | 0.000 | 0.000 | 0.000 | 0.000 | 0.000 | 0.000 | 0.000 | 0.000 | 0.001 | 0.002 | 0.004 | 0.008 | 0.014 | 0.023 | 0.033 | 0.044 | 0.056 |
| 25 | 0.000 | 0.000 | 0.000 | 0.000 | 0.000 | 0.000 | 0.000 | 0.000 | 0.000 | 0.000 | 0.000 | 0.001 | 0.001 | 0.002 | 0.005 | 0.009 | 0.015 | 0.024 | 0.034 | 0.045 |
| 26 | 0.000 | 0.000 | 0.000 | 0.000 | 0.000 | 0.000 | 0.000 | 0.000 | 0.000 | 0.000 | 0.000 | 0.000 | 0.001 | 0.001 | 0.003 | 0.006 | 0.010 | 0.016 | 0.025 | 0.034 |
| 27 | 0.000 | 0.000 | 0.000 | 0.000 | 0.000 | 0.000 | 0.000 | 0.000 | 0.000 | 0.000 | 0.000 | 0.000 | 0.000 | 0.001 | 0.002 | 0.003 | 0.006 | 0.011 | 0.017 | 0.025 |
| 28 | 0.000 | 0.000 | 0.000 | 0.000 | 0.000 | 0.000 | 0.000 | 0.000 | 0.000 | 0.000 | 0.000 | 0.000 | 0.000 | 0.000 | 0.001 | 0.002 | 0.004 | 0.007 | 0.012 | 0.018 |
| 29 | 0.000 | 0.000 | 0.000 | 0.000 | 0.000 | 0.000 | 0.000 | 0.000 | 0.000 | 0.000 | 0.000 | 0.000 | 0.000 | 0.000 | 0.000 | 0.001 | 0.002 | 0.004 | 0.008 | 0.013 |
| 30 | 0.000 | 0.000 | 0.000 | 0.000 | 0.000 | 0.000 | 0.000 | 0.000 | 0.000 | 0.000 | 0.000 | 0.000 | 0.000 | 0.000 | 0.000 | 0.001 | 0.001 | 0.003 | 0.005 | 0.008 |
| 31 | 0.000 | 0.000 | 0.000 | 0.000 | 0.000 | 0.000 | 0.000 | 0.000 | 0.000 | 0.000 | 0.000 | 0.000 | 0.000 | 0.000 | 0.000 | 0.000 | 0.001 | 0.002 | 0.003 | 0.005 |
| 32 | 0.000 | 0.000 | 0.000 | 0.000 | 0.000 | 0.000 | 0.000 | 0.000 | 0.000 | 0.000 | 0.000 | 0.000 | 0.000 | 0.000 | 0.000 | 0.000 | 0.000 | 0.001 | 0.002 | 0.003 |
| 33 | 0.000 | 0.000 | 0.000 | 0.000 | 0.000 | 0.000 | 0.000 | 0.000 | 0.000 | 0.000 | 0.000 | 0.000 | 0.000 | 0.000 | 0.000 | 0.000 | 0.000 | 0.000 | 0.001 | 0.002 |
| 34 | 0.000 | 0.000 | 0.000 | 0.000 | 0.000 | 0.000 | 0.000 | 0.000 | 0.000 | 0.000 | 0.000 | 0.000 | 0.000 | 0.000 | 0.000 | 0.000 | 0.000 | 0.000 | 0.001 | 0.001 |
| 35 | 0.000 | 0.000 | 0.000 | 0.000 | 0.000 | 0.000 | 0.000 | 0.000 | 0.000 | 0.000 | 0.000 | 0.000 | 0.000 | 0.000 | 0.000 | 0.000 | 0.000 | 0.000 | 0.000 | 0.001 |

## Table V

### Values of $e^{-x}$

| $x$ | $e^{-x}$ | $x$ | $e^{-x}$ | $x$ | $e^{-x}$ | $x$ | $e^{-x}$ |
|---|---|---|---|---|---|---|---|
| 0.00 | 1.0000 | 2.50 | 0.0821 | 5.00 | 0.0067 | 7.50 | 0.0006 |
| 0.05 | 0.9512 | 2.55 | 0.0781 | 5.05 | 0.0064 | 7.55 | 0.0005 |
| 0.10 | 0.9048 | 2.60 | 0.0743 | 5.10 | 0.0061 | 7.60 | 0.0005 |
| 0.15 | 0.8607 | 2.65 | 0.0707 | 5.15 | 0.0058 | 7.65 | 0.0005 |
| 0.20 | 0.8187 | 2.70 | 0.0672 | 5.20 | 0.0055 | 7.70 | 0.0005 |
| 0.25 | 0.7788 | 2.75 | 0.0639 | 5.25 | 0.0052 | 7.75 | 0.0004 |
| 0.30 | 0.7408 | 2.80 | 0.0608 | 5.30 | 0.0050 | 7.80 | 0.0004 |
| 0.35 | 0.7047 | 2.85 | 0.0578 | 5.35 | 0.0047 | 7.85 | 0.0004 |
| 0.40 | 0.6703 | 2.90 | 0.0550 | 5.40 | 0.0045 | 7.90 | 0.0004 |
| 0.45 | 0.6376 | 2.95 | 0.0523 | 5.45 | 0.0043 | 7.95 | 0.0004 |
| 0.50 | 0.6065 | 3.00 | 0.0498 | 5.50 | 0.0041 | 8.00 | 0.0003 |
| 0.55 | 0.5770 | 3.05 | 0.0474 | 5.55 | 0.0039 | 8.05 | 0.0003 |
| 0.60 | 0.5488 | 3.10 | 0.0450 | 5.60 | 0.0037 | 8.10 | 0.0003 |
| 0.65 | 0.5220 | 3.15 | 0.0429 | 5.65 | 0.0035 | 8.15 | 0.0003 |
| 0.70 | 0.4966 | 3.20 | 0.0408 | 5.70 | 0.0033 | 8.20 | 0.0003 |
| 0.75 | 0.4724 | 3.25 | 0.0388 | 5.75 | 0.0032 | 8.25 | 0.0003 |
| 0.80 | 0.4493 | 3.30 | 0.0369 | 5.80 | 0.0030 | 8.30 | 0.0002 |
| 0.85 | 0.4274 | 3.35 | 0.0351 | 5.85 | 0.0029 | 8.35 | 0.0002 |
| 0.90 | 0.4066 | 3.40 | 0.0334 | 5.90 | 0.0027 | 8.40 | 0.0002 |
| 0.95 | 0.3867 | 3.45 | 0.0317 | 5.95 | 0.0026 | 8.45 | 0.0002 |
| 1.00 | 0.3679 | 3.50 | 0.0302 | 6.00 | 0.0025 | 8.50 | 0.0002 |
| 1.05 | 0.3499 | 3.55 | 0.0287 | 6.05 | 0.0024 | 8.55 | 0.0002 |
| 1.10 | 0.3329 | 3.60 | 0.0273 | 6.10 | 0.0022 | 8.60 | 0.0002 |
| 1.15 | 0.3166 | 3.65 | 0.0260 | 6.15 | 0.0021 | 8.65 | 0.0002 |
| 1.20 | 0.3012 | 3.70 | 0.0247 | 6.20 | 0.0020 | 8.70 | 0.0002 |
| 1.25 | 0.2865 | 3.75 | 0.0235 | 6.25 | 0.0019 | 8.75 | 0.0002 |
| 1.30 | 0.2725 | 3.80 | 0.0224 | 6.30 | 0.0018 | 8.80 | 0.0002 |
| 1.35 | 0.2592 | 3.85 | 0.0213 | 6.35 | 0.0017 | 8.85 | 0.0001 |
| 1.40 | 0.2466 | 3.90 | 0.0202 | 6.40 | 0.0017 | 8.90 | 0.0001 |
| 1.45 | 0.2346 | 3.95 | 0.0193 | 6.45 | 0.0016 | 8.95 | 0.0001 |
| 1.50 | 0.2231 | 4.00 | 0.0183 | 6.50 | 0.0015 | 9.00 | 0.0001 |
| 1.55 | 0.2122 | 4.05 | 0.0174 | 6.55 | 0.0014 | 9.05 | 0.0001 |
| 1.60 | 0.2019 | 4.10 | 0.0166 | 6.60 | 0.0014 | 9.10 | 0.0001 |
| 1.65 | 0.1921 | 4.15 | 0.0158 | 6.65 | 0.0013 | 9.15 | 0.0001 |
| 1.70 | 0.1827 | 4.20 | 0.0150 | 6.70 | 0.0012 | 9.20 | 0.0001 |
| 1.75 | 0.1738 | 4.25 | 0.0143 | 6.75 | 0.0012 | 9.25 | 0.0001 |
| 1.80 | 0.1653 | 4.30 | 0.0136 | 6.80 | 0.0011 | 9.30 | 0.0001 |
| 1.85 | 0.1572 | 4.35 | 0.0129 | 6.85 | 0.0011 | 9.35 | 0.0001 |
| 1.90 | 0.1496 | 4.40 | 0.0123 | 6.90 | 0.0010 | 9.40 | 0.0001 |
| 1.95 | 0.1423 | 4.45 | 0.0117 | 6.95 | 0.0010 | 9.45 | 0.0001 |
| 2.00 | 0.1353 | 4.50 | 0.0111 | 7.00 | 0.0009 | 9.50 | 0.0001 |
| 2.05 | 0.1287 | 4.55 | 0.0106 | 7.05 | 0.000 | 9.55 | 0.0001 |
| 2.10 | 0.1225 | 4.60 | 0.0101 | 7.10 | 0.0008 | 9.60 | 0.0001 |
| 2.15 | 0.1165 | 4.65 | 0.0096 | 7.15 | 0.0008 | 9.65 | 0.0001 |
| 2.20 | 0.1108 | 4.70 | 0.0091 | 7.20 | 0.0007 | 9.70 | 0.0001 |
| 2.25 | 0.1054 | 4.75 | 0.0087 | 7.25 | 0.0007 | 9.75 | 0.0001 |
| 2.30 | 0.1003 | 4.80 | 0.0082 | 7.30 | 0.0007 | 9.80 | 0.0001 |
| 2.35 | 0.0954 | 4.85 | 0.0078 | 7.35 | 0.0006 | 9.85 | 0.0001 |
| 2.40 | 0.0907 | 4.90 | 0.0074 | 7.40 | 0.0006 | 9.90 | 0.0001 |
| 2.45 | 0.0863 | 4.95 | 0.0071 | 7.45 | 0.0006 | 9.95 | 0.0000 |

*Use of Table for Exponential Distribution.* The cumulative for the exponential distribution with mean $1/u$ is given by

$$F(t) = 1 - e^{-ut}$$

That is, the probability that an exponentially distributed random variable with mean $1/u$ will take on a value of $t$ or less is $F(t)$.

*Example:* What is the probability that an exponentially distributed random variable with mean 4 will take on a value between 3 and 5? ($1/u = 4$; $u = 1/4$.)

$$p(3 \leq \bar{t} \leq 5) = (1 - e^{-5/4}) - (1 - e^{-3/4}) = e^{-.75} - e^{-1.25}$$

$$= .4724 - .2865 = .1859$$

# Index

# About the Authors

D. MICHAEL WARNER, PH.D., is an Associate Professor in the Fuqua School of Business at Duke University. Previously he served on the faculty of the Duke Program in Health Administration and on the faculties of Hospital Administration and Industrial Engineering at The University of Michigan. Dr. Warner is the author of numerous books and publications in the field of Operations Research applied to Health Administration, and is an active consultant to many hospitals.

DON C. HOLLOWAY, PH.D., is Executive Vice President of a business services corporation wholly owned by the Alta Bates Health System. His previous positions include Director of Management Engineering and Information Systems at Alta Bates Hospital and Associate Professor in the School of Public Health, Hospital Administration Program, at the University of California-Berkeley. Dr. Holloway was previously a partner in the Atwork Company, providing management engineering and data processing consultation to hospitals in the San Francisco Bay area and to the Health Ministry of Portugal in Lisbon. He has published articles in *Medical Care, Health Care Management Review*, and *Health Services Research.*

KYLE L. GRAZIER, DR.P.H., is an Assistant Professor in the Department of Epidemiology and Public Health in the School of Medicine at Yale University, and a 1983 Kellogg Fellow in Health Care Financial Management. Among her many previous honors is a W. K. Kellogg Foundation Fellowship awarded by the Hospital Research and Education Trust. Dr. Grazier has served as consultant to many health care organizations, and has held research, environmental engineering, and nursing positions in several universities and health organizations. Dr. Grazier has written extensively on various aspects of health care administration.